Hematologic Malignancies

Series editor
Martin Dreyling
München, Germany

More information about this series at http://www.springernature.com/series/5416

Meletios A. Dimopoulos
Thierry Facon
Evangelos Terpos

Editors

Multiple Myeloma and Other Plasma Cell Neoplasms

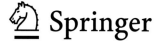

Springer

Editors
Meletios A. Dimopoulos
School of Medicine
National and Kapodistrian University
of Athens
Athens
Greece

Evangelos Terpos
School of Medicine
National and Kapodistrian University
of Athens
Athens
Greece

Thierry Facon
Service des Maladies du Sang
CHRU Lille Hôpital Claude Huriez
Lille
France

ISSN 2197-9766   ISSN 2197-9774   (electronic)
Hematologic Malignancies
ISBN 978-3-319-25584-2   ISBN 978-3-319-25586-6   (eBook)
https://doi.org/10.1007/978-3-319-25586-6

Library of Congress Control Number: 2018931877

Printed on acid-free paper

This Springer imprint is published by Springer Nature
The registered company is Springer International Publishing AG
The registered company address is: Gewerbestrasse 11, 6330 Cham, Switzerland

Contents

1 **Epidemiology and Pathophysiology of Multiple Myeloma** 1
   Malin Hultcrantz, Gareth J. Morgan, and Ola Landgren

2 **Diagnosis and Staging of Multiple Myeloma
   and Related Disorders** 17
   S. Vincent Rajkumar, Rafael Fonseca, and Jesus F. San Miguel

3 **Treatment of Transplant Eligible Patients
   with Multiple Myeloma** 29
   P. Sonneveld, H. Einsele, A. M. Brioli, and M. Cavo

4 **Treatment of Elderly Patients with Multiple Myeloma** 61
   Eileen Mary Boyle, Thierry Facon, Maria Victoria Mateos,
   and Antonio Palumbo

5 **Treatment of Relapsed/Refractory Patients
   with Multiple Myeloma** 73
   Jacob P. Laubach, Philippe Moreau, Meletios A. Dimopoulos,
   and Paul G. Richardson

6 **Minimal Residual Disease in Multiple Myeloma** 97
   Noemi Puig, Carmela Palladino, Bruno Paiva,
   and Marco Ladetto

7 **Bone Disease** 111
   Evangelos Terpos, Nikolaos Kanellias, and Noopur Raje

8 **Other Complications of Multiple Myeloma** 141
   Heinz Ludwig, Meletios-Athanasios Dimopoulos,
   and Evangelos Terpos

9 **Plasma Cell Leukemia and Extramedullary
   Plasmacytoma** 157
   Morie A. Gertz, Laura Rosinol, and Joan Bladé

10 **POEMS Syndrome** 177
    Dimitrios C. Ziogas, Angela Dispenzieri,
    and Evangelos Terpos

11   Waldenström's Macroglobulinemia 191
Steven P. Treon, Giampaolo Merlini, and
Meletios A. Dimopoulos

12   Primary Systemic Amyloidosis 221
Efstathios Kastritis, Ashutosh Wechalekar,
and Giampaolo Merlini

Epidemiology and Pathophysiology of Multiple Myeloma

Malin Hultcrantz, Gareth J. Morgan, and Ola Landgren

1.1 Introduction

Multiple myeloma is characterized by an abnormal plasma cell proliferation and in the majority of patients, production of monoclonal immunoglobulin heavy chains (M-protein) or light chains (Morgan et al. 2012). Findings of an M-protein in the blood of asymptomatic patients were first described in 1960 by Professor Jan Waldenström who called this condition "essential hypergammaglobulinemia" (Waldenstrom 1960). Kyle later observed that patients with monoclonal gammopathies were at a higher risk of developing plasma cell malignancies primarily multiple myeloma and thus concluded that this gammopathy was not always benign. They therefore coined the term monoclonal gammopathy of undetermined significance (MGUS) (Kyle 1978). More recent studies on sequential serum samples by Landgren et al. revealed that multiple myeloma is consistently preceded by MGUS (Landgren et al. 2009a). In a recent large screened study, the overall prevalence of MGUS was 2.4% with the highest prevalence observed in the African-American population (Landgren et al. 2014).

Myeloma has traditionally been associated with a poor outcome; however, the median survival has improved across all age groups after the introduction of novel agents more than 15 years old(Kristinsson et al. 2014). Importantly, survival has continued to improve with the subsequent development of second and third generations of the proteasome inhibitors and immunomodulatory drugs as well as new treatment options such as monoclonal antibodies (Kristinsson et al. 2014).

Genetically, multiple myeloma is a complex disease including multiple genetic hits and branching disease evolution. During progression from MGUS to multiple myeloma, plasma cells acquire a number of genetic hits and the ability to evade the immune system. The techniques to detect genetic aberrations and functional changes are becoming increasingly sensitive and precise. With the use of massive parallel sequencing, we have gained important insights on disease evolution during the recent years. In addition to cytogenetic changes, somatic mutations affecting various cellular mechanisms have been identified in myeloma (Manier et al. 2017). Furthermore, in myeloma there is an intense interplay with the bone marrow microenvironment and immune system acting in various ways to promote disease progression. Here we

M. Hultcrantz • O. Landgren (✉)
Myeloma Service, Department of Medicine,
Memorial Sloan Kettering Cancer Center,
New York, NY, USA
e-mail: landgrec@mskcc.org

G. J. Morgan
Myeloma Institute, University of Arkansas for
Medical Sciences, Little Rock, AR, USA

© Springer International Publishing Switzerland 2018
M. A. Dimopoulos et al. (eds.), *Multiple Myeloma and Other Plasma Cell Neoplasms*,
Hematologic Malignancies, https://doi.org/10.1007/978-3-319-25586-6_1

describe the epidemiology and pathophysiology including the genetic landscape and the role of the bone marrow microenvironment of multiple myeloma.

1.2   Epidemiology

Multiple myeloma is the second most common hematological malignancy in adults in Western countries with an age-adjusted incidence of 5/100,000 individuals in Western countries (Velez et al. 2016; Siegel et al. 2016). Myeloma is more common in the elderly population; the median age at diagnosis is 69–70 years (Kristinsson et al. 2007). Myeloma is consistently preceded by the precursor state monoclonal gammopathy of undetermined significance (MGUS) (Landgren et al. 2009a). The disease trajectory spans from MGUS which can progress to smoldering multiple myeloma and to multiple myeloma requiring therapy (Rajkumar et al. 2014). The rate of progression from MGUS to myeloma is 0.5–1% per year (Kyle et al. 2010; Turesson et al. 2014).

The etiology of MGUS and myeloma is not fully understood, but a number of host factors as well as external factors are of importance for disease evolution. Host factors include age where older individuals have a higher risk of developing myeloma. MGUS and myeloma are more common in men, and there are racial disparities in regard to incidence; MGUS and multiple myeloma are more common in African-American and African blacks compared to whites and Mexican Americans (Landgren et al. 2014; Landgren et al. 2007; Waxman et al. 2010). In a recent population-based screening study, the prevalence of MGUS was 3.7% in African-American blacks, 2.3% in whites, and 1.8% in Mexican Americans (Landgren et al. 2014). Genome-wide association studies have identified several single nucleotide polymorphisms associated with myeloma development indicating an inherited susceptibility (Morgan et al. 2014). Furthermore, exposure to certain pesticides and herbicides including Agent Orange has been correlated to an increased risk

of developing MGUS (Landgren et al. 2009b; Landgren et al. 2015).

1.3   Genetic Landscape of Multiple Myeloma

Genomic instability plays a major role in the pathogenesis of multiple myeloma and the disease including translocations, copy number abnormalities, as well as somatic mutations (Bianchi and Ghobrial 2014). The disease is heterogeneous and includes a number of subclones which evolve in a branching pattern similar to Darwinian evolution (Bolli et al. 2014; Walker et al. 2014). Initial genomic analyses captured mainly gross anatomical aberrations, while more modern techniques have rendered new insight to disease pathogenesis and individual disease patterns. The myeloma genome was first assessed using metaphase cytogenetics which is of limited value in myeloma due to limited sensitivity and the low proliferation of terminally differentiated plasma cells. Fluorescence in situ hybridization (FISH) is widely used in clinical praxis to assess translocations and copy number variations. Interphase FISH can capture also cryptic aberrations; however, FISH is hampered by several limitations; it detects only known genetic aberrations, the sensitivity is limited, and the analyses are labor intensive. Gene expression profiling was developed as a prognostic model that can be used within certain given therapies. More recently, massive parallel sequencing techniques with high-throughput sequencing of DNA have revolutionized genomic analyses. Using whole genome, whole exome, as well as targeted sequencing, great insights have been gained into the genomic landscape of multiple myeloma (Bolli et al. 2014; Chapman et al. 2011; Lohr et al. 2014; Walker et al. 2015a). Sequencing techniques have also been used to detect IgH translocations and hyperdiploidy; the modern techniques tended to be more sensitive compared to interphase FISH (Bolli et al. 2016). Here, we describe the emerging field of genomics in myeloma from cytogenetics and FISH to gene expression profiling and next-generation sequencing techniques.

1.4 Chromosomal Abnormalities

Myeloma can broadly be divided into two groups based on chromosomal aberrations; translocations involving IgH on chromosome 14 and hyperdiploidy. These events are considered initiating or primary events indicating that evolution to myeloma can follow at least two distinct pathways (Stella et al. 2015). However, these events by themselves do not seem to be sufficient for myeloma development as they are found already at the MGUS stage (Fonseca et al. 2002). IgH translocations are found in 45% of patients and hyperdiploidy in 50% of patients with myeloma (Manier et al. 2017). Approximately 10% of myeloma patients harbor both an IgH translocation and hyperdiploidy, while in 5%, neither IgH translocations nor hyperdiploidy can be detected. In addition to these primary cytogenetic events, a number of chromosomal gains and losses as well as somatic mutations are found in myeloma and can offer additional prognostic information (Stella et al. 2015).

1.4.1 IgH Translocations

Translocations occur when double-stranded DNA breaks and is aberrantly rejoined (Walker et al. 2013). During the maturation process of B-lymphocytes in the germinal center of the lymph nodes, there is genetic editing in the immunoglobulin heavy chain (IgH) gene to enhance the affinity of the antibody. First, there is a rearrangement of the hypervariable region (V-D-J) in a process called *somatic hypermutation*. Later, the cell undergoes *class-switch recombination* which results in antibodies of different isotypes (Nutt et al. 2015). Both somatic hypermutation and class-switch recombination infer double-stranded DNA breaks in the immunoglobulin locus (14q32) and require expression of activation-induced deaminase (AID). Despite rigorous control mechanisms, this genetic editing

may result in aberrant rejoining and thus chromosomal translocations (Morgan et al. 2012; Manier et al. 2017; Walker et al. 2015b). The majority of IgH translocations occur during class-switch recombination or somatic hypermutation, but translocations can also occur at various stages during B-cell development including early stages of pro-B-lymphocytes (Walker et al. 2013).

The most common IgH translocations in myeloma are *t*(4;14), *t*(6;14), *t*(11;14), *t*(14;16), and *t*(14;20), all resulting in an oncogene being placed under the strong IgH enhancer and are thus overexpressed. The net effect in the majority of these translocations is promotion of cyclin D proteins resulting in propagation of the cell cycle from G1 to S phase and a selective advance for the clone in question (Walker et al. 2013). Furthermore, the translocation partner gene is mutated in 10–25% of cases (Walker et al. 2015b). Translocations including IgH have different implications for disease prognosis and assessment for IgH rearrangement is recommended in the workup of myeloma patients (Rajkumar et al. 2014).

Translocation (11;14) between chromosome 11q13 (*CCND1*) and chromosome 14q32 is the most common translocation and is found in 15–20% of myeloma patients (Manier et al. 2017). The translocation results in the upregulation of *CCND1* and promotion of the cell cycle. Translocations between chromosome 11 and 14 are found also in mantle cell lymphoma, however, with a different breakpoints, and in 50% of patients with AL amyloidosis (REF). There is an ambiguous information on the prognostic information of *t*(11;14) in myeloma. Overall, it is considered to have a neutral impact, but there are indications that combination of *t*(11;14) translocation and *CCND1* mutations is associated with a poor prognosis (Bolli et al. 2014; Walker et al. 2015b). Concomitant *t*(11;14) translocations and CCND1 mutations are found in 10% of patients arising through a mechanism called *kataegis* (Bolli et al. 2014). Furthermore, the *t*(11;14) translocation often occurs early in B-cell development, already at the pro-B-lymphocyte stage (Walker et al. 2013), which may be an explanation behind the lymphoma-like phenotype observed in some cases. Patients with $t(11;14)$ translocations can have a lymphoplasmacytic differentiation, CD20 overexpression, and light-chain restriction. These patients may not respond as well to traditional myeloma drugs, and recently phase I/II studies indicate that these patients may respond better to treatment with novel drugs developed primarily for lymphoma (Sonneveld et al. 2016; Kumar et al. 2016; Moreau et al. 2016).

The $t(4;14)$ translocation is cryptic and is not detected by traditional metaphase cytogenetics. Therefore, FISH or polymerase chain reaction (PCR) must be performed for detection (Stella et al. 2015). Translocation (4;14) juxtaposes the genes *MMSET* and *FGFR3* from chromosome 4p16 to IgH enhancers whereby these genes are overexpressed (Sonneveld et al. 2016). The breakpoint on chromosome 4 falls between the two genes, and MMSET remains on der(4), and FGFR3 is translocated to der(14) (Walker et al. 2013). *MMSET*, which affects epigenetic regulation through histone modification, is expressed in 100% of these translocations, while sustained expression of *FGFR3*, which is an oncogenic receptor tyrosine kinase, is detected in 75% (Stella et al. 2015; Lawasut et al. 2013). There is recent data indicating that both genes are important for initial transformation but that sustained expression of *FGFR3* is not essential and this part of the der(14) is deleted in 25–30% of cases with $t(4;14)$ (Walker et al. 2013). In fact, a recent study on gene expression revealed that myeloma patients who have gene expression signature similar to those with the $t(4;14)$ translocation, i.e., *MMSET*-like signatures, have an equally poor prognosis even though they are lacking the actual translocation (Wu et al. 2016). Translocation $t(4;14)$ is associated with a poor outcome, both in regard to progression-free survival and overall survival (Sonneveld et al. 2016; Chng et al. 2014). Treatment with bortezomib and carfilzomib seems to at least partly overcome the adverse outcome in patients with $t(4;14)$ (Sonneveld et al. 2016).

Translocations $t(14;16)$ and $t(14;20)$ affect the *c-MAF* proto-oncogene and the *MAFB* oncogene, respectively, and result in their overexpression (Sonneveld et al. 2016). These in turn affect *CCND2* which also promotes proliferation by affecting the regulation of the G1/S phases of the cell cycle (Stella et al. 2015). Both $t(14;16)$ and $t(14;20)$ are associated with a poor outcome (Sonneveld et al. 2016). In addition to upregulation of *c-MAF*, the chromosome 16 breakpoints in $t(14;16)$ falls within the last intron of *WWOX*, a known tumor suppressor gene, resulting in the disruption of *WWOX* (Walker et al. 2013).

More rare translocations are $t(6;14)(q21;q32)$ and $t(12;14)(p13;q32)$ involving *CCND3* and *CCND2*, respectively, and also leading to upregulation of these cyclin D proteins and an overall promotion of the cell cycle. An alternative translocation also involving chromosome 6 is $t(6;14)(p25;q32)$ where *IRF4* is juxtaposed to IgH on chromosome 14 (Stella et al. 2015). There is limited information on the impact of the latter translocation on outcome in myeloma patients.

1.4.2 Hyperdiploidy

Patients with hyperdiploidy have gains of odd numbers of chromosomes, 3, 5, 7, 9, 11, 15, 19, and 21, and the cells harbor in total between 48 and 75 chromosomes. The mechanism behind hyperdiploidy is less clear, but the leading hypothesis is that all chromosome gains occur during one unsuccessful mitosis rather than consecutive gain of one chromosome at a time (Manier et al. 2017). Patients with hyperdiploidy are a heterogeneous group, but overall, they have a better prognosis compared to patients with IgH translocations (Stella et al. 2015; Avet-Loiseau et al. 2009). Hyperdiploidy is more often associated with IgG kappa myeloma, and patients are overall older compared to patients with IgH translocations (Stella et al. 2015). In addition to the gains of odd number of chromosomes as a probable initiating hit, these patients often have additional translocations as secondary hits. The most common are del1p, +1q, del17p, and translocations and amplifications including the *MYC* locus on 8q24.

1.4.3 Secondary Translocations in Myeloma

In addition to IgH translocations and hyperdiploidy, gains and losses of chromosomal material are seen at diagnosis and then increasingly as the disease progresses. Translocations including *MYC* on 8q24 are frequently seen in myeloma, up to 18% of newly diagnosed patients and as many as 50% of patients in the relapse setting (Stella et al. 2015; Walker et al. 2015b). *MYC* has a number of translocation partners, and *MYC* rearrangements, leading to *MYC* upregulation, are associated with a poor outcome. The most common translocation partners were the immunoglobulin heavy- and light-chain genes *IGH*, *IGL*, and *IGK* as well as additional genes frequently involved in myeloma, e.g., *FAM46C* (Walker et al. 2015b). In addition, similar to *t*(11;14) and *CCDN1* mutations, there is also evidence of *kataegis* where *MYC* translocations are combined with mutations in *MYC* (Manier et al. 2017).

1.4.4 Copy Number Variations

Gains or amplifications of 1q21 are associated with a poor overall survival and are more frequent in relapse and posttreatment samples. The minimally amplified region contains 679 genes, of which several oncogenes such as *CKS1B* and *ANP23E* have been identified. *CKS1B* encodes for a cell cycle-regulating protein which activates cyclin-dependent kinases and induces ubiquitination of inhibitory proteins, thus promoting cell proliferation (Stella et al. 2015).

Thirty percent of myeloma patients harbor deletions of the short arm of chromosome 1. Deletion 1p is associated with an adverse prognosis and can involve primarily two regions: 1p12, 1p32, or both. The first, 1p21, harbors the tumor suppressor gene *FAM46C* whose function is of importance for protein translation. Moreover, 1p32 harbors *CDKN2C* and *FAF1*. *CDKN2C* inhibits cell cycling and preserved the cell in the G1 phase. Deletion of *CDKN2C* thus results in more rapid cell cycling (Stella et al. 2015). *FAF1*

encodes for a protein involved in initiation and promotion of apoptosis (Manier et al. 2016a).

Deletion 17p is associated with a poor prognosis in myeloma as in many other hematological malignancies. *TP53*, an important DNA repair and tumor suppressor gene, is situated on 17p13, which is always included in the minimally deleted region on 17p. 17p deletions are seen in 10% of newly diagnosed myeloma patients and up to 80% of patients in later disease stages (Manier et al. 2017). Biallelic deletions of 17p or 17p deletion combined with *TP53* mutation on the remaining allele are common and associated with poor outcome (Weinhold et al. 2016a). Liu et al. recently reported from a mouse model study that 17p13 deletions were associated with a worse prognosis compared to *TP53* mutations. Their results indicated that there may be additional loci on 17p13 contributing to tumor progression through mechanisms independent of *TP53* (Liu et al. 2016).

Del13q is present in 40–50% of myeloma patients and is more common in IgH-translocated myelomas. In the majority of cases, the whole long arm of chromosome 13 is deleted. The minimally deleted region includes the tumor suppressor gene *Rb1* which has a role in cell cycle regulation. *DIS3* which is often mutated or deleted in myeloma is also located on the long arm of chromosome 13, however, not in the minimally deleted region (Manier et al. 2017). Historically, del13q has been associated with a poor prognosis; however, the majority of patients with 13q also harbor *t*(4;14) translocations. Therefore, it is currently not obvious whether del13q has a prognostic implication independent of *t*(4;14) translocations (Tables 1.1 and 1.2) (Manier et al. 2016a).

Table 1.1 High-risk and standard-risk cytogenetic aberrations (Sonneveld et al. 2016)

High-risk cytogenetic aberrations	Standard-risk cytogenetic aberrations
t(4;14)	*t*(11;14)
t(14;16)	*t*(6;14)
t(14;20)	
del(17/17p)	
gain(1q)	
Non-hyperdiploidy	

Table 1.2 Most common cytogenetic aberrations in myeloma and the genes involved

Chromosomal aberration	Genes involved
t(4;14)(p16;q32)	MMSET/FGFR3-IGH
t(6;14)(p25;q32)	IRF4/IGH
t(6;14)(p21;q32)	CCND3/IGH
t(11;14)(q13;q32)	CCND1/IGH
t(14;16)(q32;q23)	IGH/c-MAF. WWOX disrupted
t(14;20)(q32;q11)	MAFB/IGH
8q24	MYC
del(17/17p13)	TP53
gain(1q)	CSK1B
del(13q)	Rb1, DIS3

1.5 Somatic Mutations

Through massive parallel sequencing, a number of recurrent somatic mutations have been identified in multiple myeloma by using next-generation sequencing (Bolli et al. 2014; Chapman et al. 2011; Lohr et al. 2014; Walker et al. 2015a). So far, no unique disease-specific gene mutation has been identified, but a number of the recurrently mutated driver genes have been described. The frequently mutated genes affect various cellular functions including the MAPK and NFKB signaling pathways as well as DNA repair, RNA editing, and cell cycling.

Mutations in *KRAS* and *NRAS* are observed in 50% of patients and are in the majority of cases mutually exclusive (Bolli et al. 2014; Lohr et al. 2014; Walker et al. 2015a). *KRAS* and *NRAS* are oncogenes which are mutated in a large spectrum of tumors and affect intracellular signaling through the RAS/MAPK pathway. Activation of the RAS/MAPK pathway alters gene expression ultimately affecting cell differentiation, proliferation, and survival. *BRAF* is also part of this signaling pathway and is mutated in 10% of myeloma patients. *BRAF* mutations are primarily found in codon 600 (V600E), same as in hairy cell leukemia, but additional mutations in *BRAF* have also been observed (Walker et al. 2015a). Walker et al. reported the mean clonal cancer fraction of *KRAS*, *NRAS*, and *BRAF* mutations to be around 30% suggesting that these mutations

are secondary subclonal events associated with progression rather than being founder mutations (Walker et al. 2015a). The NFKB pathway is upregulated in myeloma cells leading to gene transcription and cell proliferation. This signaling pathway is important in myeloma cells which also is reflected in frequent mutations in a number of genes involved in this signaling pathway, e.g., *TRAF3*, *CYLD*, *MAP3K14*, *BIRC2*, *BIRC3*, *IKBKB*, and more (Lohr et al. 2014; Walker et al. 2015a).

DNA repair mechanisms are altered by somatic mutations and gene deletions of *TP53* and deletions of the short arm of 17p. Mutations and deletions affecting the 17p region become more frequent as the disease progresses and are associated with a poor prognosis (Manier et al. 2017). Mutations and deletions in *ATM* and *ATR*, which are part of the same DNA repair mechanism as TP53, are also commonly observed in myeloma (Walker et al. 2015a). Mutations involving genes associated with regulation of RNA editing and protein translation are common in myeloma. FAM46C and DIS3, both involved in RNA regulation and protein translation, are affected by inactivating mutations and/or deletions (Bianchi and Ghobrial 2014; Bolli et al. 2014; Lohr et al. 2014; Walker et al. 2015a).

In addition to several translocations and mutations affecting the cyclin D proteins, cell cycle regulation is affected through events resulting in the loss of function of negative cell cycle regulatory genes such as *CSKN2C*, *CDKN2A*, and *RB1*. These genomic events can be inactivating mutations, gene deletions, or a combination of both (Weinhold et al. 2016a). The most frequently mutated genes in myeloma are listed in Table 1.3.

Weinhold et al. recently observed that biallelic inactivating events are common in myeloma. These include deletions and/or inactivating mutations in known tumor suppressor genes such as *TP53*, *FAM46C*, *TRAF3*, *CYLD*, and more (Weinhold et al. 2016a). Biallelic events were more common in the relapse setting compared to newly diagnosed patients and are associated with adverse gene expression profiling signatures. Especially biallelic events including 17p deletion

Table 1.3 Most frequent genetic mutations in multiple myeloma

Gene	Frequency (%) (Bolli et al. 2014; Lohr et al. 2014; Walker et al. 2015a; Kortuem et al. 2016)
KRAS	20–23
NRAS	19–20
BRAF	6–12
FAM46C	6–11
TP53	3–12
DIS3	1–11
PRDM1	5
EGR1	2–6
SP140	4–6
TRAF3	2–5
CCND1	2–4
ATM	2–4
HISTH1E	3
CYLD	1–5
LTB	1–4
RB1	2–3
IRF4	3
STAT3	3
MAX	1–3
ATR	1–2

and *TP53* mutations were associated with a poor prognosis (Weinhold et al. 2016a).

1.5.1 Clonal Evolution

Chromosomal translocations are necessary but not sufficient for developing myeloma. MGUS and smoldering myeloma are similar to myeloma in regard to translocations, but myeloma is more genetically complex and has a higher mutational load (Walker et al. 2014; Malek et al. 2016). There is so far limited information on the genomic landscape and clonal evolution during transition from MGUS to smoldering myeloma to myeloma. Progression from MGUS to myeloma may be caused by acquisition of additional genetic events or the expansion of pre-existing clones already present at the MGUS stage. In the myeloma stage, there are often multiple disease clones present at diagnosis. Lohr et al. reported that most myeloma patients have at least three subclones and many patients had up to seven clones

(Lohr et al. 2014). Their study was able to detect subclones that were at least 10% of the tumor sample, while in reality, the number of subclones per myeloma patients is likely far greater (Lohr et al. 2014). Furthermore, some mutations in myeloma tend to be clonal, e.g., *RB1*, *CCND1*, and *TP53*, while others are more often subclonal, e.g., *KRAS/NRAS* and *FAM46C*, indicating early vs later acquisition (Manier et al. 2017; Walker et al. 2015a).

Myeloma evolution has been shown to proceed according to a branching disease evolution driven by competing subclones (Morgan et al. 2012). Bolli et al. observed four different patterns of disease progression in patients where they had sequential samples. These included lineal evolution, branching evolution where there was a different dominant subclone at relapse, a new subclone had emerged in parallel with the original dominant clone, or the emergence of a new subclone while the original clone was not detectable (Bolli et al. 2014).

1.5.2 Prognostic Impact

So far, approximately 900 patients in four published studies have been sequenced using whole exome or targeted sequencing. Thus, there is currently no robust information on the prognostic effect of specific gene mutations. In these studies, mutations in *TP53*, *KRAS*, *STAT3*, *PTPN11*, *PRDM1*, *CXCR4*, *IRF4*, *MAFB*, *ZFHX4*, *NCKAP5*, and *SP140* were associated with a shorter overall and/or progression-free survival (Bolli et al. 2014; Lohr et al. 2014; Walker et al. 2015a; Kortuem et al. 2016). *TRAF3* was on the other hand associated with a longer progression-free survival (Kortuem et al. 2016); however, as mentioned, there is so far limited data to support these findings.

1.5.3 Relapse

Regarding chromosomal aberrations, high-risk features such as gain1q, del 17p, and genetic events involving MYC are more common in relapse samples (Walker et al. 2015b; Kortum et al. 2016). Moreover, Weinhold et al. described higher frequencies of del(1p) and loss of heterozygosity at 6q and 16q (Weinhold et al. 2016a). Furthermore, mutations affecting specific treatment pathways such as cereblon, the target of immunomodulatory drugs (IMiDs), are more common in relapse samples compared to samples analyzed at diagnosis. In a recent study on 50 heavily pretreated myeloma patients, Kortuem et al. found cereblon-associated mutation in 25% of the relapse patients. All of these patients were refractory to IMIDs. These mutations included *CRBN*, *CUL4B*, *IRF4*, and *IKZF1*. In some of these, pretreatment samples were available for comparison. None of the pretreatment samples harbored the *CRBN*-associated mutations even with increased sequencing depth supporting that the resistance was indeed acquired over the course of the disease (Kortum et al. 2016).

In addition to *CRBN*, mutations were also found in the proteasome 19S subunit in patients that were refractory to proteasome inhibitors and immunomodulatory drugs. Kortum et al. also reported mutations in genes coding for proteasome subunits, i.e., *PSMB8* and *PSMD1*. In addition, mutations in *XBP1*, also found in one patient, have also been associated with PI resistance (Kortum et al. 2016). In the study by Kortuem et al., the majority of patients with *CRBN* mutation were found to be refractory to IMiDs (Kortum et al. 2016).

Weinhold et al. recently reported on sequential sequencing at diagnosis and relapse of 33 myeloma patients. The majority of the relapse samples showed a pattern of branching disease evolution. In the relapse samples, there were increasing proportions of 17p deletions, *TP53* mutations, as well as *MYC* translocations. There was also a higher mutational load in the relapse samples compared to the diagnostic samples, on average 43 nonsynonymous somatic mutations at presentation versus 60 at relapse. Furthermore, there were more biallelic events in tumor suppressor genes, e.g., *TP53*, *FAM46C*, and *TRAF3*, at relapse. No increase in *CRBN* mutations was observed (Weinhold et al. 2016a). These 33 patients were all treated on the total therapy protocols with a combination of alkylating agents and proteasome inhibitors. Weinhold et al. did observe any *CRBN* mutations; however, none of the patients were reported to be IMiDs refractory (Weinhold et al. 2016a).

1.6 Gene Expression

The first molecular classification in myeloma was performed using gene expression profiling. Assessing gene expression through microarray has provided a tool for prognostication that can contribute with additional information to conventional risk stratification using FISH. These analyses have revealed over- as well as underexpression of various genes including oncogenes, tumor suppressor genes, and cell signaling and transcription factor genes. The Arkansas group, the IFM group, and the HOVON group have all published gene expression signature that can predict favorable versus unfavorable outcome (Decaux et al. 2008; Kuiper et al. 2012; Shaughnessy et al. 2007).

Initially, Shaughnessy et al. within the Arkansas group identified a 70-gene signature (GEP70) based on myeloma patients treated within the total therapy protocols (Shaughnessy et al. 2007). Depending on the level of expression of these 70 genes, patients were classified into seven separate subgroups with high or low risk of disease progression. These seven subtypes largely corresponded to the most common chromosomal translocations and hyperdiploidy (Shaughnessy et al. 2007; Zhan et al. 2006). The seven subtypes were abbreviated MS, reflecting the activation of *MMSET* in the t(4;14) translocation, MF reflecting translocations t(14;16) and t(14;20) and activations of *c-MAF* and *MAFB*, CD-1 corresponding to t(11;14) and *CCND1* activation and CD-2 corresponding to t(6;14) translocation and activation of *CCDN3*, HY corresponding to the hyperdiploid karyotype, PR reflecting a subset of patients with a high disease proliferation, and LB which includes patients with a low prevalence of bone disease (Shaughnessy et al. 2007). In the newly diagnosed setting, around 10–15% had high-risk signatures, while in the relapse setting, a significantly higher proportion of patients had gene expression profiles associated with a high risk of progression (Weinhold et al. 2016a; Shaughnessy et al. 2007; Weinhold et al. 2016b). The most common upregulated genes are found on 1q, and the majority of the downregulated genes are located on 1p (Shaughnessy et al. 2007; Zhan et al. 2006). The GEP70 model was able to predict outcome independently of the International Staging System (Shaughnessy et al. 2007).

Similarly, the EMC92 is based on a 92-gene signature, and the IFM model is based on a 15-gene signature. Of note, there is a little overlap in the genes included in the different models. Even though the gene expression profiles are powerful prognostic tools, the signature models have been developed in specific patient cohorts that were uniformly treated with clinical trials. The models perform well within their respective patient population, but overall, not all gene expression profiling models have held true when cross-validated between patient cohorts. In addition, gene expression profiling generates large amounts of data and requires complex analyses. This, together with issues getting sufficient RNA for the microarrays, has hampered the implementation of gene expression profiling in the general clinical praxis (van Laar et al. 2014).

Recently, a simplified subgroup classification was presented, which is based on gene expression profiles as well as DNA sequencing data in a subset of patients. The new classification includes five translocation cyclin (TC) subgroups identified as the name implies through translocations and deregulation of cyclin D (Stein et al. 2016). There were clear associations between chromosomal aberrations (TC subtypes), somatic mutations, and RNA expression. Interestingly, activation of the NFKB pathway and MAPK pathway was inversely associated, and activation of these pathways was different between the TC subtypes (Stein et al. 2016).

Looking forward, gene expression is being assessed using high-throughput RNA sequencing of bone marrow samples and single-cell analyses of circulating tumor cells in the peripheral blood (Lohr et al. 2016). Additionally, RNA assessment

can identify subsets of patients with gene expression profiles mimicking those in the high-risk groups, such as the MMSET-like profile leading to a poor prognosis similar to patients who harbor the actual $t(4;14)$ translocation as mentioned earlier (Wu et al. 2016). Studies including analyses of transcriptome modifiers such as alternative splicing, microRNAs, and epigenetic profiles are also ongoing (Szalat and Munshi 2015). Gene expression, particularly using RNA sequencing in combination with DNA sequencing will be of great interest to further delineate myeloma pathogenesis.

1.7 Bone Marrow Microenvironment

In addition to genomic aberrations and changes in gene expression, there is growing evidence that the bone marrow environment plays an important role in the pathogenesis of myeloma. There are multiple interactions, e.g., through direct cell–cell interactions and adhesion molecules, secretion of cytokines and chemokines as well as exosomes with miRNA, between the bone marrow niche and the malignant plasma cells. These interactions result in the promotion of tumor cells survival and proliferation. The bone marrow environment consists of a cellular component including hematopoietic and non-hematopoietic cells and a noncellular component including the extracellular matrix, liquid milieu, and oxygen level. There is a dense interplay including multiple feedback loops between all compartments with an overall effect of promoting malignant plasma cell growth and survival (Landgren 2013).

The hematopoietic cells within the cellular component are hematopoietic stem cells, myeloid cells, B- and T-lymphocytes, natural killer (NK) cells, dendritic cells, and macrophages. Several of these cells have an altered function in myeloma resulting in either immunosuppressive effects allowing the malignant plasma cell to evade the immune system or various mechanisms to support growth and survival of the myeloma clone (Manier et al. 2016b; Balakumaran et al. 2010).

The immunosuppressive mechanisms, often induced by the tumor cells, are mediated through expansion of regulatory/inhibitory immune cells, primarily myeloid-derived stem cells (MDSCs) and regulatory T-cells (Tregs). MDSCs are immature cells that under normal circumstances develop into granulocytes, macrophages, and dendritic cells. In myeloma, however, they remain in this early form with immunosuppressive properties and may enable immune escape and inhibit the T-cell response and thus facilitate myeloma cell growth (Malek et al. 2016; Gorgun et al. 2013; Kawano et al. 2015). Through bidirectional interaction, MDSCs assist in protecting the MM cells against chemotherapy and promote angiogenesis and metastasis (Malek et al. 2016). In addition, the MDSCs can contribute to bone destruction in myeloma by directly serving as osteoclast precursors (Kawano et al. 2015; Zhuang et al. 2012). IMiDs and bortezomib both act on myeloma cells and on the bone marrow microenvironment, however, they have not been shown to be effective in reversing the immunosuppressive effect of MDSCs (Gorgun et al. 2013; Kawano et al. 2015). Tregs are CD4+ T-cells characterized by the expression of the transcription factor FOXP3. In myeloma, Tregs accumulate in the blood and bone marrow, and an increasing number of Tregs have been associated with a poorer prognosis. Like MDSCs, Tregs also suppress an effective anti-myeloma immune response; the effect is mediated through inhibiting the function of normal antigen-presenting cells and effector T-cells either by direct contact or through cytokine secretion (Moschetta et al. 2016). In addition, dendritic cells, which promote either immunity or tolerance, and natural killer cells (NK cells) are observed to be functionally defective in myeloma further aiding myeloma cells to proliferate and evade the immune system (Kawano et al. 2015). In addition, NK cells expresses PD-1 which binds to PDL-1 on myeloma cells, not on normal plasma cells, thereby suppressing the antitumoral effect of NK cells in myeloma (Manier et al. 2016b; Moschetta et al. 2016).

Taken together, these effects result in immune escape and tumor growth through the direct stimulation and loss of effective antigen presentation, effector cell dysfunction, deletion of myeloma-specific T-cells, and increasing presence of inhibitory cells (Tregs and MDSCs).

Macrophages interact with malignant plasma cells through contact as well as non-contact mechanisms, thereby stimulating cell growth and tumor cell invasion as well as protecting myeloma cells from therapy-induced apoptosis (Kawano et al. 2015; Moschetta et al. 2016). Macrophages secrete several pro-angiogenic cytokines including vascular endothelial growth factor (VEGF), interleukin-8 (IL-8), fibroblast growth factor, as well as the cytokines IL-1b, IL-10, TNFa, and IL-6 with net effects of promoting angiogenesis and myeloma cell growth (Figs. 1.1 and 1.2) (Kawano et al. 2015).

The cells within the non-hematopoietic cellular compartment are stromal cells including mesenchymal stem cells, fibroblasts, bone marrow adipocytes, osteoclasts, osteoblasts, and endothelial cells. Bone marrow stromal cells (BMSCs) bind closely to the plasma cells through various adhesion molecules such as intercellular adhesion molecule 1 (ICAM-1) and vascular cell adhesion molecule 1 (VCAM-1). This adhesion triggers signaling through a number of pathways in the plasma cells, e.g., the RAS/MAPK, NFKB, and PI3K signaling pathways, resulting in cell proliferation and drug resistance (Manier et al. 2016b). The BMSCs secrete cytokines, e.g., IL-6, which is a key cytokine in myeloma as it promotes proliferation and survival of myeloma cells (Kawano et al. 2015). The plasma cells in turn secrete growth factors such as VEGF, fibroblast growth factor, and many more to stimulate proliferation of BMSCs, endothelial cells, and neoangiogenesis (Kawano et al. 2015). This creates a loop of cytokine secretion between the bone marrow plasma cells and the bone marrow niche which is essential for the survival of the myeloma cells (Manier et al. 2016b). Furthermore, BMSCs secrete stromal cell-derived factor 1 (SDF-1) belonging to the CRCX4 axis which is critical for stromal-myeloma interaction in the bone marrow niche and for dissemination of myeloma cells within the bone marrow as well as to extramedullary sites (Manier et al. 2016b;

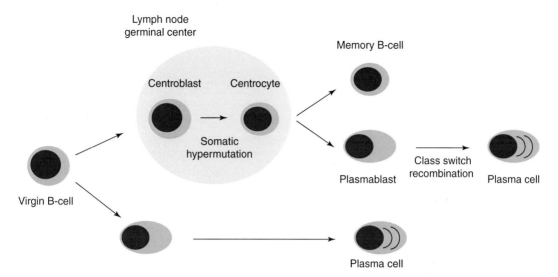

Fig. 1.1 Origin of malignant plasma cell

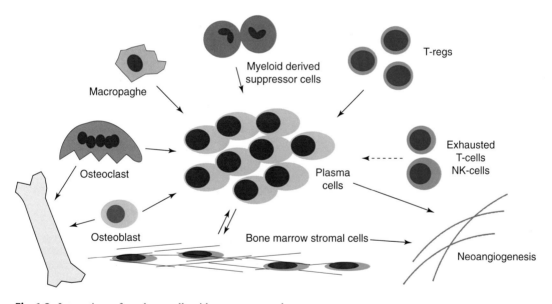

Fig. 1.2 Interactions of myeloma cells with marrow stromal

Kuiper et al. 2012; Stein et al. 2016; Lohr et al. 2016; Szalat and Munshi 2015). In addition, BMSCs release exosome with miRNA and specific proteins that are taken up by the plasma cells and have the potential to affect gene expression and tumor growth (Kawano et al. 2015). Bortezomib can reverse many of the interactions between myeloma and stromal cell interactions as well as inhibit cytokine production and secretion (Manier et al. 2016b).

In patients with myeloma, there is an ongoing neovascularization within the bone marrow. This process is gradually increased from MGUS to smoldering myeloma to multiple myeloma, and elevated microvascular density has been correlated to a worse prognosis (Rajkumar et al. 2002). Within the bone marrow, myeloma cells secrete VEGF and stimulating endothelial cells which in turn secrete IL-6 resulting in simultaneous proliferation of both myeloma cells and neoangiogenesis

(Munshi and Wilson 2001; Rajkumar and Kyle 2001). Treatment with IMiDs has a negative effect on angiogenesis (Kawano et al. 2015).

In myeloma, the balance between bone formation and bone resorption is altered favoring bone resorption and suppression of osteoblast activity. Osteoblasts, which normally are responsible for bone formation, are suppressed via Dickkopf-1 (DKK1), a Wnt signaling inhibitor, contributing to lytic lesions. Osteoblasts also secrete IL-6 and osteoprotegerin blocking TRAIL-mediated programmed cell death MM by secreting (Manier et al. 2016b). In myeloma, the balance is tipped toward osteoclast activation leading to lytic lesions. Myeloma cells produce receptor activator of nuclear factor kappa-B ligand (RANKL), macrophage inflammatory protein 1a (MIP-1a), IL-3, and IL-6, all contributing to an increased osteoclast activity. RANKL is in the TNF family and plays a major role in osteoclast activation in myeloma. Blocking RANKL with the monoclonal antibody denosumab, which is a soluble form of RANK, has been shown to modulate bone loss and improve overall survival in in vivo models (Manier et al. 2016b). Furthermore, bisphosphonates can inhibit osteoclasts but also target feedback loop with osteoclasts and myeloma cells (Manier et al. 2016b).

The noncellular compartment can be divided into the extracellular matrix component and the soluble component. The extracellular matrix consists of fibrous proteins including collagenous proteins to 90%; the remaining 10% is made up of proteoglycans, glycosaminoglycans, and small integrin-binding ligand N-linked glycoproteins (SIBLINGs) (Balakumaran et al. 2010). These proteins constitute a supporting structure for bone marrow cells but also interact with myeloma cells directly promoting cell proliferation (Balakumaran et al. 2010). Remodeling of the extracellular matrix by BMSC may be important in the progression from MGUS to myeloma (Slany et al. 2014).

The soluble component includes a variety of cytokines, growth factors, and adhesion molecules produced by the myeloma cells and nontumor cells in the bone marrow (Balakumaran et al. 2010). As mentioned, IL-6 is primarily produced

by BMSCs and osteoblasts and is a key growth factor in myeloma cell growth. IL-6 stimulates osteoclasts formation as well as affects gene expression in myeloma cells through the MAPK, JAK/STAT, and PI3K/Akt signaling pathways resulting in the expression of transcription factors and activation of antiapoptotic proteins (Balakumaran et al. 2010). SDF-1α produced by BMSCs upregulates adhesion between myeloma cells to fibronectin and VCAM-1 resulting in proliferation, migration, and protection against drug-induced apoptosis. SDF-1 also affects BMSCs leading to upregulated secretion of IL-6 and VEGF. TNFα and members of the TNF superfamily including CD40L, BAFF, and APRIL all mediate myeloma cell growth, through either direct mechanisms or upregulation of IL-6. RANKL, also a member of the TNF family, as mentioned increases osteoclastogenesis through binding to RANK on the osteoclasts (Balakumaran et al. 2010). Additional growth factors include VEGF from myeloma cells stimulating endothelial cells and angiogenesis. Insulin-like growth factor-1 (IGF-1) which also is found in the liquid milieu of myeloma patients promotes cell growth, survival, and migration (Balakumaran et al. 2010). Moreover, matrix metalloproteinases act through growth factors resulting in neovascularization and osteoclast activity leading to myeloma progression (Balakumaran et al. 2010).

The liquid milieu is physiologically hypoxic and organized with varying oxygen content near the trabecular bone and near the vascular niche near sinusoids (Moschetta et al. 2016). The hypoxia of the endosteal niche supports myeloma cells primarily mediated through HIF-1 and HIF-2. In addition to promoting myeloma clone growth, hypoxia also decreases CD138 expression and induces a more immature and stem cell-like expression program in myeloma cells (Moschetta et al. 2016).

1.8 Future Perspective

The field of genomic assessment in multiple myeloma has over a short period of time gone from gross anatomical assessment using cytogenetics and FISH to more advanced techniques which has led to great insights to the genomic landscape of myeloma. The first of these modern techniques was gene expression profiling where relative upregulation and downregulation of mRNA are analyzed which may contribute with prognostic information. As mentioned, there are caveats with these techniques not being fully generalizable outside of the setting they were developed in (Szalat and Munshi 2015). More recently, next-generation sequencing including whole genome, whole exome, or targeted sequencing techniques have been utilized in myeloma. When applying bioinformatics processing tools and filtering out intronic and silent mutations, thus focusing on nonsynonymous exons coding for RNA and later protein products, the average number of mutation in multiple myeloma tumor cells is around 50 (Kortum et al. 2016; Mailankody et al. 2016).

These techniques enable DNA sequencing with a high resolution but are also associated with technical limitations. For instance, the polymerase chain reaction of the sequencing process and possible sequencing misreads result in an error rate of around 1% for next-generation sequencing platforms. In emerging techniques such as duplex sequencing with DNA strand-specific bar coding, the error rate can be reduced to 1 in 10^9 bases (Schmitt et al. 2012).

Going forward, the clinical implications of the various somatic mutations need to be confirmed across clinical datasets. Unanswered questions include whether the mutational landscape is affected by treatment or if treatment drives specific mutations, for instance, in treatment pathways such as cereblon? How is the clonal evolution and subclone dominance affected by treatment and does treatment select for more aggressive subclones? Furthermore, emerging techniques such as analysis of circulating tumor cells, cell-free DNA, RNA expression, and proteomics will most likely lead to additional insights to myelomagenesis. How do findings from sequencing and functional studies correlate with the bone marrow picture, and can these techniques be used for diagnostic and prognostic assessment going forward? Interestingly, in a recent study by Lohr et al., the DNA and RNA sequencing data from circulating tumor cells corresponded well with the findings from the malignant plasma cells in the bone marrow suggesting that the assessment of circulating tumor cells could be a reliable and noninvasive option in the near future (Lohr et al. 2016). Larger patient cohorts and combination of findings from several techniques are desired to explore differences in the genetic landscape between patients as well as within individual patients, e.g., intra-tumor difference and spatial and temporal difference, as well as to decipher the clinical implications.

References

Avet-Loiseau H, Li C, Magrangeas F, Gouraud W, Charbonnel C, Harousseau JL et al (2009) Prognostic significance of copy-number alterations in multiple myeloma. J Clin Oncol 27(27):4585–4590

Balakumaran A, Robey PG, Fedarko N, Landgren O (2010) Bone marrow microenvironment in myelomagenesis: its potential role in early diagnosis. Expert Rev Mol Diagn 10(4):465–480

Bianchi G, Ghobrial IM (2014) Biological and clinical implications of clonal heterogeneity and clonal evolution in multiple myeloma. Curr Cancer Ther Rev 10(2):70–79

Bolli N, Avet-Loiseau H, Wedge DC, Van Loo P, Alexandrov LB, Martincorena I et al (2014) Heterogeneity of genomic evolution and mutational profiles in multiple myeloma. Nat Commun 5:2997

Bolli N, Li Y, Sathiaseelan V, Raine K, Jones D, Ganly P et al (2016) A DNA target-enrichment approach to detect mutations, copy number changes and immunoglobulin translocations in multiple myeloma. Blood Cancer J 6(9):e467

Chapman MA, Lawrence MS, Keats JJ, Cibulskis K, Sougnez C, Schinzel AC et al (2011) Initial genome sequencing and analysis of multiple myeloma. Nature 471(7339):467–472

Chng WJ, Dispenzieri A, Chim CS, Fonseca R, Goldschmidt H, Lentzsch S et al (2014) IMWG consensus on risk stratification in multiple myeloma. Leukemia 28(2):269–277

Decaux O, Lode L, Magrangeas F, Charbonnel C, Gouraud W, Jezequel P et al (2008) Prediction of survival in multiple myeloma based on gene expression profiles reveals cell cycle and chromosomal instability signatures in high-risk patients and hyperdiploid signatures in low-risk patients: a study of the Intergroupe francophone du Myelome. J Clin Oncol 26(29):4798–4805

Fonseca R, Bailey RJ, Ahmann GJ, Rajkumar SV, Hoyer JD, Lust JA et al (2002) Genomic abnormalities in monoclonal gammopathy of undetermined significance. Blood 100(4):1417–1424

Gorgun GT, Whitehill G, Anderson JL, Hideshima T, Maguire C, Laubach J et al (2013) Tumor-promoting immune-suppressive myeloid-derived suppressor cells in the multiple myeloma microenvironment in humans. Blood 121(15):2975–2987

Kawano Y, Moschetta M, Manier S, Glavey S, Gorgun GT, Roccaro AM et al (2015) Targeting the bone marrow microenvironment in multiple myeloma. Immunol Rev 263(1):160–172

Kortuem KM, Braggio E, Bruins L, Barrio S, Shi CS, Zhu YX et al (2016) Panel sequencing for clinically oriented variant screening and copy number detection in 142 untreated multiple myeloma patients. Blood Cancer J 6:e397

Kortum KM, Mai EK, Hanafiah NH, Shi CX, Zhu YX, Bruins L et al (2016) Targeted sequencing of refractory myeloma reveals a high incidence of mutations in CRBN and Ras pathway genes. Blood 128(9):1226–1233

Kristinsson SY, Landgren O, Dickman PW, Derolf AR, Bjorkholm M (2007) Patterns of survival in multiple myeloma: a population-based study of patients diagnosed in Sweden from 1973 to 2003. J Clin Oncol 25(15):1993–1999

Kristinsson SY, Anderson WF, Landgren O (2014) Improved long-term survival in multiple myeloma up to the age of 80 years. Leukemia 28(6):1346–1348

Kuiper R, Broyl A, de Knegt Y, van Vliet MH, van Beers EH, van der Holt B et al (2012) A gene expression signature for high-risk multiple myeloma. Leukemia 26(11):2406–2413

Kumar S, Vij R, Kaufman JL, Mikhael J, Facon T, Pegourie B et al (2016) Phase 1 study of venetoclax monotherapy for relapsed/refractory multiple myeloma. Haematologica 101:328

Kyle RA (1978) Monoclonal gammopathy of undetermined significance. Natural history in 241 cases. Am J Med 64(5):814–826

Kyle RA, Durie BG, Rajkumar SV, Landgren O, Blade J, Merlini G et al (2010) Monoclonal gammopathy of undetermined significance (MGUS) and smoldering (asymptomatic) multiple myeloma: IMWG consensus perspectives risk factors for progression and guidelines for monitoring and management. Leukemia 24(6):1121–1127

Landgren O (2013) Monoclonal gammopathy of undetermined significance and smoldering multiple myeloma: biological insights and early treatment strategies. Hematology Am Soc Hematol Educ Program 2013:478–487

Landgren O, Katzmann JA, Hsing AW, Pfeiffer RM, Kyle RA, Yeboah ED et al (2007) Prevalence of monoclonal gammopathy of undetermined significance among men in Ghana. Mayo Clin Proc 82(12):1468–1473

Landgren O, Kyle RA, Pfeiffer RM, Katzmann JA, Caporaso NE, Hayes RB et al (2009a) Monoclonal gammopathy of undetermined significance (MGUS) consistently precedes multiple myeloma: a prospective study. Blood 113(22):5412–5417

Landgren O, Kyle RA, Hoppin JA, Beane Freeman LE, Cerhan JR, Katzmann JA et al (2009b) Pesticide exposure and risk of monoclonal gammopathy of undetermined significance in the agricultural health study. Blood 113(25):6386–6391

Landgren O, Graubard BI, Katzmann JA, Kyle RA, Ahmadizadeh I, Clark R et al (2014) Racial disparities in the prevalence of monoclonal gammopathies: a population-based study of 12,482 persons from the national health and nutritional examination survey. Leukemia 28(7):1537–1542

Landgren O, Shim YK, Michalek J, Costello R, Burton D, Ketchum N et al (2015) Agent orange exposure and monoclonal gammopathy of undetermined significance: an operation ranch hand veteran cohort study. JAMA Oncol 1(8):1061–1068

Lawasut P, Groen RW, Dhimolea E, Richardson PG, Anderson KC, Mitsiades CS (2013) Decoding the pathophysiology and the genetics of multiple myeloma to identify new therapeutic targets. Semin Oncol 40(5):537–548

Liu Y, Chen C, Xu Z, Scuoppo C, Rillahan CD, Gao J et al (2016) Deletions linked to TP53 loss drive cancer through p53-independent mechanisms. Nature 531(7595):471–475

Lohr JG, Stojanov P, Carter SL, Cruz-Gordillo P, Lawrence MS, Auclair D et al (2014) Widespread genetic heterogeneity in multiple myeloma: implications for targeted therapy. Cancer Cell 25(1):91–101

Lohr JG, Kim S, Gould J, Knoechel B, Drier Y, Cotton MJ et al (2016) Genetic interrogation of circulating multiple myeloma cells at single-cell resolution. Sci Transl Med 8(363):363ra147

Mailankody S, Korde N, Roschewski MJ, Christofferson A, Boateng M, Zhang Y et al (2016) Genetic plasma cell signatures in high-risk smoldering myeloma versus multiple myeloma patients. ASCO Meet Abstr 34(15 Suppl):8003

Malek E, de Lima M, Letterio JJ, Kim BG, Finke JH, Driscoll JJ et al (2016) Myeloid-derived suppressor cells: the green light for myeloma immune escape. Blood Rev 30(5):341–348

Manier S, Salem K, Glavey SV, Roccaro AM, Ghobrial IM (2016a) Genomic aberrations in multiple myeloma. Cancer Treat Res 169:23–34

Manier S, Kawano Y, Bianchi G, Roccaro AM, Ghobrial IM (2016b) Cell autonomous and microenvironmental regulation of tumor progression in precursor states of multiple myeloma. Curr Opin Hematol 23(4):426–433

Manier S, Salem KZ, Park J, Landau DA, Getz G, Ghobrial IM (2017) Genomic complexity of multiple myeloma and its clinical implications. Nat Rev Clin Oncol 14(2):100–113

Moreau P, Chanan-Khan A, Roberts AW, Agarwal A, Facon T, Kumar S et al (2016) Phase 1b study of venetoclax combined with bortezomib and dexamethasone in relapsed/refractory multiple myeloma. Haematologica 101:81–82

Morgan GJ, Walker BA, Davies FE (2012) The genetic architecture of multiple myeloma. Nat Rev Cancer 12(5):335–348

Morgan GJ, Johnson DC, Weinhold N, Goldschmidt H, Landgren O, Lynch HT et al (2014) Inherited genetic susceptibility to multiple myeloma. Leukemia 28(3):518–524

Moschetta M, Kawano Y, Podar K (2016) Targeting the bone marrow microenvironment. Cancer Treat Res 169:63–102

Munshi NC, Wilson C (2001) Increased bone marrow microvessel density in newly diagnosed multiple myeloma carries a poor prognosis. Semin Oncol 28(6):565–569

Nutt SL, Hodgkin PD, Tarlinton DM, Corcoran LM (2015) The generation of antibody-secreting plasma cells. Nat Rev Immunol 15(3):160–171

Rajkumar SV, Kyle RA (2001) Angiogenesis in multiple myeloma. Semin Oncol 28(6):560–564

Rajkumar SV, Mesa RA, Fonseca R, Schroeder G, Plevak MF, Dispenzieri A et al (2002) Bone marrow angiogenesis in 400 patients with monoclonal gammopathy of undetermined significance, multiple myeloma, and primary amyloidosis. Clin Cancer Res 8(7):2210–2216

Rajkumar SV, Dimopoulos MA, Palumbo A, Blade J, Merlini G, Mateos MV et al (2014) International myeloma working group updated criteria for the diagnosis of multiple myeloma. Lancet Oncol 15(12):e538–e548

Schmitt MW, Kennedy SR, Salk JJ, Fox EJ, Hiatt JB, Loeb LA (2012) Detection of ultra-rare mutations by next-generation sequencing. Proc Natl Acad Sci U S A 109(36):14508–14513

Shaughnessy JD Jr, Zhan F, Burington BE, Huang Y, Colla S, Hanamura I et al (2007) A validated gene expression model of high-risk multiple myeloma is defined by deregulated expression of genes mapping to chromosome 1. Blood 109(6):2276–2284

Siegel RL, Miller KD, Jemal A (2016) Cancer statistics, 2016. CA Cancer J Clin 66(1):7–30

Slany A, Haudek-Prinz V, Meshcheryakova A, Bileck A, Lamm W, Zielinski C et al (2014) Extracellular matrix remodeling by bone marrow fibroblast-like cells correlates with disease progression in multiple myeloma. J Proteome Res 13(2):844–854

Sonneveld P, Avet-Loiseau H, Lonial S, Usmani S, Siegel D, Anderson KC et al (2016) Treatment of multiple myeloma with high-risk cytogenetics: a consensus of the international myeloma working group. Blood 127(24):2955–2962

Stein CK, Pawlyn C, Chavan SS, Weinhold N, Walker BA, Rosenthal A et al (2016) The mutational and signaling landscape of multiple myeloma varies dependent upon Translocation Cyclin D (TC) subgroup. Blood 128(22):4441

Stella F, Pedrazzini E, Agazzoni M, Ballester O, Slavutsky I (2015) Cytogenetic alterations in multiple myeloma: prognostic significance and the choice of frontline therapy. Cancer Investig 33(10):496–504

Szalat R, Munshi NC (2015) Genomic heterogeneity in multiple myeloma. Curr Opin Genet Dev 30:56–65

Turesson I, Kovalchik SA, Pfeiffer RM, Kristinsson SY, Goldin LR, Drayson MT et al (2014) Monoclonal gammopathy of undetermined significance and

risk of lymphoid and myeloid malignancies: 728 cases followed up to 30 years in Sweden. Blood 123(3):338–345

van Laar R, Flinchum R, Brown N, Ramsey J, Riccitelli S, Heuck C et al (2014) Translating a gene expression signature for multiple myeloma prognosis into a robust high-throughput assay for clinical use. BMC Med Genet 7:25

Velez R, Turesson I, Landgren O, Kristinsson SY, Cuzick J (2016) Incidence of multiple myeloma in Great Britain, Sweden, and Malmo, Sweden: the impact of differences in case ascertainment on observed incidence trends. BMJ Open 6(1):e009584

Waldenstrom J (1960) Studies on conditions associated with disturbed gamma globulin formation (gammopathies). Harvey Lect 56:211–231

Walker BA, Wardell CP, Johnson DC, Kaiser MF, Begum DB, Dahir NB et al (2013) Characterization of IGH locus breakpoints in multiple myeloma indicates a subset of translocations appear to occur in pregerminal center B cells. Blood 121(17):3413–3419

Walker BA, Wardell CP, Melchor L, Brioli A, Johnson DC, Kaiser MF et al (2014) Intraclonal heterogeneity is a critical early event in the development of myeloma and precedes the development of clinical symptoms. Leukemia 28(2):384–390

Walker BA, Boyle EM, Wardell CP, Murison A, Begum DB, Dahir NM et al (2015a) Mutational spectrum, copy number changes, and outcome: results of a sequencing study of patients with newly diagnosed myeloma. J Clin Oncol 33(33):3911–3920

Walker BA, Wardell CP, Murison A, Boyle EM, Begum DB, Dahir NM et al (2015b) APOBEC family mutational signatures are associated with poor prognosis translocations in multiple myeloma. Nat Commun 6:6997

Waxman AJ, Mink PJ, Devesa SS, Anderson WF, Weiss BM, Kristinsson SY et al (2010) Racial disparities in incidence and outcome in multiple myeloma: a population-based study. Blood 116(25):5501–5506

Weinhold N, Ashby C, Rasche L, Chavan SS, Stein C, Stephens OW et al (2016a) Clonal selection and double-hit events involving tumor suppressor genes underlie relapse in myeloma. Blood 128(13):1735–1744

Weinhold N, Heuck CJ, Rosenthal A, Thanendrarajan S, Stein CK, Van Rhee F et al (2016b) Clinical value of molecular subtyping multiple myeloma using gene expression profiling. Leukemia 30(2):423–430

Wu SP, Pfeiffer RM, Ahn I, Mailankody S, Sonneveld P, van Duin M et al (2016) Impact of genes highly correlated with MMSET myeloma on survival of non-MMSET myeloma patients. Clin Cancer Res 22(16):4039–4044

Zhan F, Huang Y, Colla S, Stewart JP, Hanamura I, Gupta S et al (2006) The molecular classification of multiple myeloma. Blood 108(6):2020–2028

Zhuang J, Zhang J, Lwin ST, Edwards JR, Edwards CM, Mundy GR et al (2012) Osteoclasts in multiple myeloma are derived from Gr-1+CD11b+myeloid-derived suppressor cells. PLoS One 7(11):e48871

Diagnosis and Staging of Multiple Myeloma and Related Disorders

S. Vincent Rajkumar, Rafael Fonseca, and Jesus F. San Miguel

2.1   Disease Definition

Multiple myeloma (MM) was defined until recently based on a combination of pathologic and clinical features. Specifically, in addition to demonstration of a neoplastic plasma cell clone, the definition also required the presence of specific end-organ damage (hypercalcemia, renal failure, anemia, or bone lesions, referred to as CRAB features) attributable to the underlying clonal process (Rajkumar 2011; Rajkumar et al. 2011a). Patients with a neoplastic clone who did not have end-organ damage were considered to have either monoclonal gammopathy of undetermined significance (MGUS) or smoldering multiple myeloma (SMM) depending on the extent of bone marrow plasmacytosis or the level of the monoclonal (M) protein. The disorders MGUS and SMM were split based on the risk of progression to malignancy, and this distinction is critical for clinical care, counseling, prognostic assessment, and management. SMM carries a much higher risk of progression to malignancy (approximately 10% per year) than MGUS (approximately 1% per year) (Kyle et al. 2002, 2007).

Until the late 1990s, there were few drugs to treat MM, and the ones that were available (alkylators and corticosteroids) were not very effective and carried long-term risks. Thus, it made sense to require a strict definition for MM, in order to limit therapy only to those who were symptomatic. Further, many patients with MGUS and SMM can be asymptomatic and progression free for years without any therapy. But this meant that early therapy was not possible and that end-organ damage had to occur by definition before treatment can be instituted. In 2014, the International Myeloma Working Group (IMWG) revised the disease definition of MM to enable early diagnosis before end-organ damage occurred (Rajkumar et al. 2014). This paradigm shift was made possible by four key developments in the field. First, several new highly active drugs are now available to treat MM, and these agents have more than doubled the survival of patients with MM (Kumar et al. 2014). Second, specific biomarkers were identified that accurately distinguished patients with SMM who have a high probability ($\geq$80%) or progression to MM within 2 years, thereby

S. V. Rajkumar (✉)
Division of Hematology, Mayo Clinic, Rochester, MN, USA
e-mail: rajkumar.vincent@mayo.edu

R. Fonseca
Division of Hematology and Oncology, Mayo Clinic, Scottsdale, AZ, USA
e-mail: fonseca.rafael@mayo.edu

J. F. San Miguel
Clinica Universidad de Navarra, Centro de Investigacion Medica Aplicada (CIMA), IDISNA, Pamplona, Spain
e-mail: sanmiguel@unav.es

© Springer International Publishing Switzerland 2018
M. A. Dimopoulos et al. (eds.), *Multiple Myeloma and Other Plasma Cell Neoplasms*,
Hematologic Malignancies, https://doi.org/10.1007/978-3-319-25586-6_2

providing the opportunity to deliver therapy only to patients with the highest risk, while patients with true MGUS and SMM could continue to be observed, with the exception of high-risk SMM that could be considered as candidates for early treatment but only within clinical trials (Rajkumar et al. 2012). Third, advanced imaging modalities to detect disease early became available, especially low-dose whole-body computed tomography (CT) and positron emission tomography/computed tomographic scans (PET/CT) (Zamagni et al. 2007). This also meant that patients who are being observed could potentially be diagnosed when bone lesions are still small and nondestructive (Regelink et al. 2013). Finally, a randomized trial conducted by the Spanish Myeloma Group in patients with

high-risk SMM showed a survival advantage to early therapy with lenalidomide and low-dose dexamethasone (Rd) (Mateos et al. 2013). This trial greatly reduced long-standing fears that prevented SMM from being treated.

2.1.1 New Diagnostic Criteria for MM

The revised IMWG criteria for the diagnosis of MM and related disorders are shown on Table 2.1 (Rajkumar et al. 2014). The diagnosis of MM now requires evidence of either 10% or more clonal plasma cells on bone marrow examination or a biopsy-proven plasmacytoma *plus* one or more myeloma defining events (MDE) in

Table 2.1 International Myeloma Working Group diagnostic criteria for multiple myeloma and related plasma cell disorders

Disorder	Disease definition
Non-IgM monoclonal gammopathy of undetermined significance (MGUS)	All three criteria must be met: • Serum monoclonal protein (non-IgM type) <3 gm/dL • Clonal bone marrow plasma cells <10%[a] • Absence of end-organ damage such as hypercalcemia, renal insufficiency, anemia, and bone lesions (CRAB) that can be attributed to the plasma cell proliferative disorder
Smoldering multiple myeloma	Both criteria must be met: • Serum monoclonal protein (IgG or IgA) ≥3 gm/dL, or urinary monoclonal protein ≥500 mg per 24 h, and/or clonal bone marrow plasma cells 10–60% • Absence of myeloma defining events or amyloidosis

Multiple myeloma	Both criteria must be met:
	• Clonal bone marrow plasma cells ≥10% or biopsy-proven bony or extramedullary plasmacytoma
	• Any one or more of the following myeloma defining events:
	 – Evidence of end-organ damage that can be attributed to the underlying plasma cell proliferative disorder, specifically:
	   Hypercalcemia: serum calcium >0.25 mmol/L (>1 mg/dL) higher than the upper limit of normal or >2.75 mmol/L (>11 mg/dL)
	   Renal insufficiency: creatinine clearance <40 mL per minute or serum creatinine >177 μmol/L (>2 mg/dL)
	   Anemia: hemoglobin value of >2 g/dL below the lower limit of normal, or a hemoglobin value <10 g/dL
	   Bone lesions: one or more osteolytic lesions on skeletal radiography, computed tomography (CT), or positron emission tomography-CT (PET-CT)
	 – Clonal bone marrow plasma cell percentage ≥60%
	 – Involved: uninvolved serum free light chain (FLC) ratio ≥100 (involved free light chain level must be ≥100 mg/L)
	 – >1 focal lesions on magnetic resonance imaging (MRI) studies (at least 5 mm in size)

Table 2.1 (continued)

Disorder	Disease definition
IgM monoclonal gammopathy of undetermined significance (IgM MGUS)	All three criteria must be met: • Serum IgM monoclonal protein <3 gm/dL • Bone marrow lymphoplasmacytic infiltration <10% • No evidence of anemia, constitutional symptoms, hyperviscosity, lymphadenopathy, or hepatosplenomegaly that can be attributed to the underlying lymphoproliferative disorder
Light chain MGUS	All criteria must be met: • Abnormal FLC ratio (<0.26 or >1.65) • Increased level of the appropriate involved light chain (increased kappa FLC in patients with ratio >1.65 and increased lambda FLC in patients with ratio <0.26) • No immunoglobulin heavy chain expression on immunofixation • Absence of end-organ damage that can be attributed to the plasma cell proliferative disorder • Clonal bone marrow plasma cells <10% • Urinary monoclonal protein <500 mg/24 h
Solitary plasmacytoma	All four criteria must be met: • Biopsy-proven solitary lesion of bone or soft tissue with evidence of clonal plasma cells • Normal bone marrow with no evidence of clonal plasma cells • Normal skeletal survey and MRI (or CT) of the spine and pelvis (except for the primary solitary lesion) • Absence of end-organ damage such as hypercalcemia, renal insufficiency, anemia, or bone lesions (CRAB) that can be attributed to a lympho-plasma cell proliferative disorder
Solitary plasmacytoma with minimal marrow involvement[b]	All four criteria must be met: • Biopsy-proven solitary lesion of bone or soft tissue with evidence of clonal plasma cells • Clonal bone marrow plasma cells <10% • Normal skeletal survey and MRI (or CT) of the spine and pelvis (except for the primary solitary lesion) • Absence of end-organ damage such as hypercalcemia, renal insufficiency, anemia, or bone lesions (CRAB) that can be attributed to a lympho-plasma cell proliferative disorder

POEMS syndrome	All four criteria must be met:
	• Polyneuropathy
	• Monoclonal plasma cell proliferative disorder (almost always *lambda*)
	• Any one of the following three other major criteria:
	  – Sclerotic bone lesions
	  – Castleman's disease
	  – Elevated levels of vascular endothelial growth factor (VEGF)[c]
	• Any one of the following six minor criteria
	  – Organomegaly (splenomegaly, hepatomegaly, or lymphadenopathy)
	  – Extravascular volume overload (edema, pleural effusion, or ascites)
	  – Endocrinopathy (adrenal, thyroid, pituitary, gonadal, parathyroid, pancreatic)[d]
	  – Skin changes (hyperpigmentation, hypertrichosis, glomeruloid hemangiomata, plethora, acrocyanosis, flushing, white nails)
	  – Papilledema
	  – Thrombocytosis/polycythemia
	Note: Not every patient meeting the above criteria will have POEMS syndrome; the features should have a temporal relationship to each other and no other attributable causes. Anemia and/or thrombocytopenia are distinctively unusual in this syndrome unless Castleman's disease is present

(continued)

Table 2.1 (continued)

Disorder	Disease definition
Systemic AL amyloidosis[e]	All four criteria must be met: • Presence of an amyloid-related systemic syndrome (such as renal, liver, heart, gastrointestinal tract, or peripheral nerve involvement) • Positive amyloid staining by Congo red in any tissue (e.g., fat aspirate, bone marrow, or organ biopsy) • Evidence that amyloid is light chain related established by direct examination of the amyloid using mass spectrometry (MS)-based proteomic analysis or immunoelectron microscopy • Evidence of a monoclonal plasma cell proliferative disorder (serum or urine M protein, abnormal free light chain ratio, or clonal plasma cells in the bone marrow) Note: Approximately 2–3% of patients with AL amyloidosis will not meet the requirement for evidence of a monoclonal plasma cell disorder listed above; the diagnosis of AL amyloidosis must be made with caution in these patients

Reproduced from Rajkumar SV, Dimopoulos MA, Palumbo A, et al. International Myeloma Working Group updated criteria for the diagnosis of multiple myeloma. Lancet Oncol 2014; 15: e538–e548

MGUS monoclonal gammopathy of undetermined significance, *AL* immunoglobulin light chain amyloidosis, *AHL* immunoglobulin heavy and light chain amyloidosis, *AH* immunoglobulin heavy chain amyloidosis, *FLC* free light chain

[a]A bone marrow can be deferred in patients with low-risk MGUS (IgG type, M protein <15 gm/L, normal free light chain ratio) in whom there are no clinical features concerning for myeloma

[b]Solitary plasmacytoma with 10% or more clonal plasma cells is considered as multiple myeloma

[c]The source data do not define an optimal cutoff value for considering elevated VEGF level as a major criterion. We suggest that VEGF measured in the serum or plasma should be at least threefold to fourfold higher than the normal reference range for the laboratory that is doing the testing to be considered a major criterion

[d]In order to consider endocrinopathy as a minor criterion, an endocrine disorder other than diabetes or hypothyroidism is required since these two disorders are common in the general population

[e]Patients with AL amyloidosis who also meet criteria for multiple myeloma are considered to have both diseases

addition to. The MDE includes established CRAB features attributable to a plasma cell proliferative disorder, as well as three new biomarkers: clonal bone marrow plasma cells ≥60%, serum free light chain (FLC) ratio ≥100 (provided involved FLC level is ≥100 mg/L), and more than one focal lesion on magnetic resonance imaging (MRI). The new biomarkers were added to the definition of MM since they are associated with a very high (approximately 80% within 2 years) risk of progression to symptomatic end-organ damage in two or more independent studies.

cells ≥60% (Rajkumar et al. 2011b). These patients had rapid progression to symptomatic malignancy with a median progression-free survival (PFS) of 7.7 months (Rajkumar et al. 2011b). In another Mayo Clinic cohort of 651 patients with SMM, only 21 (3.2%) had clonal bone marrow plasma cells ≥60% (Rajkumar et al. 2011b). Of these, 95% progressed to MM within 2 years of diagnosis with a median time to progression (TTP) of 7 months. These results were confirmed by the Greek Myeloma Group (Kastritis et al. 2012) and by the University of Pennsylvania (Waxman et al. 2014).

2.1.1.1 Clonal Bone Marrow Plasma Cells ≥60%

Clonal bone marrow plasma cell involvement of ≥60% is very uncommon without concomitant CRAB features. If it does occur, however, there is a high probability of end-organ damage within a few months. In a Mayo Clinic study, only 6 of 276 patients (2%) had clonal bone marrow plasma

2.1.1.2 Elevated Serum Involved/Uninvolved FLC Ratio ≥100

In SMM, an abnormal involved/uninvolved FLC ratio (≥8) is known to be associated with a higher risk of progression to MM (Dispenzieri et al. 2008). The risk is proportional to the ratio. Thus, Larsen and colleagues investigated whether extreme abnormalities of the serum FLC ratio will result in a risk of progression that meets the threshold for definition of malignancy (Larsen et al. 2013). In a study of 586 patients with SMM, an involved/uninvolved FLC ratio ≥100 was seen in 90 patients (15%). The risk of progression to MM within the first 2 years with an FLC ratio ≥100 was 72%. If progression to AL amyloidosis was added, the risk of progression within 2 years increased to 79%. This risk increased further if one considered risk over a 3-year period. Kastritis et al. studied 96 patients with SMM and found an involved/uninvolved FLC ratio of ≥100 in 7% of patients; almost all of these patients progressed to MM within 18 months (Kastritis et al. 2012). In a third study, at the University of Pennsylvania, SMM patients with an involved/uninvolved FLC ratio ≥100 had a 64% risk of progression within 2 years (Waxman et al. 2014). To reduce possibility of error, in addition to the FLC ratio ≥100, the IMWG also added a requirement for a minimal involved FLC level of at least 100 mg/L in order to be considered as an MDE (Rajkumar et al. 2014).

2.1.1.3 More than One Focal Lesion on MRI

Diffuse and focal lesions on MRI have been associated with an increased risk of progression in SMM. But sample sizes were small to determine if the risk was high enough to consider them as biomarkers of malignancy. In a study by Hillengass et al., 23 of 149 (15%) patients with SMM had more than one focal lesion on whole-body MRI (Hillengass et al. 2010). In these patients, the risk of progression to symptomatic MM was 70% within 2 years, with a median time to progression of 13 months. These results were confirmed later by Kastritis et al. They found >1 focal lesion on spinal MRI in 9 of 65 patients (14%) with SMM (Kastritis et al. 2014). The risk of progression within 2 years was 69%, with a median time to progression of 15 months. The IMWG added a requirement that focal lesions need to be at least 5 mm or more in size and recommended follow-up examinations in 3–6 months in patients who had a solitary focal lesion, equivocal findings, or diffuse infiltration (Rajkumar et al. 2014).

2.1.1.4 Imaging Requirements

The updated IMWG criteria state that in addition to whole-body skeletal radiographs, CT scans, low-dose whole-body CT, and positron emission tomography with PET-CT can be used to diagnose lytic bone disease in MM (Rajkumar et al. 2014). These modalities are more sensitive and will enable early and more accurate diagnosis of MM (Zamagni et al. 2007; Bartel et al. 2009; Siontis et al. 2015). In order to qualify as an MDE, one or more sites of osteolytic bone destruction of at least 5 mm or more in size felt secondary to the plasma cell disorder are required. In terms of PET-CT scans, increased focal or diffuse FDG uptake is alone not adequate for the diagnosis. There must be evidence of actual osteolytic bone destruction on the CT portion of the PET-CT. The revised IMWG criteria were made more strict in terms of other bone lesions; thus, the presence of osteoporosis, vertebral compression fractures, or bone densitometric changes in the absence of lytic lesions is not a sufficient evidence of MM bone disease. As with skeletal radiographs, biopsy of one of the bone lesions should be considered if there is any doubt about the diagnosis of MM.

2.1.1.5 Other Miscellaneous Changes

Besides the revisions discussed above, the revised IMWG criteria also clarified several areas of controversy. Hyperviscosity, systemic AL amyloidosis, peripheral neuropathy, and recurrent bacterial infections are not considered as MDE (Rajkumar et al. 2014). In terms of renal disease, only suspected or proven light chain cast nephropathy is considered as an MDE (Rajkumar et al. 2014). Other renal disorders associated with M proteins such as light chain deposition disease, membranoproliferative glomerulonephritis, and AL amyloidosis are considered unique diseases and not MM. An accurate diagnosis of light chain cast nephropathy is essential (Gonsalves et al. 2015). A renal biopsy to clarify the underlying cause of the renal failure is recommended in patients with suspected cast nephropathy, especially if the serum involved FLC levels are less than 500 mg/L (Hutchison et al. 2012).

2.2 New Diagnostic Criteria for SMM

Changes to the disease definition of MM automatically result in a revision to the diagnostic criteria for SMM. SMM is now defined by the presence of a serum monoclonal (M) protein of ≥3 g/dl and/or 10–60% clonal bone marrow plasma cells with no evidence of MDE or amyloidosis (Table 2.1) (Rajkumar et al. 2014). SMM should be distinguished from MGUS, MM, and other related plasma cell disorders using the criteria listed on Table 2.1. At least one advanced imaging exam (PET-CT, low-dose whole-body CT, or MRI of the whole body or spine) is recommended in patients with suspected SMM or solitary plasmacytoma (Rajkumar et al. 2014; Siontis et al. 2015; Dimopoulos et al. 2015).

Despite the changes to the criteria which reclassify some patients with the highest risk of progression as MM based on biomarkers, SMM remains a major clinical dilemma with an overall risk of progression of approximately 10% per year for the first 5 years (Rajkumar et al. 2015).

2.3 Molecular Classification of Myeloma

There are several molecular subtypes of MM, associated with several unique differences in disease presentation and prognosis (Table 2.2) (Kumar et al. 2012). Most patients with MM can be classified into one of the three groups: primary immunoglobulin heavy chain (IgH) translocations, trisomies (40%), or a combination of IgH translocations and trisomies. There are five common primary IgH translocations; each of these involves the IgH locus on chromosome 14q32, and one of the five recurrent partner chromosome loci: 11q13 (CCND1 [cyclin D1 gene]), 4p16.3 (FGFR-3 and MMSET), 6p21 (CCND3 [cyclin D3 gene]), 16q23 (c-maf), and 20q11 (mafB). The resultant five IgH translocations, namely, $t(11;14)$, $t(4;14)$, $t(6;14)$, $t(14;16)$, and $t(14;20)$, are considered nonoverlapping. Thus, a given patient with MM will not have two different types of IgH translocation. The molecular subtype of MM does influence clinical features and prognosis. For example, trisomic MM responds

Table 2.2 Primary molecular cytogenetic classification of multiple myeloma

Subtype	Gene(s)/chromosomes affected[a]	Percentage of myeloma patients
Trisomic MM	Recurrent trisomies involving odd-numbered chromosomes with the exception of chromosomes 1, 13, and 21	42
IgH-translocated MM		30
$t(11;14)$ (q13;q32)	CCND1 (cyclin D1)	15
$t(4;14)$ (p16;q32)	FGFR-3 and MMSET	6
$t(14;16)$ (q32;q23)	C-MAF	4
$t(14;20)$ (q32;q11)	MAFB	<1
Other IgH translocations[a]	CCND3 (cyclin D3) in $t(6;14)$ MM	5
Combined IgH translocated/trisomic MM	Presence of trisomies and any one of the recurrent IgH translocations in the same patient	15
Isolated monosomy 14	Few cases may represent 14q32 translocations involving unknown partner chromosomes	4.5
Other cytogenetic abnormalities in the absence of IgH translocations or trisomy or monosomy 14		5.5
Normal		3

Modified from Kumar S et al. Trisomies in multiple myeloma: impact on survival in patients with high-risk cytogenetics. Blood 2012; 119:2100. © American Society of Hematology

[a]Includes the $t(6;14)(p21;q32)$ translocation and, rarely, other IgH translocations involving uncommon partner chromosomes

particularly well to lenalidomide-based therapy (Pandey et al. 2013; Vu et al. 2015). In contrast, *t*(4;14) MM requires bortezomib-based induction, stem cell transplantation, and maintenance therapy for good outcome (Sonneveld et al. 2012; Cavo et al. 2010). At diagnosis, *t*(4;14) MM is less likely to be associated with bone disease at diagnosis, while *t*(14;16) MM is often associated with high levels of serum free light chains (FLC) and a higher risk of acute renal failure (Greenberg et al. 2014). In general, *t*(4;14), *t*(14;16), and *t*(14;20) are considered high-risk features.

In addition to molecular classification based on specific cytogenetic abnormalities, patients with MM may also be grouped into two major categories according to ploidy status assessed by karyotyping: the hyperdiploid group (more than 46/47 chromosomes) and the non-hyperdiploid group, composed of hypodiploid (up to 44/45 chromosomes), pseudodiploid (44/45 to 46/47), and near-tetraploid (more than 74) cases. As expected, non-hyperdiploid MM is characterized by a very high prevalence of IGH translocations involving the five recurrent chromosome partners. Besides primary cytogenetic abnormalities, there are several recurrent abnormalities that occur in MM that have prognostic significance. Conventional cytogenetics, FISH, and comparative genomic hybridization analysis have all demonstrated that lesions of chromosome 1 are the most common abnormalities in MM; these include gain(1q) (as the result of tandem duplications and jumping segmental duplications of the chromosome 1q band) and del(1p). Both these abnormalities are thought to confer an adverse prognosis, but their independent impact is still controversial. The loss of chromosome 13 is the most frequent monosomy in MM, occurring in 40–50% of newly diagnosed patients. This abnormality shows a strong association with *t*(4;14) and *t*(14;16) and deletion of 17p and gain(1q). Although monosomy 13/del(13q) was initially considered as an adverse prognostic feature, this was mainly due to associations with other adverse prognostic factors. Del(17p), which includes loss of *TP53*, occurs at a lower frequency in newly diagnosed MM (5–10%). The prevalence of del(17p) increases in more advanced stages of

MM, but the proportion is higher in advanced stages. Del(17p) probably represents the most adverse prognostic genetic feature in MM and is frequently associated with extramedullary disease.

2.4 Staging and Risk Stratification

Being able to predict outcome is critical not only for counseling patients but also in terms of deciding treatment strategy (choice of drugs, duration of therapy, aggressiveness of the intervention, etc.). Besides the molecular subtype of MM which represents disease biology, there are several other factors that affect prognosis. These include host factors (age, performance status, comorbidities), disease stage, and response to therapy (Palumbo et al. 2015a; Russell and Rajkumar 2011). Moreover, disease biology is also affected by secondary cytogenetic abnormalities such as del(17p) and gain(1q). These secondary cytogenetic abnormalities can occur in any of the molecular subtypes as additional events, and they generally carry a more adverse prognosis.

Staging of MM has been traditionally done using the Durie-Salmon Staging (DSS) (Durie and Salmon 1975) or the International Staging System (ISS) (Greipp et al. 2005; Hari et al. 2009). The DSS primarily classified patients based on tumor burden, while the ISS also includes a host factor determinant, namely, serum albumin. The main disadvantage of these older staging systems is that outcome in MM unlike many other malignancies is dependent more on disease biology. To rectify this, a Revised International Staging System (RISS) has been adopted by the IMWG that combines the ISS with determinants of disease biology (Palumbo et al. 2015b).

2.4.1 Revised International Staging System for MM

Recently, a Revised International Staging System (RISS) has been adopted by the IMWG (Palumbo

Table 2.3 Revised International Staging System for myeloma (Palumbo et al. 2015b)

Stage	Frequency (% of patients)	5-year survival rate (%)
Stage I		
• ISS stage I (serum albumin >3.5, serum beta-2-microglobulin <3.5) • No high-risk cytogenetics • Normal LDH	28	82
Stage II		
• Neither stage I or III	62	62
Stage III		
• ISS stage III (serum beta-2-microglobulin >5.5) • High-risk cytogenetics [t(4;14), t(14;16), or del(17p)] or elevated LDH	10	40

Derived from: Palumbo A, et al. J Clin Oncol 2015; 33: 2863–2869

et al. 2015b). The RISS incorporates determinants of disease biology (the presence of high-risk cytogenetic abnormalities or elevated lactate dehydrogenase level) into the former ISS to create three disease stages (Table 2.3). The cytogenetic abnormalities considered as high risk in the RISS include t(4;14), t(14;16), and del(17p). In a study of 4445 patients with newly diagnosed MM from 11 international trials, the 5-year survival rate of patients with stage I, II, and III RISS was 82%, 62%, and 40%, respectively.

2.4.2 Risk Stratification of SMM

The risk of progression of SMM is approximately 10% per year for the first 5 years; after 5 years (cumulative 50% at 5 years), the risk decreases to 3% per year for the next 5 years (cumulative 65% at 10 years) and further decreases to approximately 1% per year thereafter (Kyle et al. 2007). Patients with SMM who have a median time to progression of 2 years should be considered to have high-risk SMM (25% per year risk of progression in the first 2 years). Several studies have identified important prognostic markers that can identify such patients (Kyle et al. 2007; Dispenzieri et al. 2008; Hillengass et al. 2010; Perez-Persona et al. 2007; Rosinol et al. 2003; Rajkumar et al. 2013; Neben et al. 2013; Dhodapkar et al. 2014; Bianchi et al. 2013). Importantly the underlying cytogenetic subtype

does affect outcome in SMM. Patients with t(4;14) translocation, del 17p, and gain 1q have a higher risk of progression from SMM to MM. Table 2.4 provides the criteria for high-risk SMM (Rajkumar et al. 2015). Based on encouraging results of the Spanish clinical trial in high-risk SMM (Mateos et al. 2013), certain patients with multiple risk factors can be considered candidates for MM therapy after a careful discussion of risks and benefits, particularly within clinical trials. In contrast, patients with low-risk SMM likely have a risk of progression of 5% per year or less and can be observed.

2.5 Response Assessment and Monitoring

Response to therapy in MM is done using the International Myeloma Working Group uniform response criteria (Table 2.5) (Durie et al. 2006). In order to assess response and identify relapse in a timely manner, patients require periodic monitoring as outlined in Table 2.6. Besides history and examination, and basic aboratory tests (complete blood count, calcium, and 404 creatinine measurements), the mainstay of monitoring include serial measurements of M protein levels by serum protein electrophoresis (SPEP) and urine protein electrophoresis (UPEP). The serum FLC assay is an alternative to the UPEP; but even it is a good

Table 2.4 Definition of high-risk smoldering multiple myeloma[a]

Bone marrow clonal plasma cells ≥10% and any one or more of the following:
Serum M protein ≥30 g/L
IgA SMM
Immunoparesis with reduction of two uninvolved immunoglobulin isotypes
Serum involved/uninvolved free light chain ratio ≥8 (but less than 100)
Progressive increase in M protein level (evolving type of SMM)[b]
Bone marrow clonal plasma cells 50–60%
Abnormal plasma cell immunophenotype (≥95% of bone marrow plasma cells are clonal) and reduction of one or more uninvolved immunoglobulin isotypes
t(4;14) or del 17p or 1q gain
Increased circulating plasma cells
MRI with diffuse abnormalities or one focal lesion
PET-CT with focal lesion with increased uptake without underlying osteolytic bone destruction

SMM smoldering multiple myeloma, *M* monoclonal, *MRI* magnetic resonance imaging, *PET-CT* positron emission tomography-computed tomography

Reproduced from Rajkumar SV, Landgren O, Mateos MV. Smoldering Multiple Myeloma. Blood. 2015 Apr 2. pii: blood-2014-09-568899 © American Society of Hematology

[a]Note that the term smoldering multiple myeloma excludes patients without end-organ damage who meet revised definition of multiple myeloma, namely, clonal bone marrow plasma cells ≥60% or serum free light chain (FLC) ratio ≥100 (plus measurable involved FLC level ≥100 mg/L) or more than one focal lesion on magnetic resonance imaging. The risk factors listed in this table are not meant to be indications for therapy; they are variables associated with a high risk of progression of SMM and identify patients who need close follow-up and consideration for clinical trials

[b]Increase in serum monoclonal protein by ≥25% on two successive evaluations within a 6-month period

Table 2.5 International Myeloma Working Group uniform response criteria for multiple myeloma

Response subcategory	Response criteria
Complete response[a] (CR)	• Negative immunofixation of serum and urine • Disappearance of any soft tissue plasmacytomas • <5% plasma cells in the bone marrow
Stringent complete response (sCR)[b]	CR as defined above plus • Normal FLC ratio • Absence of clonal PC by immunohistochemistry or 2–4 color flow cytometry
Very good partial response (VGPR)[a]	• Serum and urine M-component detectable by immunofixation but not on electrophoresis • ≥90% or greater reduction in serum M-component plus urine M-component <100 mg per 24 h
Partial response (PR)	• ≥50% reduction of serum M protein and reduction in 24-h urinary M protein by ≥90% or to <200 mg per 24 h • If the serum and urine M protein are unmeasurable, a ≥50% decrease in the difference between involved and uninvolved FLC levels is required in place of the M protein criteria • If serum and urine M protein are unmeasurable, and serum free light assay is also unmeasurable, ≥50% reduction in bone marrow plasma cells is required in place of M protein, provided baseline percentage was ≥30% • In addition to the above criteria, if present at baseline, ≥50% reduction in the size of soft tissue plasmacytomas is also required
Stable disease (SD)	• Not meeting criteria for CR, VGPR, PR, or progressive disease

(continued)

Table 2.5 (continued)

Response subcategory	Response criteria
Progressive disease (PD)[b]	• Increase of 25% from lowest response value in any one or more of the following: – Serum M-component (absolute increase must be ≥0.5 g/dl)[c] and/or – Urine M-component (absolute increase must be ≥200 mg/24 h) and/or – Only in patients without measurable serum and urine M protein levels: the difference between involved and uninvolved FLC levels (absolute increase must be >100 mg/L) – Only in patients without measurable serum and urine M protein levels and without measurable disease by FLC levels, bone marrow plasma cell percentage (absolute % must be ≥10%) • Definite development of new bone lesions or soft tissue plasmacytomas or definite increase in the size of existing bone lesions or soft tissue plasmacytomas • Development of hypercalcemia (corrected serum calcium >11.5 mg/dl) that can be attributed solely to the plasma cell proliferative disorder

All response categories (CR, sCR, VGPR, PR, and PD) require two consecutive assessments made at any time before the institution of any new therapy; complete response and PR and SD categories also require no known evidence of progressive or new bone lesions if radiographic studies were performed. VGPR and CR categories require serum and urine studies regardless of whether disease at baseline was measurable on serum, urine, both, or neither. Radiographic studies are not required to satisfy these response requirements. Bone marrow assessments need not be confirmed
Reproduced from Kyle RA, Rajkumar SV. Criteria for diagnosis, staging, risk stratification and response assessment of multiple myeloma. Leukemia 2009; 23: 3–9
[a]Note clarifications to IMWG criteria for coding CR and VGPR in patients in whom the only measurable disease is by serum FLC levels: CR in such patients is a normal FLC ratio of 0.26–1.65 in addition to CR criteria listed above. VGPR in such patients requires in addition a >90% decrease in the difference between involved and uninvolved free light chain (FLC) levels
[b]Note clarifications to IMWG criteria for coding PD: bone marrow criteria for progressive disease are to be used only in patients without measurable disease by M protein and by FLC levels. Clarified that "25% increase" refers to M protein, FLC, and bone marrow results and does not refer to bone lesions, soft tissue plasmacytomas, or hypercalcemia. Note that the "lowest response value" does not need to be a confirmed value

clinical practice to assess UPEP once every few months even in patients with stable serum FLC levels. Most patients without measurable disease in serum or urine, defined as less than 1 gm/dL M protein on SPEP and <200 mg/24 h M protein on UPEP, can be followed using the serum FLC assay provided the FLC ratio is abnormal and the level of the involved FLC is ≥10 mg/dL (Dispenzieri et al. 2009).

In general, these laboratory tests and M protein measurements are done monthly during active therapy, and once every 3 months when patients are being observed without therapy or using maintenance therapy (Table 2.6). Radiographic tests are typically done when symptoms indicate their need. Bone marrow studies are repeated if needed to confirm complete response or when clinically indicated to assess relapse.

Further refinements to the response criteria are ongoing. These proposed revisions will stipulate new definitions for minimal residual disease (MRD)

negative status. MRD negative can be ascertained up to the level of 1 in 10^{-5} using next-generation flow cytometry or next-generation sequencing. At present MRD negative status is clearly known to confer a favorable prognosis in MM, even in patients who are in complete response. However, it is still not known whether treatment decisions should be based on MRD results. Randomized trials in this regard are needed.

Acknowledgements Supported in part by grants CA 107476 and CA 168762 from the National Cancer Institute, Rockville, MD, USA, and Asociación Española Contra el Cáncer (GCB120981SAN), Spain.

Authorship Contribution Statement SVR, RF, and JFS conceived the paper, researched the literature, and wrote the manuscript.

Disclosure of Conflicts of Interest SVR and JSM declare no conflict of interest. RF has received a patent for the prognostication of MM based on genetic categorization by FISH of the disease.

Table 2.6 Disease monitoring

	Recommendations
Monoclonal protein studies	• Serum protein electrophoresis and serum free light chain assay monthly while on therapy and every 3–4 months when off therapy • Urine protein electrophoresis every 3–6 months • Serum and urine immunofixation to document complete response • In patients with IgA M proteins, quantitative IgA immunoglobulin level should also be measured
Bone marrow studies	• Bone marrow studies to document complete response and to assess relapse as clinically indicated • At relapse, bone marrow studies should include FISH studies for del 17p and gain 1q and should also include probes to detect immunoglobulin heavy chain translocations and trisomies if informative results are not available from baseline marrow studies • Bone marrow studies should also include multiparameter flow cytometry to assess clonality and to determine proportion of aberrant vs. normal PCs
Imaging studies	• Skeletal survey or low-dose whole-body CT should be considered once a year • PET-CT is an alternative and may be helpful if extramedullary disease is suspected. Response to therapy on PET-CT may also have prognostic value and should be considered in patients with oligo-secretory or nonsecretory disease • MRI of the spine/pelvis or whole body is needed in patients with suspected disease in the spine. MRI may be particularly helpful in smoldering myeloma or solitary plasmacytoma
MRD monitoring	• MRD assessment is still investigational. It should be considered in patients in complete response • Next-generation flow cytometry or next-generation sequencing using standard methods that are sensitive to at least 1×10^{-5} or greater can help in the detection of MRD • MRD negativity has prognostic value, but more studies are needed to determine if assessment is of value in changing therapy

PCs plasma cells, *FISH* fluorescence in situ hybridization, *MRI* magnetic resonance imaging, *CT* computed tomography, *PET-CT* positron emission tomography/computed tomography, *MRD* minimal residual disease

References

Bartel TB, Haessler J, Brown TL et al (2009) F18-fluorodeoxyglucose positron emission tomography in the context of other imaging techniques and prognostic factors in multiple myeloma. Blood 114:2068–2076

Bianchi G, Kyle RA, Larson DR et al (2013) High levels of peripheral blood circulating plasma cells as a specific risk factor for progression of smoldering multiple myeloma. Leukemia 27:680–685

Cavo M, Tacchetti P, Patriarca F et al (2010) Bortezomib with thalidomide plus dexamethasone compared with thalidomide plus dexamethasone as induction therapy before, and consolidation therapy after, double autologous stem-cell transplantation in newly diagnosed multiple myeloma: a randomised phase 3 study. Lancet 376:2075–2085

Dhodapkar MV, Sexton R, Waheed S et al (2014) Clinical, genomic, and imaging predictors of myeloma progression from asymptomatic monoclonal gammopathies (SWOG S0120). Blood 123:78–85

Dimopoulos MA, Hillengass J, Usmani S et al (2015) Role of magnetic resonance imaging in the management of patients with multiple myeloma: a consensus statement. J Clin Oncol Off J Am Soc Clin Oncol 33:657–664

Dispenzieri A, Kyle RA, Katzmann JA et al (2008) Immunoglobulin free light chain ratio is an independent risk factor for progression of smoldering (asymptomatic) multiple myeloma. Blood 111:785–789

Dispenzieri A, Kyle R, Merlini G et al (2009) International myeloma working group guidelines for serum-free light chain analysis in multiple myeloma and related disorders. Leukemia 23:215–224

Durie BG, Salmon SE (1975) A clinical staging system for multiple myeloma. Correlation of measured myeloma cell mass with presenting clinical features, response to treatment, and survival. Cancer 36:842–854

Durie BGM, Harousseau J-L, Miguel JS et al (2006) International uniform response criteria for multiple myeloma. Leukemia 20:1467–1473

Gonsalves WI, Leung N, Rajkumar SV et al (2015) Improvement in renal function and its impact on survival in patients with newly diagnosed multiple myeloma. Blood Cancer J 5:e296

Greenberg AJ, Rajkumar SV, Therneau TM, Singh PP, Dispenzieri A, Kumar SK (2014) Relationship between initial clinical presentation and the molecular cytogenetic classification of myeloma. Leukemia 28:398–403

Greipp PR, San Miguel JF, Durie BG et al (2005) International staging system for multiple myeloma. J Clin Oncol 23:3412–3420

Hari PN, Zhang MJ, Roy V et al (2009) Is the international staging system superior to the Durie-Salmon staging system? A comparison in multiple myeloma patients undergoing autologous transplant. Leukemia 23:1528–1534

Hillengass J, Fechtner K, Weber MA et al (2010) Prognostic significance of focal lesions in whole-body magnetic resonance imaging in patients with asymptomatic multiple myeloma. J Clin Oncol Off J Am Soc Clin Oncol 28:1606–1610

Hutchison CA, Batuman V, Behrens J et al (2012) The pathogenesis and diagnosis of acute kidney injury in multiple myeloma. Nat Rev Nephrol 8:43–51

Kastritis E, Terpos E, Moulopoulos L et al (2012) Extensive bone marrow infiltration and abnormal free light chain ratio identifies patients with asymptomatic myeloma at high risk for progression to symptomatic disease. Leukemia 27:947–953

Kastritis E, Moulopoulos LA, Terpos E, Koutoulidis V, Dimopoulos MA (2014) The prognostic importance of the presence of more than one focal lesion in spine MRI of patients with asymptomatic (smoldering) multiple myeloma. Leukemia 28:2402–2403

Kumar S, Fonseca R, Ketterling RP et al (2012) Trisomies in multiple myeloma: impact on survival in patients with high-risk cytogenetics. Blood 119:2100–2105

Kumar SK, Dispenzieri A, Lacy MQ et al (2014) Continued improvement in survival in multiple myeloma: changes in early mortality and outcomes in older patients. Leukemia 28:1122–1128

Kyle RA, Therneau TM, Rajkumar SV et al (2002) A long-term study of prognosis of monoclonal gammopathy of undetermined significance. N Engl J Med 346:564–569

Kyle RA, Remstein ED, Therneau TM et al (2007) Clinical course and prognosis of smoldering (asymptomatic) multiple myeloma. N Engl J Med 356:2582–2590

Larsen JT, Kumar SK, Dispenzieri A, Kyle RA, Katzmann JA, Rajkumar SV (2013) Serum free light chain ratio as a biomarker for high-risk smoldering multiple myeloma. Leukemia 27:941–946

Mateos M-V, Hernández M-T, Giraldo P et al (2013) Lenalidomide plus dexamethasone for high-risk smoldering multiple myeloma. N Engl J Med 369:438–447

Neben K, Jauch A, Hielscher T et al (2013) Progression in smoldering myeloma is independently determined by the chromosomal abnormalities del(17p), $t(4;14)$, gain 1q, hyperdiploidy, and tumor load. J Clin Oncol Off J Am Soc Clin Oncol 31:4325–4332

Palumbo A, Bringhen S, Mateos MV et al (2015a) Geriatric assessment predicts survival and toxicities in elderly myeloma patients: an international myeloma working group report. Blood 125:2068–2074

Palumbo A, Avet-Loiseau H, Oliva S et al (2015b) Revised international staging system for multiple myeloma: a report from international myeloma working group. J Clin Oncol Off J Am Soc Clin Oncol 33:2863–2869

Pandey S, Rajkumar SV, Kapoor P et al (2013) Impact of FISH abnormalities on response to lenalidomide in patients with multiple myeloma. Blood 122:3210

Perez-Persona E, Vidriales MB, Mateo G et al (2007) New criteria to identify risk of progression in monoclonal gammopathy of uncertain significance and

smoldering multiple myeloma based on multiparameter flow cytometry analysis of bone marrow plasma cells. Blood 110:2586–2592

Rajkumar SV (2011) Treatment of multiple myeloma. Nat Rev Clin Oncol 8:479–491

Rajkumar SV, Gahrton G, Bergsagel PL (2011a) Approach to the treatment of multiple myeloma: a clash of philosophies. Blood 118:3205–3211

Rajkumar SV, Larson D, Kyle RA (2011b) Diagnosis of smoldering multiple myeloma. N Engl J Med 365:474–475

Rajkumar SV, Merlini G, San Miguel JF (2012) Redefining myeloma. Nat Rev Clin Oncol 9:494–496

Rajkumar SV, Gupta V, Fonseca R et al (2013) Impact of primary molecular cytogenetic abnormalities and risk of progression in smoldering multiple myeloma. Leukemia 27:1738–1744

Rajkumar SV, Dimopoulos MA, Palumbo A et al (2014) International myeloma working group updated criteria for the diagnosis of multiple myeloma. Lancet Oncol 15:e538–e548

Rajkumar SV, Landgren O, Mateos MV (2015) Smoldering multiple myeloma. Blood 125:3069–3075

Regelink JC, Minnema MC, Terpos E et al (2013) Comparison of modern and conventional imaging techniques in establishing multiple myeloma-related bone disease: a systematic review. Br J Haematol 162:50–61

Rosinol L, Blade J, Esteve J et al (2003) Smoldering multiple myeloma: natural history and recognition of an evolving type. Br J Haematol 123:631–636

Russell SJ, Rajkumar SV (2011) Multiple myeloma and the road to personalised medicine. Lancet Oncol 12:617–619

Siontis B, Kumar S, Dispenzieri A et al (2015) Positron emission tomography-computed tomography in the diagnostic evaluation of smoldering multiple myeloma: identification of patients needing therapy. Blood Cancer J 5:e364

Sonneveld P, Schmidt-Wolf IGH, van der Holt B et al (2012) Bortezomib induction and maintenance treatment in patients with newly diagnosed multiple myeloma: results of the randomized phase III HOVON-65/GMMG-HD4 trial. J Clin Oncol 30:2946–2955

Vu T, Gonsalves W, Kumar S et al (2015) Characteristics of exceptional responders to lenalidomide-based therapy in multiple myeloma. Blood Cancer J 5:e363

Waxman AJ, Mick R, Garfall AL et al (2014) Modeling the risk of progression in smoldering multiple myeloma. J Clin Oncol 32:A8607

Zamagni E, Nanni C, Patriarca F et al (2007) A prospective comparison of 18F-fluorodeoxyglucose positron emission tomography-computed tomography, magnetic resonance imaging and whole-body planar radiographs in the assessment of bone disease in newly diagnosed multiple myeloma. Haematologica 92:50–55

Treatment of Transplant Eligible Patients with Multiple Myeloma

P. Sonneveld, H. Einsele, A. M. Brioli, and M. Cavo

3.1 Part 1: High-Dose Therapy

3.1.1 Introduction

The treatment outcome of patients with multiple myeloma (MM) has been invariably poor until the 1960s. With the introduction of the alkylating agent melphalan, later combined with prednisone it became possible to reduce tumor burden and thereby to effectively improve the patient's quality of life. However, the duration of remission was usually short and prolonged dosing proved difficult because of bone marrow suppression. In 1983 McElwain investigated the concept of dose escalation based on the fact that the anti-tumor effect of melphalan is dose-dependent. Seven patients with plasma-cell leukemia and (refractory) MM were treated with a single high-dose of intravenous melphalan (HDM) without stem-cell support (McElwain and Powles 1983). The same group expanded this concept in a larger group of

patients still with obvious and lasting responses (Selby et al. 1988). Because of the severe hematologic toxicity that was observed, further treatments with high-dose melphalan were performed with autologous stem-cell support (ASCT) in eligible patients with multiple myeloma.

The group of Barlogie investigated the concept of autologous stem-cell support in order to reduce the risk of long myelosuppression and/or incomplete bone marrow recovery (Barlogie et al. 1987).

After initial studies in relapsed MM, it became clear that HDM is more effective in previously untreated patients. Since the 1990s, high-dose therapy with ASCT has been the standard of care for younger (≤65 years) patients who are eligible for this procedure and have no significant co-morbidities (Harousseau and Moreau 2009). Through these efforts HDM became a backbone of treatment in younger patients, to which other therapies could be added. Current treatment protocols include sequential blocks of therapy, namely induction, consolidation, and maintenance. All of these components are widely investigated in numerous ongoing international clinical trials, aimed at identifying the most effective treatment combination and the optimal therapeutic sequence. In most countries this treatment is now recommended for newly diagnosed MM (NDMM), while more recently its delayed use in relapsed and/or refractory MM (RRMM) has received renewed interest.

P. Sonneveld
Erasmus MC Cancer Institute,
Rotterdam, The Netherlands

H. Einsele (✉)
Department of Internal Medicine II, University Hospital,
Julius Maximilians University Würzburg, Germany
e-mail: Einsele_H@ukw.de

A. M. Brioli • M. Cavo
Seràgnoli Institute of Hematology, Bologna
University School of Medicine, Bologna, Italy

© Springer International Publishing Switzerland 2018
M. A. Dimopoulos et al. (eds.), *Multiple Myeloma and Other Plasma Cell Neoplasms*,
Hematologic Malignancies, https://doi.org/10.1007/978-3-319-25586-6_3

Allogeneic transplantation for MM has been developed in the 1980s and its clinical application is currently concentrated in high-risk RRMM and in clinical trials.

In this chapter the role of high-dose treatment with autologous stem cell rescue in newly diagnosed, transplant-eligible patients will be discussed in the context of the era of *novel* drugs for induction, consolidation, and maintenance treatment. The role of high-dose therapy as salvage treatment will be discussed elsewhere. In addition the role of allogeneic transplantation will be discussed.

3.1.1.1 HDT and ASCT: The Principle

Since the introduction of HDT supported by ASCT as a concept to improve response and long-term outcome, several cooperative trial groups have investigated this question. Early development concentrated on salvage treatment in patients with RRMM. Since 1990 HDT was investigated in NDMM, showing a higher response rate of 30% complete response (CR) as compared with standard dose melphalan combined with prednisone. Later, prospective randomized Phase 3 trials were performed, comparing HDT + ASCT with various schedules of conventional chemotherapy in newly diagnosed transplant-eligible patients. As an induction regimen prior to HDT, usually vincristine, doxorubicin, dexamethasone (VAD) was used based on the regimen for refractory disease, however still before the introduction of *novel* drugs (Attal et al. 1996; Fermand et al. 1998, 2005; Child et al. 2003; Palumbo et al. 2004; Blade et al. 2005; Segeren et al. 2003; Barlogie et al. 2006a). In the majority of these trials, response rate, quality of response, and event-free survival were superior with HDT/ASCT, while an overall survival (OS) benefit was observed in only 3/8 trials (Table 3.1). An important aspect of dose-intensification with HDT has been the reproducible observation that the associated higher "very good" response rates (VGPR) or better (CR) correlate with longer progression-free survival (PFS) and possibly OS (Harousseau et al. 2009). These data indicate that HDT when given without effective pretreatment that reduces tumor burden has

Table 3.1 ASCT vs conventional chemotherapy: results of randomized studies

Author	Patients (n)	Age	CR/ VGPR	EFS	OS
Attal et al. (1996)	200	≤65	Yes	Yes	Yes
Fermand et al. (1998)	202	<55	Yes	Yes	No
Child et al. (2003)	401	≤65	Yes	Yes	Yes
Palumbo et al. (2004)	194	<70	Yes	Yes	Yes
Fermand et al. (2005)	190	55–65	Yes	Yes	No
Blade et al. (2005)	164	≤65	Yes	Yes	No
Barlogie et al. (2006a)	516	≤70	No	No	No

only a limited benefit for long-term outcome, i.e. OS. While there may be several explanations for this lack of OS improvement, the most likely explanation is the availability of HDT as salvage treatment in patients progressing from conventional chemotherapy. Also, over time the use of total body irradiation (TBI) combined with cyclophosphamide as HDT was omitted in favor of high-dose melphalan (HDM) based on a French trial that showed better tolerability and superior efficacy of the latter (Moreau et al. 2002). Hence, HDM 200 mg/m^2 became the standard conditioning regimen for HDT + ASCT. In general, HDM with ASCT is used as part of a front-line treatment in transplant-eligible patients. However, the consensus is that it can also be used as a salvage treatment in patients who have not received this before, or in patients who had a favorable response and longer time to progression after prior HDM (Giralt et al. 2015; Ludwig et al. 2014).

3.1.2 Induction Treatment Prior to HDT

While high-dose melphalan was initially developed as a stand-alone treatment, it soon became clear that remission-induction treatment was required before this procedure for several reasons. First, newly diagnosed patients and/or patients with a fulminant relapse had to be stabilized and disease symptom control was needed prior to intensive treatment. Second, in order to be able to collect good quality hematopoietic stem cells with little contamination of myeloma cells, pre-emptive non-hemato-toxic chemotherapy was required. Finally, it became evident that achieving a good response after induction treatment plus intensification with high-dose melphalan incurred a better overall survival (Lahuerta et al. 2008).

During the 1990s VAD was the induction regimen of choice in nearly all HDT trials.

With the introduction of thalidomide in 1999, it became possible to include thalidomide in induction regimens and later lines of therapy. Thalidomide was combined with dexamethasone (TD), doxorubicin/dexamethasone (TAD), or cyclophosphamide/dexamethasone (CTD) in several randomized trials in transplant eligible NDMM (Cavo et al. 2005; Lokhorst et al. 2010; Morgan et al. 2011; Spencer et al. 2009; Barlogie et al. 2006b). While complete response rates in comparison with VAD are not necessarily higher, the very good partial response (VGPR) rate and overall response rate with thalidomide after induction were superior. The main endpoints of these trials were progression-free survival (PFS) and/or overall survival (OS). While PFS was better with thalidomide, OS was similar in some of these trials. The main obstacles towards a general routine use of thalidomide in this setting have been the high incidence of serious complications such as thrombosis and peripheral neuropathy as well as the introduction of proteasome inhibitors (PI).

Bortezomib was the first PI that was introduced in induction regimens for transplant eligible NDMM. The drug was combined with dexamethasone (BD) by the French IFM group or with doxorubicin/dexamethasone (PAD) by the HOVON65/GMMG-HD4 group and compared with VAD (Harousseau et al. 2010; Sonneveld et al. 2012). In both trials CR rate after induction was significantly higher with the bortezomib combination. In the HOVON65/GMMG-HD4 trial bortezomib induction followed by HDM plus ASCT and bortezomib maintenance for 2 years resulted in a superior PFS and OS when compared with standard treatment and

thalidomide maintenance. Other regimens currently used include bortezomib, cyclophosphamide, dexamethasone (VCD), lenalidomide, bortezomib, dexamethasone (VRD), and other combinations (Kumar et al. 2012). Several trials have combined the 2 *novel* agents bortezomib and thalidomide with dexamethasone (VTD) as a regimen for induction prior to HDM/ASCT (Cavo et al. 2010; Rosiñol et al. 2012; Moreau et al. 2011a). In these trials the VTD combination when compared to TD showed superior overall response rate, CR + VGPR before and after ASCT as well as PFS (Cavo et al. 2015). More recently, it was demonstrated that VTD is also superior to VCD (Cavo et al. 2015; Moreau et al. 2015). Currently, VCD and VTD are widely used as induction regimens in Europe, since they combine good CR + VGPR rates with good tolerability. Generally 4–6 cycles are administered before stem cell collection is performed. In general it can be concluded that from a cross-comparison between available regimens triplet combinations are more effective and give higher response rates than doublet combinations. An overview of available induction regimens is given in Fig. 3.1.

3.1.2.1 Conditioning Regimens Prior to ASCT

In transplant-eligible patients with myeloma the standard conditioning regimen prior to transplantation is high-dose intravenous melphalan (HDM) at a dose of 200 mg/m^2. In the past lower dosages of melphalan 140, 70, 100 mg/m^2 as well as higher dosages have been used; however, these were not compared in a prospective way (Segeren et al. 2003). Alternative conditioning regimens include Total Body Irradiation (TBI), oral busulfan, intravenous busulfan, and combinations of these. TBI is no longer used because of the transplant-related morbidity and mortality. HDM 140 mg/m^2 plus oral busulfan was evaluated in comparison with HDM 200 mg/m^2 in the Spanish Pethema trial and proved to be more toxic, while not improving survival (Lahuerta et al. 2010). Intravenous busulfan lacks this toxic profile, but unlike in acute leukemia, it is rarely used in myeloma. Other attempts to improve the efficacy of HDM followed by ASCT include the addition

	Thalidomide based	Lenalidomide based	Bortezomib based	Bortezomib + IMiD based
2-drug combinations	TD	RD Rd	VD	
3-drug combinations	TAD CTD	RAD RCD BiRD	PAD VCD	VTD VRD
4-drug combinations				VTDC RVDC

Fig. 3.1 Induction regimens prior to HDM in previously untreated multiple myeloma (Ludwig et al. 2012a). Note: Not all agents may be indicated for listed combinations or settings. *BiRD* clarithromycin, lenalidomide, dexamethasone, *CTD* cyclophosphamide, thalidomide, dexamethasone, *IMiD* immunomodulatory drug, *PAD* bortezomib, doxorubicin, dexamethasone, *RAD* lenalidomide, adriamycin, dexamethasone, *RCD* lenalidomide, cyclophosphamide, dexamethasone, *Rd* lenalidomide, low-dose dexamethasone, *RD* lenalidomide, high-dose dexamethasone, *RVDC* lenalidomide, bortezomib, dexamethasone, cyclophosphamide, *TAD* thalidomide, adriamycin, dexamethasone, *TD* thalidomide, dexamethasone, *VCD* bortezomib, cyclophosphamide, dexamethasone, *VD* bortezomib, dexamethasone, *VRD* bortezomib, lenalidomide, dexamethasone, *VTD* bortezomib, thalidomide, dexamethasone, *VTDC* bortezomib, thalidomide, dexamethasone, cyclophosphamide

Table 3.2 Results of induction regimens incorporating novel agents

Author	Induction regimens	Patients (n)	Overall response after induction	CR/≥VGPR	Overall response after ASCT	CR/≥VGPR	PFS (months)
Cavo et al. (2010)	VTD vs TD	236 238	93 79	19/63 5/28	93 84	42/82 30/64	68 at 3 year 56 at 3 year
Moreau et al. (2011a)	VTD vs VD	100 99	88 81	13/49 12/36	89 86	29/74 31/58	26 30
Rosiñol et al. (2012)	TD vs VTD vs VBMCP/ VBAD/Bort	127 130 129	62 85 75	14/29 35/60 21/36	– – –	40 57 48	28 56 35
Sonneveld et al. (2012)	VAD PAD	414 413	54 78	5/20 11/53	77 88	15/51 30/91	24 36
Roussel et al. (2014)	RVD	31	93	23/35	93	47/23	NR

of bortezomib during the first days after stem cell reinfusion. In a phase 2 trial performed by the French IFM group this regimen resulted in a higher CR rate compared with matched controls (Roussel et al. 2010) (Table 3.2).

3.1.2.2 Single Versus Double ASCT

In an attempt to improve the outcome of HDM followed by ASCT, several groups have treated patients with tandem (double) transplantation. The Arkansas group has made the tandem transplantation a standard procedure as part of their intensified treatment program. Indeed, overall survival is superior to many other regimens (Barlogie et al. 2010). Several groups have prospectively compared single versus double intensive therapy (Segeren et al. 2003; Attal et al. 2003). In all studies PFS or EFS was better with double intensive, but not OS. The extra impact of a second intensified regimen is especially evident in patients who achieve less than CR or VGPR with the first transplant. Still, tandem transplant has not become a standard regimen in most countries. Recently the HOVON65/ GMMG-HD4 trial evaluated a single HDM/ ASCT strategy with a double HDM/ASCT in two different countries (Sonneveld et al. 2012). OS and PFS were superior with the double transplant. Although this was not the primary study question, these results have renewed interest in a tandem transplantation.

In conclusion, high-dose therapy will remain the standard backbone of treatment in newly diagnosed patients with multiple myeloma. The introduction of *novel* agents like proteasome inhibitors and IMiDs has contributed to achieving higher response rates and also deeper responses. However, so far there are no indications that combinations of these drugs may replace the standard approach. The insight that deeper CRs can be achieved has raised the awareness that the goals of treatment should be CR for all patients and that new response criteria are needed, which are based on minimal residual disease assessment. Other new agents such as the antibodies daratumumab, elotuzumab, and new proteasome inhibitors will be included in this backbone.

3.2 Part 2: Consolidation and Maintenance

3.2.1 Consolidation

The recent availability of different classes of drugs with different mechanism of action and good tolerability, as well as their proved effectiveness as induction treatment for newly diagnosed multiple myeloma (MM), has dramatically changed the therapeutic paradigm of this still incurable hematologic malignancy. Although the concept of sequential treatment is not new in MM, having already been explored by some groups at the beginning of 2000 (Barlogie et al. 1999, 2006c), only recently, with the new insight in the biology of myeloma (Brioli et al. 2014a), the concept of consolidation and maintenance treatment is becoming more widely accepted.

A first important distinction has to be made between the two concept of consolidation and maintenance. Although the two terms are often used synonymously, the rationale supporting these two strategies is different. Consolidation treatment is generally short-term and aims to increase the frequency and depth of response obtained with the previous treatment phases. Conversely maintenance therapy is given for a prolonged time period with the goal of keeping the disease under control, decreasing the risk of relapse while ensuring a good quality of life.

3.2.2 Transplantation as Consolidation Therapy

The existence of a dose response to melphalan formed the basis of the development of melphalan high dose therapy (HDT) followed by autologous stem cell rescue (or stem cell transplantation, ASCT). Based on the results of phase III clinical trials, reporting and increased rate of complete response (CR) and consequently prolonged overall survival (OS) in comparison with conventional chemotherapy, HDT and ASCT is still considered as one of the mainstays of up-front treatment for younger patients with newly diagnosed MM (Attal et al. 1996; Child et al. 2003). A systematic review and meta-analysis of randomized clinical trials comparing ASCT with standard-dose therapy has confirmed that a single ASCT can significantly prolong progression-free survival (PFS), although an advantage in OS could not be demonstrated (Koreth et al. 2007).

In order to improve the results of ASCT, efforts were made to increase the cytotoxic dose intensity: the administration of two sequential courses of melphalan followed by double, or tandem, ASCT was explored in several studies. Following demonstration that such a procedure was feasible and effective, five randomized trials addressed the question of single versus double ASCT as up-front therapy for MM (Segeren et al. 2003; Attal et al. 2003; Cavo et al. 2007; Mai et al. 2016; Goldschmidt 2005; Fermand 2005). Results of these trials were not homogeneous. In particular, while extended event-free survival (EFS) with double ASCT was observed in most of the studies, an OS benefit was not consistently shown (Segeren et al. 2003; Attal et al. 2003; Cavo et al. 2007; Mai et al. 2016; Goldschmidt

2005; Fermand 2005). A meta-analysis of data pooled from controlled clinical trials confirmed that double ASCT was associated with improved response rates and EFS in comparison with a single ASCT (Kumar et al. 2009). Post-hoc analyses of several subgroups of patients further suggested that the second ASCT was of major benefit for those patients who failed to achieve either a CR or at least a very good partial response (VGPR) after the first ASCT (Attal et al. 2003; Cavo et al. 2007). It has to be noted, however, that one of the major limitations of these studies was their lack of power to demonstrate the equivalence of one versus two transplants for patients achieving high-quality responses after the first course of HDT. Another major limitation was the fact that all the studies were conducted before the novel agents thalidomide, lenalidomide, and bortezomib were included in the induction treatment of transplant eligible newly diagnosed MM patients.

With the recent incorporation of novel agents into the transplantation sequence, the role of single versus double ASCT still remains undetermined.

Recently an integrated analysis of 606 newly diagnosed myeloma patients enrolled in 3 phase III studies evaluating the role of bortezomib as induction therapy before ASCT showed that patients with adverse prognostic factors were those benefitting the most form a double ASCT approach. Patients were differentiated into four different risk groups, based on the presence or absence of known adverse prognostic variables (ISS3, high risk cytogenetic and failure to achieve a CR after induction therapy). Double ASCT significantly prolonged PFS and OS in comparison with a single ASCT for those patients presenting with two adverse prognostic factors (Cavo et al. 2013a). To further evaluate which group of patients can gain the highest advantage in terms of prolonged survival from a double transplant approach three studies are currently ongoing in Europe and in the USA, one headed by the European Myeloma Network, the German GMMS XIV Study and the American study chaired by the Blood and Marrow Transplant Clinical Trials Network.

3.2.3 Novel Agents as Consolidation Therapy After ASCT

The novel agents thalidomide, lenalidomide, and bortezomib have been successfully combined with one another and/or with cytotoxic drugs to form various doublet, triplet, and quadruplet regimens that have been widely investigated as induction therapy before ASCT. More recently the second generation PI carfilzomib and the monoclonal antibodies elotuzumab and daratumumab are also being investigated in the newly diagnosed setting. Based on the favorable results obtained with the use of these drugs as induction treatment, a three-drug regimen incorporating bortezomib combined with an IMiD or a cytotoxic drug, like cyclophosphamide or doxorubicin, is currently considered the standard of care in preparation for ASCT (Cavo et al. 2010, 2011; Ludwig et al. 2012a). In several phase III studies the gain offered by novel agents incorporated into the ASCT sequence in terms of enhanced high-quality responses translated into extended PFS (Sonneveld et al. 2012; Cavo et al. 2010; Rosiñol et al. 2012) and, albeit less frequently, OS (Sonneveld et al. 2012).

It is widely recognized that the achievement of a deep response is associated with improved outcomes. Therefore achieving the deeper possible CR (to the level of undetectable minimal residual disease, MRD) and attaining a sustained response represents a major endpoint of current treatment strategies incorporating autotransplantation upfront (Barlogie et al. 2008a; Chanan-Khan and Giralt 2010). To reach these objectives, over the last years the novel agents have been extensively investigated as part of post-ASCT consolidation and maintenance strategies (Barlogie et al. 2008b). The main studies with consolidation regimen with novel agents after ASCT are summarized in Table 3.3.

3.2.3.1 Conventional Chemotherapy with or Without Thalidomide

The use of consolidation therapy after ASCT was pioneered by Barlogie et al. as part of Total Therapy 2 (TT2), an intensified treatment

Table 3.3 Major studies exploring the role of consolidation after ASCT

Type of trial	No. of patients	Treatment scheme	Response rate	EFS or PFS	OS	Reference
Conventional chemotherapy						
Retrospective comparison	345 vs 231	DCEP/CAD/DPACE (TT2) vs no treatment (TT1)	CR: 43% vs 41% (P = ns)	5 years EFS 43% vs 28% $P < 0.001$	5 years OS 62% vs 57% P = ns	Barlogie et al. (2006c)
Bortezomib-based						
Phase III	370	Bortezomib consolidation vs no treatment	≥VGPR pre-consolidation: 40% vs 39% ≥VGPR post-consolidation: 71% vs 57% ($P = 0.009$)	Median PFS 27 vs 20 m $P = 0.05$	2 years OS 80% vs 80% P = ns	Mellqvist et al. (2013)
Phase III	160 vs 161	VTD vs TD (as induction and consolidation)	nCR/CR pre-consolidation: 63% vs 55% (P = ns) nCR/CR post-consolidation: 73% vs 61% ($P = 0.020$)	3 years PFS 60% vs 48% $P = 0.042$	3 years OS 90% vs 88% P = ns	Cavo et al. (2012)
Retrospective comparison	121 vs 96	VTD consolidation vs no consolidation	CR: 52% vs 30% ($P = 0.001$)	Median TTP not reached vs 25 m	4 years OS 84% vs 91% P = ns	Leleu et al. (2013)
Phase II	39	VTD consolidation	CR pre-VTD: 15% CR post-VTD: 49%	Median PFS 60 m	3 years OS 89%	Ladetto et al. (2010)
Lenalidomide-based						
Phase III	307 vs 307	Len consolidation + Len maintenance vs Len consolidation + placebo	CR pre-consolidation: 58% CR post-consolidation: 69% $P < 0.001$	41 vs 23 m $P < 0.001$ (after maintenance)	3 years OS 80% vs 84% P = ns (after maintenance)	Attal et al. (2012)
Phase II	31	VRD consolidation	sCR pre-VRD: 27% sCR post-VRD: 40%	3 years PFS 77%	3 years OS 100%	Roussel et al. (2014)

CR complete response, *EFS* event-free survival, *ns* not significant, *vs* versus, *OS* overall survival, *PFS* progression-free survival, *VGPR* very good partial response, *sCR* stringent complete response, *DCEP* cyclophosphamide, etoposide, cisplatin, dexamethasone, *CAD* cyclophosphamide, adriamycin, dexamethasone, *DPACE* dexamethasone, cisplatin, adriamycin, cyclophosphamide, etoposide, *Thal* thalidomide, *VTD* bortezomib, thalidomide, dexamethasone, *TD* thalidomide, dexamethasone, *Len* lenalidomide, *VRD* bortezomib, lenalidomide, dexamethasone program that was primarily aimed at evaluating in a randomized fashion the role of thalidomide incorporated into double ASCT (Barlogie et al. 2006b, c). In addition, TT2 introduced post-transplant consolidation therapy, initially with DCEP (dexamethasone plus 4-day continuous infusions of cyclophosphamide, etoposide and cisplatin) for four cycles versus DCEP alternating with CAD (4-day continuous infusions of cyclophosphamide, doxorubicin, dexamethasone) for eight cycles and, in a later phase, with D-PACE (dexamethasone plus 4-day continuous infusions of cisplatin, doxorubicin, cyclophosphamide, etoposide) for four cycles. Pulsing HD-dex was offered as an alternative consolidation strategy to those patients who failed platelet recovery or response to DCEP induction. In a post-hoc analysis, the outcomes of patients randomized to the nonthalidomide-based arm of TT2 were compared with those of patients enrolled in the previous TT1 program that did not include thalidomide and post-ASCT consolidation therapy (Barlogie et al. 2006c). Despite similar rates of CR with the two treatments when considering the overall patient population, TT2 was associated with a higher 5-year probability of EFS (43%) and sustained CR (45%) than TT1 (28% and 32%, respectively; $P < 0.001$ for both comparisons). In comparison with TT1, TT2 extended both EFS and OS for patients whose tumors lacked chromosomal abnormalities. Among patients who were enrolled in TT2 and had abnormal metaphases in their bone marrow plasma cells, those receiving post-ASCT consolidation chemotherapy had a longer OS (measured from a 6-month landmark after the second auto-transplantation) at 4 years (76%) compared with those treated with HD-dex (34%) ($P < 0.020$). The 4-year OS estimate for patients who were enrolled in TT1 and did not have cytogenetic changes was 69%, suggesting that consolidation chemotherapy in TT2 improved the outcome of the high-risk cytogenetic subgroup to the level obtained with TT1 in the low-risk group. However, results of this retrospective analysis should be cautiously interpreted due to differences between studies with respect to the treatment program that included a more intensive induction chemotherapy in TT2 and the lack of post-transplant consolidation therapy in TT1 (Barlogie et al. 2006c).

3.2.3.2 Bortezomib

The role of single agent bortezomib as consolidation therapy after ASCT was evaluated in a phase 3 study in patients not previously exposed to the proteasome inhibitor (Mellqvist et al. 2013). A total of 370 patients were randomized 3 months after a single ASCT to receive no consolidation therapy or standard-dose bortezomib given twice-weekly for the first two 3-week cycles and then once weekly on day 1, 8, and 15 for four additional 4-week cycles. Roughly 39% of patients in both treatment arms had achieved at least VGPR at the time of randomization. After bortezomib consolidation therapy, the probability of achieving CR plus VGPR was 71%, a value significantly higher than the 57% seen in the control group ($P = 0.008$). As a result, median PFS measured from the time of randomization was 27 months for bortezomib-treated patients compared to 20 months ($P = 0.05$) for those randomly assigned to the observation arm, although no significant advantage in OS could be seen. It has to be noted, however, that the benefit of bortezomib consolidation treatment in terms of prolonged PFS was seen only in those patients failing to achieve at least a VGPR after ASCT. Patients achieving at least a VGPR had a significantly longer PFS, irrespective of the time of VGPR achievement (post ASCT or post consolidation) (Mellqvist et al. 2013).

3.2.3.3 Bortezomib in Combination with IMiDs

Bortezomib combined with thalidomide and dexamethasone (VTD) has been reported to yield profound and quick tumor cell mass reduction before ASCT. Based on these data, several groups have explored the activity of this triplet regimen as consolidation therapy after a single or double ASCT.

A large phase 3 study designed to compare VTD versus TD as induction therapy prior to ASCT evaluated also the role of the two regimens as consolidation therapy (Cavo et al. 2010).

Of the 480 patients enrolled in the trial, 321 patients entered the consolidation phase. Patients who were initially randomized to the VTD ($n = 160$) or TD ($n = 161$) arms of the study were planned to receive two 35-day cycles of the same triplet or doublet regimens as consolidation following double autotransplantation. In both arms, thalidomide and dexamethasone as part of consolidation therapy were given at the dose of 100 mg daily and 320 mg per cycle, respectively, while bortezomib, 1.3 mg/m^2 once a week on days 1, 8, 15 and 22, was incorporated into VTD. At the landmark of starting consolidation therapy, the rates of CR were similar in the two treatment groups. However, after consolidation the frequency of CR was significantly higher with VTD (61%) than TD (47%) ($P = 0.012$). Overall, the probability of upgrading from less than CR before consolidation to CR after consolidation therapy was two times higher for the VTD-treated group compared with TD (31 vs 17%, $P = 0.030$). With a median follow-up of 30 months from start of consolidation therapy, the estimated 3-year PFS rate was significantly longer with VTD versus TD (60% vs. 48%, $P = 0.042$), a gain retained across subgroups of patients with poor prognosis (such as the presence of $t(4;14)$ or del17p) and confirmed in a multivariate analysis (Cavo et al. 2012). Importantly, with an extended follow-up of 5 years, the post relapse OS was similar between the two randomization arms, and the PFS2 (defined as the time from initial randomization to second disease progression or death from any cause) was higher in patients receiving VTD (76% vs. 63% at 5 years, respectively; HR 0.64, $P = 0.009$) as compared to patients randomized to TD. This advantage was seen regardless of second line therapy, i.e. irrespective to the use of bortezomib or an IMiD as part of treatment after relapse, suggesting that induction and consolidation therapy with VTD does not select the emergence of bortezomib-resistant clones at the time of relapse (Tacchetti et al. 2014a).

The activity of VTD consolidation after a single ASCT preceded by VTD induction was also reported by French IFM Group (Leleu et al. 2013). Consolidation was given for two 3-week cycles and included standard-dose, twice weekly, bortezomib combined with thalidomide, 100 mg daily. Clinical outcomes of these patients were retrospectively compared with those of a control group who received the same treatment without consolidation therapy. Results confirmed the benefits of consolidation therapy in terms of increased rate of CR (52% vs 30%, $P = 0.001$) and reduced probability of relapse (21% vs 45%, $P = 0.001$), although no difference in PFS was seen between the two groups (Leleu et al. 2013).

An additional phase 2 study was designed to enroll patients who had achieved at least a VGPR after double ASCT and had an available molecular marker to detect MRD (Ladetto et al. 2010). Thirty-nine bortezomib-naïve patients were included and received four 35-day cycles of bortezomib (1.6 mg/m^2 on days 1, 8, 15, and 22), thalidomide (up to the maximum daily dose of 200 mg), and dexamethasone (20 mg on days 1-4, 8-11, and 15-18). The CR rate increased from 15% after double ASCT to 49% after VTD consolidation therapy. MRD, as evaluated by qualitative polymerase chain reaction (PCR) using tumor-clone-specific primers, was undetectable in a single patient (3%) before the start of consolidation therapy and in 6 patients out of 37 (16%) who were assessed after consolidation. In these latter patients, consolidation therapy yielded a quantitative tumor cell mass reduction in the range of approximately four natural logarithms. Patients achieving a low residual tumor mass measured by quantitative PCR had a significantly longer PFS in comparison with those who failed this objective. The benefit of achieving an MRD negative CR was confirmed with an extended median follow-up of 93 months. With a median follow-up of 8 years the OS was 72% for patients MRD negative as compared to 48% for those with MRD persistence ($P = 0.041$). In addition, MRD kinetics resulted predictive for relapse: patients with persistent MRD negativity had a longer duration of remission (DOR) as compared to those patients in which MRD negativity was lost. Patients never achieving an MRD negativity showed the worst outcome, with a DOR of less than 1 year (DOR NR vs 38 vs

9 months for MRD negative patients, patient losing MRD negativity and patient persistent MRD positive, respectively, $P < 0.001$) (Ferrero et al. 2015).

Interestingly a consolidation treatment with the VTD regimen showed a positive effect not only in improving survival outcomes, but also in preventing myeloma-related complications such as the development of bone disease. In a prospective open label study two consolidation blocks of four cycles of VTD were administered after ASCT (Terpos et al. 2014). The first consolidation block was given 100 days after ASCT and the second 100 days after the first consolidation. VTD consolidation resulted in a significant reduction of bone resorption (evaluated as a reduction in circulating C-terminal cross-linking telopeptide of collagen type I, soluble receptor activator of NF-kB and osteocalcin) leading the authors to conclude that VTD consolidation has positive effects in reducing myeloma-related bone disease. Importantly patients enrolled in the study did not receive any bisphosphonate treatment (Terpos et al. 2014).

Given the impressive results of bortezomib consolidation when combined with thalidomide and dexamethasone, the further step was the evaluation of bortezomib consolidation in combination with the second generation IMiD lenalidomide.

In a phase II study, lenalidomide (25 mg/day for 21 days) was combined with standard-dose, twice weekly, bortezomib and dexamethasone to form a triplet regimen (VRD) that was given as induction therapy before, and consolidation after, a single ASCT (Roussel et al. 2014). The primary study endpoint was the rate of best responses achieved after two 3-week cycles of VRD as consolidation therapy. The rate of at least a VGPR increased from 58% after induction to 70% after ASCT to 87% after consolidation. Although the increase in the rate of CR after consolidation was marginal (47–50%), sCR improved from 27% to 40%, highlighting the role of consolidation treatment in improving the depth of response. Furthermore the study was able to show that at the end of consolidation treatment 58% of the patients were MRD negative as evaluated by flow cytometry (Roussel et al. 2014). The role of VRD as consolidation therapy is further being explored in the ongoing phase III trial chaired by the European Myeloma Network that will be discussed later.

3.2.3.4 Lenalidomide

Due to its oral formulation, the lack of neurological toxicity and its immunomodulatory mechanism of action lenalidomide has so far been regarded as the ideal agent to be use in a maintenance context rather than being explored as single agent in a consolidation setting. In a phase III trial, patients with nonprogressive disease after a single ASCT were randomized to receive consolidation therapy with lenalidomide followed by lenalidomide maintenance or lenalidomide consolidation followed by placebo (Attal et al. 2012). The consolidation phase of the study included two cycles of lenalidomide given at the dose of 25 mg/day for 3 weeks every 28 days. Although the primary study endpoint was PFS for patients randomized to lenalidomide maintenance or placebo, results of consolidation therapy were briefly reported. Overall, consolidation with standard-dose lenalidomide improved the rate of CR plus VGPR, which increased from 58% before consolidation to 69% after consolidation therapy ($P < 0.0001$).

3.2.3.5 Ongoing Studies Exploring the Role of Novel-Agent-Based Consolidation Therapy

The role of novel agents as (part of) consolidation therapy after ASCT needs to be prospectively explored in the context of randomized clinical trials before routine consolidation can be recommended. Furthermore the availability of many promising novel target treatment questions the role of ASCT as consolidation therapy in comparison with novel agents. In a recently reported phase III clinical trial a tandem ASCT after lenalidomide/dexamethasone (Rd) induction was compared with six cycles of melphalan, prednisolone, and lenalidomide (MPR) after the same induction regimen. Lenalidomide was given at the normal dose of 25 mg/day for

1 day of a 28-day cycle, in association with dexamethasone 40 mg weekly. In the MPR arm lenalidomide was given at a reduced dose of 10 mg/day for 21 days in association with melphalan 0.18 mg/kg and prednisone 2 mg/kg for day 1–4 for 6 28 days cycles. Patients were then further randomized to receive maintenance with lenalidomide versus observation. The results were in favor of a double transplant approach, with a median PFS of 43 months for patients receiving transplant versus 22.4 months for patients randomized to MPR ($P < 0.001$). The double ASCT group also showed a longer OS as compared to the experimental treatment arm (OS 81.6 vs 65.3%, $P < 0.02$) (Palumbo et al. 2014a).

The role of ASCT as consolidation treatment was further explored in another trial with a similar design. After an induction treatment with Rd for four cycles, 389 patients were randomized to receive either two courses of high dose melphalan with stem cell support, or a consolidation therapy with 6 cycles of cyclophosphamide (cyclophosphamide 300 mg/m^2, days 1, 8, and 15), dexamethasone (40 mg, days 1, 8, 15, and 22), and lenalidomide (25 mg/day consecutively for 21 days of a 28-day cycle). Patients were then further randomized between two maintenance arms, lenalidomide (10 mg/day) or lenalidomide plus prednisone (50 mg every other day). As already seen with the previous study survival data were in favor of the double transplant arm, with a median PFS of 28.6 months (95% CI 20.6–36.7) for patients receiving chemotherapy plus lenalidomide as compared to 43.3 months (95% CI 33.2–52.2) for patients receiving ASCT (HR for the first 24 months 2.51, 95% CI 1.60–3.94; $P < 0.0001$) (Gay et al. 2015). However one of the limits of the abovementioned trials is the nonoptimal induction treatment, with a two-drug combination instead of one the more widely agreed and effective three-drug combinations.

Another trial exploring the value of a transplant consolidation versus a treatment regimen including novel agents is the IFM/DFCI 2009 trial, evaluating the role of ASCT plus VRD consolidation (two cycles) as compared to 5 VRD cycles on 700 patients. Patients in both treatment arms are to receive an induction phase with VRD for three cycles. With a median follow-up of 39 months, patients receiving ASCT had a significantly higher rate of CR, which translated into a significant advantage in terms of PFS (PFS 3 years post randomization 61% vs 48% for ASCT and VRD arm, respectively, $P < 0.0002$; HR 1.5, 95% CI 1.2–1.9), whilst an advantage on OS could not be demonstrated. Importantly the PSF benefit obtained by patients randomized in the ASCT group was not influenced by the presence of risk factors (patients >60 years, ISS stage III, high risk cytogenetic, less than CR after induction) (Attal et al. 2015).

Further trials are currently ongoing and investigating the role of ASCT and consolidation therapy in the context of novel agents. One of these trials is the already mentioned phase III study headed by the European Myeloma Network (EMN02 study). Patients with newly diagnosed MM are randomized to an intensive therapy arm including single or double ASCT up-front or to a non-intensive treatment comprising bortezomib-melphalan-prednisone (VMP) eventually followed by salvage ASCT at the time of relapse. In the USA the fully recruited BMT CTN 0702 trial did not show an improvement for consolidation with 4 cycles of VRD or with a second transplantation in patients with newly diagnosed MM after extensive induction therapy and a first ASCT who also receive lenalidomide maintenance until progression.

Recently the proved effectiveness of monoclonal antibodies in the treatment of relapsed/refractory and newly diagnosed MM patients not candidate to ASCT has opened a further treatment possibility for MM patients. An ongoing clinical trial chaired by the French IFM and the Netherlander HOVON groups (IFM2015/HOVON131) is currently exploring the role of the monoclonal antibody anti-CD38 daratumumab in combination with VTD as induction before and consolidation after ASCT. Furthermore those patients receiving induction and consolidation with VTD-Daratumumab will receive additional daratumumab as maintenance treatment for up to 2 years.

3.2.4 Toxicities Related to Consolidation Therapy

Based on data so far reported, consolidation treatment appears to be generally safe and well tolerated, regardless of the class and number of agents used as part of the treatment program.

The most common adverse event reported with the use of thalidomide- and bortezomib-based treatment is peripheral neuropathy (PN), a complication that can impair patients' quality of life. Thalidomide-induced PN (TiPN) is typically dose-dependent (more prevalent with daily doses higher than 200 mg) and duration-dependent (more likely to occur after 6–12 months of treatment). Bortezomib-induced PN (BiPN) is more frequently sensory, often painful, rarely presenting with motor signs. It is dose-dependent and reaches a plateau at a threshold dose ranging between 30 and 45 mg/m^2. Because consolidation is short-term and treatment intensity is frequently lower in comparison with other phases of the ASCT sequence, in many studies the frequency and severity of treatment-emergent or -worsening PN was low. In a study of bortezomib as single agent, grade 2 or higher PN was observed in 5% of patients (Mellqvist et al. 2013). In two studies investigating the triplet VTD regimen with standard-dose bortezomib, either once or twice a week, and thalidomide 100 mg daily, the rate of grade 3–4 PN did not exceed 1% (Cavo et al. 2012; Leleu et al. 2013; Tacchetti et al. 2014b). In an additional study in which four cycles of VTD as consolidation were planned using higher doses of bortezomib ($1.6 mg/m^2$, once a week) and thalidomide (up to 200 mg/daily), grade 3–4 neuropathic pain was reported in 13% of cases (Ladetto et al. 2010). Grade 2 PN was observed in 13% of patients treated with two cycles of VRD (Roussel et al. 2014), while 8% of patients receiving two VTD cycles had grade 2–3 neurological toxicity (Cavo et al. 2012; Tacchetti et al. 2014b).

Myelosuppression is the most common toxicity related to lenalidomide therapy. In a study designed to administer three cycles of VRD induction and two cycles of VRD consolidation with bortezomib at the standard dose and lenalidomide at 25 mg daily for 3 weeks, grade 3–4 neutropenia and thrombocytopenia (evaluated as incidence in induction or consolidation) were seen in 35% and 13% of patients, respectively (Roussel et al. 2014). As expected, severe thrombocytopenia (grade 3–4) was observed more frequently in comparison with that reported with the triplet VTD regimen (5.5% all grades) (Ladetto et al. 2010). Notably, no major infectious complications were reported with VRD (Roussel et al. 2014).

In one study designed to compare no consolidation with six cycles of bortezomib as single-agent consolidation therapy, the planned number of bortezomib infusions was 20 and the median number of infusions actually received was 19, corresponding to a median given dose of 90% (calculated as the total given dose divided by the total planned dose for each patient) (Mellqvist et al. 2013).

In another study of VTD versus TD consolidation, 93% of the patients in the VTD arm received the planned doses of bortezomib and thalidomide; in TD arm 97% of patients received the planned dose of thalidomide (Ladetto et al. 2010).

The impact of consolidation therapy on patients' quality of life was prospectively evaluated in a phase 3 study (Mellqvist et al. 2013). In comparison with no consolidation, fatigue was reported more frequently after the first two cycles of bortezomib given twice weekly and was not registered when the once weekly schedule was used.

The major toxicities of consolidation therapy reported in the abovementioned trials are summarized in Table 3.4.

3.2.5 Conclusion and Open Issues

Overall, all available studies demonstrate that novel agent-based consolidation therapy enhances the frequency and depth of response achieved with the previous treatment phases, including induction with novel agents and ASCT (either single or double). In several trials, the depth of response was improved up to the molecular level, a finding previously seen only after

Table 3.4 Major toxicities of consolidation treatment

Reference	Type of trial	Treatment scheme	No. of patients	Hematologic toxicity	Nonhematologic toxicity
Cavo et al. (2012)	Phase III	VTD vs TD	160 vs 161	NR	Infections: 1.2% vs 3.1% (P = ns) HZV: 0.6% vs 0.6% (P = ns) GI: 1.8% vs 0.6% (P = ns) PN: 0.6% vs 0% (P = ns) DVT: 0.6% vs 0.6% (P = ns)
Mellqvist et al. (2013)	Phase III	Bortezomib consolidation vs no consolidation	187 vs 183	NR	PN grade >2: 5% vs 1% (P < 0.04)
Ladetto et al. (2010)	Phase II	VTD	39	Thrombocytopenia 5%	Infections: 12% HZV: 5% GI: 7% PN: 7% Fatigue: 8%
Leleu et al. (2013)	Retrospective comparison	VTD-ASCT VTD vs VTD-ASCT	131 vs 96	Hematological AE 6% vs 4% (P = ns)	PN 1% during consolidation (overall 5 vs 3%)
Roussel et al. (2014)	Phase II	VRD	31	Neutropenia: 35% Thrombocytopenia: 13%	Grade 2 PN: 16%

VTD bortezomib, thalidomide, dexamethasone, *TD* thalidomide, dexamethasone, *NR* not reported, *HZV* herpes zoster virus, *PN* peripheral neuropathy, *GI* gastrointestinal, *DVT* deep vein thrombosis, *ns* not significant, *vs* versus, *ASCT* autologous stem cell transplantation, *VRD* bortezomib, lenalidomide, dexamethasone

allogeneic stem-cell transplantation. Enhanced rates and quality of responses offered by consolidation therapy translated into an extended PFS, suggesting that this treatment phase contributed to the improved clinical outcomes seen on an intention-to-treat analysis of the entire ASCT sequence. Nevertheless, the role of consolidation needs to be formally demonstrated before this treatment strategy is routinely recommended (Cavo et al. 2013b).

Notably, in several trials the superior activity of a particular induction regimen was retained despite re-administration of the same therapy as post-ASCT consolidation, suggesting that a switch from one class to another class of novel agents is not necessary moving from induction to consolidation therapy (Cavo et al. 2010, 2012; Roussel et al. 2014; Leleu et al. 2013). As previously demonstrated in the induction phase, it is likely that combining two different agents with different mechanisms of action, like a proteasome inhibitor with an immunomodulatory drug, may help to maximize the activity of consolidation therapy.

Consolidation treatment appears to be generally safe, with a substantial reduction of toxic events in comparison with those frequently seen with the same regimen in the induction phase, a finding possibly related to a reduction in treatment intensity and changes in the schedule of the drugs (Cavo et al. 2013b). Recent availability of subcutaneous bortezomib as well as of novel proteasome inhibitors that have little neurological toxicity would potentially allow a higher dose-intensity and/or more prolonged consolidation therapy. Whether more intensive consolidation regimens might ultimately result in improved activity and reduced toxicity compared with previous ones remains an open issue.

Additional, not yet addressed, issues include the choice of the best consolidation therapy, the need, if any, to use consolidation therapy in all patients or, by the opposite, to plan a risk- and/or response-adapted consolidation strategy and the interface of consolidation with subsequent maintenance therapy. All these issues should be addressed in the context of future prospective randomized trials designed to further improve long-term clinical outcomes, while retaining a good quality of life.

3.3 Maintenance

3.3.1 Introduction

It is widely recognized that not only achieving the deepest level of response is an important step towards MM cure, but also maintaining a sustained remission has a pivotal importance (Lonial and Anderson 2014). To achieve this goal, a sequential treatment strategy including consolidation and/or maintenance is currently being actively studied and incorporated into most of the running phase II-III clinical trials. It is likely that consolidation and maintenance therapies will be implemented in the modern therapeutic paradigm and will become of clinical praxis for patients with MM. Both consolidation and maintenance therapies are ultimately aimed at prolonging OS, without impairing the quality of life. In particular maintenance treatment is regarded as a long lasting treatment that should keep the disease under control, without significantly impairing the quality of life.

The excellent activity shown by IMiDs and/or bortezomib as part of induction treatment for MM has led to their investigational use as maintenance therapy both in younger patients who are eligible to receive autologous stem-cell transplantation (ASCT) and in elderly, nontransplant candidates (Sonneveld et al. 2012; Attal et al. 2012; McCarthy et al. 2012; Palumbo et al. 2012; Mateos et al. 2012). More specifically a long lasting treatment with lenalidomide and dexamethasone is now regarded as a new standard of care for elderly nontransplant eligible myeloma patients, based on the results of an international phase III clinical study. However, despite promising results obtained with continuous treatment with the novel agents, consensus regarding maintenance therapy, especially on the post-ASCT setting, is still lacking. The difficulty to provide a definite answer to the "maintenance question" is highlighted by a consensus

manuscript provided by the International Myeloma Working Group that failed to identify a widely agreed standard for maintenance therapy. Based on the available data the authors concluded that any patient's and physician's decision regarding maintenance should rely upon a careful balance of potential benefits and risks (Ludwig et al. 2012b).

3.3.2 Maintenance Treatment in the Pre-Novel Agent Era: Chemotherapy and Steroids

The first attempts to use maintenance therapy in MM patients date back to the late 1970 and early 1980s, when melphalan and prednisone (MP) was continued after response had been achieved. Despite PFS being significantly shorter in patients who did not receive maintenance, the study failed to show an improvement in OS (Belch et al. 1988).

Over the same years, the role of α-interferon as a maintenance treatment was assessed, however, with conflicting results in the different studies. Barlogie et al. compared the outcomes of 116 patients who were enrolled in Total Therapy (TT) 1 treatment program, including α-interferon maintenance following double ASCT, with those of matched controls who received standard chemotherapy and no maintenance treatment. Results of the paired comparison showed better responses for the TT-treated group, which ultimately translated in an extended event-free survival (EFS) (49 vs 22 months; $P = 0.0001$) and OS (median not reached at 62 vs 48 months; $P = 0.01$). A pitfall of the study is, however, that patients receiving maintenance were treated with a different and more intensive regimen compared to patients not receiving α-interferon, and therefore a formal comparison between maintenance and no maintenance therapy in this subset is not possible (Barlogie et al. 1997). Two meta-analyses evaluating the outcomes of approximately 4000 patients demonstrated a survival benefit of nearly 6 months with α-interferon maintenance compared with observation alone (Fritz and Ludwig 2000; Myeloma Trialists'

Collaborative Group 2001). However, the limited survival advantage and the unfavorable toxicity profile of α-interferon, mainly characterized by mood swings and flu like symptoms, lead to a progressive decrease in the interest for using this treatment strategy and interferon maintenance treatment was abandoned.

Corticosteroids have a significant activity against the malignant plasma cells. This beneficial effect has led to their investigational use not only as partner drug for many myeloma treatments, but also alone and in combination in the maintenance setting, with a particular focus on the role of dexamethasone. Studies on dexamethasone maintenance versus observation after MP induction therapy demonstrated a significant improvement in PFS (2.8 vs 2.1 years; $P = 0.0002$), but no OS benefit (4.1 vs 3.8 years; $P = 0.4$) (Shustik et al. 2007). Different doses of steroids were also tested, and a randomized trial comparing two different doses of prednisolone (e.g., 50 mg every other day versus 10 mg every other day) showed an increased benefit for patients receiving the higher dose in terms of extended PFS (14 vs 5 months; $P = 0.003$) and OS (37 vs 26 months; $P = 0.05$) (Berenson et al. 2002). However, it has to be noted that no comparison between prednisolone maintenance and observation alone was planned in this trial. A randomized comparison between two different maintenance approaches including α-interferon and dexamethasone showed similar outcomes in terms of PFS (Alexanian et al. 2000). The role of dexamethasone as maintenance after ASCT was explored in two studies from the Italian group. In the phase II Bologna 2002 study patients received thalidomide-dexamethasone (thalidomide at the dose of 100 mg for the first 15 days, then 200 mg daily and dexamethasone 320 mg per cycle) for four cycles in preparation to two courses of high-dose melphalan (HMD) with stem cell support (Cavo et al. 2005, 2009). In the GIMEMA 26866138-MMY-3006 trial 480 patients were randomized to receive bortezomib-thalidomide-dexamethasone (VTD) or thalidomide-dexamethasone (TD) as induction before and consolidation after double ASCT (Cavo et al. 2010). In both studies dexamethasone

maintenance at the dose of 320 mg/month was given after completion of study treatment. Unfortunately in both studies a maintenance randomization was not foreseen, so that, even if TD implemented in double ASCT improved the outcomes compared with conventional chemotherapy and ASCT (PFS 51 vs 31% at 4 years for TD+ASCT and ASCT respectively, $P = 0.001$) and patients receiving VTD had a significantly longer PFS as compared to patients receiving TD (3 years PFS 68% vs 56% respectively, $P = 0.0057$), a definitive conclusion on the role of maintenance dexamethasone after ASCT cannot be drawn. Furthermore both studies failed to demonstrate an advantage for the experimental arm in terms of OS survival, even if a trend towards a better OS with the treatments including one or two novel agents could be seen (Cavo et al. 2005, 2009, 2010). Based on the lack of efficacy in prolonging OS and the not clear benefit on PFS, the use of maintenance therapy with steroids has not been recommended by the International Myeloma Working Group (Ludwig et al. 2012b).

3.3.3 Maintenance Treatment in the Era of Novel Agents

3.3.3.1 Thalidomide

The immunomodulatory drug thalidomide has been extensively investigated as a maintenance treatment. Generally, most of these studies demonstrated a PFS advantage, in the range between 6 and 12 months, with thalidomide maintenance, while its impact on OS was less clear (Lokhorst et al. 2010; Spencer et al. 2009; Barlogie et al. 2006b; Morgan et al. 2012; Attal et al. 2006; Stewart et al. 2013).

In the autotransplant setting, the combination of thalidomide (100–200 mg daily) and prednisolone (50 mg every other day) was more effective than prednisolone alone both in increasing the rate of at least very good partial response (VGPR) after a single ASCT (63% vs 40%, $P < 0.001$) and in prolonging both PFS (42% vs 23% at 3 years, $P < 0.001$) and OS (86% vs 75% at 3 years, $P = 0.004$). Furthermore, thalidomide maintenance did not seem to affect survival after relapse (79% vs 77% at 1 year for the control treatment, $P = 0.244$) (Spencer et al. 2009).

The Intergroupe Francophone du Myélome (IFM) reported an OS benefit for patient receiving thalidomide maintenance as well. In the French trial patients who had received double ASCT were randomized to either no maintenance or to receive maintenance treatment with pamidronate alone or pamidronate plus thalidomide at 400 mg daily. Thalidomide maintenance increased the rate of at least VGPR (67%) in comparison with both pamidronate alone (57%) and no maintenance (55%) ($P = 0.03$), a gain which ultimately resulted in significantly prolonged PFS ($P = 0.009$) and OS ($P = 0.04$) (Attal et al. 2006). Based on these findings and the observation that PFS benefit with thalidomide was limited to those patients who failed VGPR after ASCT, the authors hypothesized that the most relevant activity of the drug was that of a consolidation rather than of maintenance effect, improving the quality of response, rather than keeping under control the residual tumor burden after high-dose therapy. Notably, the OS benefit initially reported with thalidomide maintenance was not confirmed with a longer follow-up of 5.7 years ($P = 0.39$) (Barlogie et al. 2010).

Total Therapy 2 (TT2) was an intensified treatment program designed by Barlogie et al. to primarily compare thalidomide maintenance versus no maintenance after double ASCT followed by post-transplant consolidation chemotherapy. Patients randomized to receive thalidomide maintenance experienced a higher rate of CR (62% vs 43%, $P = 0.001$) and a longer PFS (56 vs 44% at 5 years, $P = 0.01$) compared to the control arm (Barlogie et al. 2006b). Although an OS benefit with thalidomide maintenance could not be demonstrated at the time of the first analysis, it became evident at a later analysis in patients with adverse metaphase cytogenetics and was significantly longer in the total group of patients after more than 7 years of follow-up. The survival advantage was seen despite 80% of the patients discontinuing maintenance treatment within 2 years due to side effects (Barlogie et al. 2008c, 2010).

Three additional independent trials confirmed a significant improvement in PFS with thalidomide maintenance compared to observation or interferon in ASCT eligible patients, but failed to demonstrate an OS benefit (Lokhorst et al. 2010; Morgan et al. 2012; Stewart et al. 2013).

Finally, the BMT CTN 0102 study comparing thalidomide and dexamethasone as maintenance therapy for 1 year versus no maintenance after double ASCT failed to demonstrate any benefit in terms of PFS (49% vs 43% at 3 years) and OS (80% vs 81% at 3 years) for patients randomized to the maintenance arm of the trial. These results, however, are likely due to the poor toxicity profile of thalidomide-dexamethasone ultimately leading to premature treatment discontinuation in 84% of patients and inability to complete the planned therapy in 77% of subjects (Krishnan et al. 2011).

To more carefully evaluate the role of thalidomide maintenance in the ASCT setting three meta-analyses of published trials were recently performed. Results revealed a significant PFS and OS advantage for patients treated with thalidomide maintenance (Ludwig et al. 2012b; Morgan et al. 2012; Hahn-Ast et al. 2011). Incorporation of thalidomide into both induction and maintenance treatment phases did not adversely affect clinical outcomes in comparison with thalidomide maintenance alone. However, due to a major effect of heterogeneity between trials on OS benefit, caution in interpreting positive results of thalidomide maintenance is recommended.

3.3.3.2 Bortezomib

The first-in-class proteasome inhibitor bortezomib has been investigated as maintenance treatment in six phase III clinical trials, of whom four were designed for elderly, transplant ineligible, patients and two for younger, ASCT eligible, patients.

The HOVON-65/GMMG0-HD4 study jointly conducted by the Dutch (Hemato-Oncologie voor Volwassenen Nederland, HOVON) and German (German-Speaking Myeloma Multicenter Group, GMMG) cooperative groups was designed to compare VAD induction therapy followed by post-ASCT maintenance with bortezomib (1.3 mg/m^2 every 2 weeks) for 2 years versus bortezomib-doxorubicin-dexamethasone as induction therapy followed by thalidomide maintenance (50 mg daily). Patients were planned to receive a single or double ASCT according to the policy of HOVON and GMMG groups, respectively. With a median follow-up of 42 months, patients randomized to the bortezomib arm of the study had prolonged PFS (35 vs 28 months; $P = 0.002$) compared to the non-bortezomib-treated group. Analysis of PFS from the landmark of last ASCT suggested that bortezomib maintenance contributed more to improved outcomes than thalidomide (median, 31 vs 26 months, $P = 0.05$). In a multivariate analysis, a borderline OS advantage for bortezomib-treated patients could also be demonstrated ($P = 0.049$) (Sonneveld et al. 2012). With a longer follow-up no difference between the two maintenance arms was seen in terms of PFS from the landmark of starting maintenance therapy, but OS was superior for patients randomized to receive bortezomib maintenance ($p = 0.035$) (Sonneveld et al. 2013). However, these data on an improved OS could not be confirmed in a further update with a median follow-up of 91.4 months. A landmark analysis starting at 12 months showed a significant PFS advantage for bortezomib treated patients that had achieved at least a VGPR ($p = 0.02$), whilst no difference between treatment arms was seen for patients already in CR ($p = 0.19$). With a longer follow-up the significant difference in OS could not be confirmed, with 9 years OS of 42% for both treatment groups (Sonneveld et al. 2015). Interestingly bortezomib gave an OS advantage for patients with del17p cytogenetic abnormalities and for those patients who presented in renal failure (Sonneveld et al. 2015; Neben et al. 2012). However, due to the design of the study which did not include a randomization to receive different strategies after ASCT, no definitive conclusion regarding the impact of bortezomib maintenance can be drawn.

Bortezomib was also included as part of post-ASCT maintenance therapy in Total Therapy 3A (TT3A) and Total Therapy 3B (TT3B) conducted by the Arkansas Group. In the TT3A trial bortezomib combined with thalidomide and dexamethasone (VTD) was administered for 1 year after a multi-drug sequential approach including induction with VTD-PACE (cisplatin, doxorubicin, cyclophosphamide, etoposide), ASCT and VTD-PACE consolidation. TD maintenance was continued for two additional years after bortezomib was stopped. The TT3B trial had the same induction and consolidation phases as TT3A, but the planned maintenance treatment included bortezomib, lenalidomide, and dexamethasone (VRD) for 3 years. Results of the two trials were comparable in terms of both EFS (88% vs 86% at 2 years) and OS (91% vs 90% at 2 years), despite a higher number of patients with advanced ISS stage and adverse gene expression profiling (GEP) signature were enrolled in the TT3B study. According to the authors' hypothesis, similar outcomes observed with the two treatment programs may be due to the superior activity of VRD maintenance regimen (Nair et al. 2010).

In an additional study conducted by the Spanish PETHEMA/GEM group, transplant eligible MM patients were randomized after a single ASCT to receive 3-year maintenance therapy with either bortezomib-thalidomide (VT), thalidomide alone or α-interferon. Bortezomib was administered at the dose of 1.3 mg/m^2 on days 1, 4, 8, and 11 every 3 months, thalidomide at 100 mg daily, and α-interferon at the standard dose of 3 MU three times per week. No difference between the three arms was seen in terms of upgraded responses to CR (19%, 15% and 17% for VT, thalidomide and α-interferon, respectively). However, with a median follow-up of 34.9 months, PFS was significantly longer for patients receiving VT maintenance ($p = 0.0009$), while OS was similar between the three arms (Rosiñol et al. 2015).

3.3.3.3 Lenalidomide

Lenalidomide, a second generation IMiD, is likely to be an ideal drug for maintenance treatment, due to the advantages of oral administration and the favorable toxicity profile. In particular lenalidomide lacks of neurological toxicity that is the most dreadful side effect of thalidomide and bortezomib.

Lenalidomide has first proven its remarkable anti-MM efficacy as salvage treatment for patients with relapsed/refractory disease; in this setting, the drug is approved as a continuous therapy until relapse or progression occurs (Dimopoulos et al. 2007; Weber et al. 2007). Based on these favorable results, two double-blind phase III studies were designed to address the specific question of efficacy and toxicity of lenalidomide maintenance after ASCT in newly diagnosed patients (Attal et al. 2012; McCarthy et al. 2012). Two additional trials investigated the role of continuous treatment with lenalidomide in transplant ineligible newly diagnosed MM patients (Palumbo et al. 2012; Benboubker et al. 2014).

In the IFM 05-02 study, patients having received previous induction therapy with either vincristine-doxorubicin-dexamethasone (VAD) or bortezomib-dexamethasone (VD) followed by one or two ASCT were treated with two cycles of lenalidomide consolidation therapy and were thereafter randomized to lenalidomide maintenance (10–15 mg daily) or placebo until disease progression. After a median follow-up of 45 months from randomization, the 4-year estimates of PFS were 43% for the lenalidomide group and 22% for the placebo group ($P < 0.001$), while no difference in OS was seen between the two groups (73% vs 75%). Maintenance treatment was stopped in all patients after 32 months, due to concerns regarding an increased risk of developing second primary malignancies (SPMs) in patients randomized to lenalidomide maintenance (Attal et al. 2012). With a longer follow-up of 60 months, the PFS benefit with lenalidomide maintenance was confirmed ($P < 0.0001$), but no gain in OS was appreciated (68% at 5 years for the lenalidomide group vs 67% for the placebo group) as a result of the significantly shorter time from first to second relapse/progression observed for patients randomized to lenalidomide maintenance (10 vs 18 months for the placebo group, $P < 0.0001$), a finding that ultimately translated into a shorter OS after the first relapse (29 vs 48 months, $P < 0.0001$) (Attal et al. 2013).

The Cancer and Leukemia Group B (CALGB) designed a similar study (CALGB 1000104) for patients treated with one ASCT following thalidomide- or lenalidomide-based induction therapy. No consolidation was planned. As for the IFM study, patients receiving lenalidomide maintenance had a significantly longer time to progression (TTP) compared to those in the placebo arm (46 vs 27 months, $p < 0.001$). With a median follow-up of 34 months, a significantly longer OS was observed for patients in the maintenance arm (85% vs 77% for those randomized to receive placebo, $p = 0.028$). Notably, the OS benefit with lenalidomide was retained although 67% of the patients in the placebo arm who did not have progressive disease were allowed to cross over to lenalidomide therapy after the primary end point (TTP) was met and the study was unblinded (McCarthy et al. 2012).

A meta-analysis of three studies using lenalidomide maintenance (Attal et al. 2012; McCarthy et al. 2012; Palumbo et al. 2012) performed on 1380 patients confirmed that maintenance therapy was associated with a 65% reduction of the risk of progression (Ludwig et al. 2012b). However, concerns regarding the routine use of lenalidomide maintenance were raised by the increased risk of SPMs observed in the lenalidomide arm of all the trials.

More recently, in a prospective randomized trial comparing a nonintensive treatment including MPR with double ASCT, patients in both treatment arms were further randomized to receive lenalidomide maintenance (10 mg on days 1–21, every 28 days) or no maintenance. In comparison with the no maintenance group, randomization to lenalidomide maintenance was associated with a significantly longer PFS (21.6 vs 41.9 months; $P < 0.001$) from the landmark of starting maintenance therapy. However, OS was not significantly improved as compared to the nonmaintenance arm OS (79.2% vs 88% at 3 years; $p = 0.14$) (Palumbo et al. 2014a). The beneficial effect of lenalidomide maintenance on PFS was homogeneous in all subgroups with the only exception of patients with stage III disease at the time of diagnosis ($P = 0.04$ for the interaction between stage and treatment).

A similarly designed study randomized 389 patients to receive consolidation therapy with two courses of high dose melphalan plus ASCT or intensification chemotherapy with lenalidomide, cyclophosphamide, and dexamethasone after induction therapy with lenalidomide and dexamethasone. Patients were further randomized between to maintenance regimen, either lenalidomide alone (at the standard dose of 10 mg daily for day 1–21 of a 28 day cycle) or lenalidomide plus prednisone (50 mg every other day). Patients eligible for the maintenance treatment were 223. Progression-free survival did not differ between the two maintenance treatments (median 28.5 months vs 37·5 months respectively, HR 0.84, 95% CI 0.59–1.20; $p = 0.34$), as did the adverse events that were comparable between the two treatment arms (Gay et al. 2015).

The Myeloma XI trial currently on going in the United Kingdom will further address the issue of lenalidomide maintenance either alone (10 mg daily for 21 consecutive days of a 28-days cycle) or in combination with the histone deacetylase inhibitor vorinostat (300 mg on days 1–7 and 15–21 of a 28-days cycle) versus observation in newly diagnosed MM patients of all age.

Based on its efficacy seen in randomized phase III clinical trials lenalidomide maintenance has currently been incorporated in phase III trials evaluating the role of consolidation therapy with novel agents as compared with ASCT as consolidation strategy. In the IFM/DFCI 2009 trial patients will receive maintenance with lenalidomide (10–15 mg/days) after being randomized to consolidation treatment with RVD for five cycles or ASCT plus two VRD cycles. All patients will receive an induction phase with three courses of RVD. Patients in the European part of the trial will be on maintenance for 2 years, whilst patients randomized in the USA will receive maintenance until disease progression. The European EMN2 trial will randomize patients to ASCT or VMP treatment after an induction with four cycles of VCD. Patients in both arms will be further randomized to consolidation with two courses of VRD versus observation. All patients will receive maintenance with lenalidomide 10 mg/day until disease progression.

3.3.3.4 Monoclonal Antibodies

The proven efficacy of monoclonal antibodies in the treatment of relapsed/refractory MM patients, together with their favorable toxicity's profile, makes them a very attractive option also in the setting of maintenance after ASCT (Lokhorst et al. 2015; Lonial et al. 2015, 2016). The currently ongoing phase III trial IFM2015/HOVON131 is exploring the role of the monoclonal antibody anti-CD38 daratumumab in combination with VTD as induction before and consolidation after ASCT. Patient randomized in the daratumumab arm will receive additional daratumumab as maintenance treatment for up to 2 years.

3.3.4 Toxicity and Secondary Primary Malignancies

The mainstay of a maintenance treatment is the ease of administration and limited side effects, both allowing the drug(s) to be given over a long period of time, as a chronic therapy, without impairing patients' quality of life.

In this respect thalidomide, despite being orally available, is the less promising candidate for a maintenance treatment, due to its unfavorable toxicity profile. Studies with thalidomide maintenance differed in terms of treatment duration, ranging from 7 to 24 months. The major and most wearisome side effect of thalidomide is peripheral neuropathy (PN), which is known to be both dose- and time-dependent, the higher prevalence being observed at daily doses above 200 mg and after 6–12 months of treatment. During the years, thalidomide doses have been progressively decreased from 400 mg daily (Attal et al. 2006) to 50 mg daily (Lokhorst et al. 2010), with an improvement in tolerability and duration of treatment. It is, however, interesting to note that the trial with the shortest median duration of thalidomide maintenance (i.e. 7 months) is the MRC IX trial, in which thalidomide was delivered at the dose of 50–100 mg daily (Morgan et al. 2012). Other important side effects of thalidomide include an increased risk of developing deep vein thrombosis and pulmonary embolism, constipation, somnolence, and loss of balance. Elderly patients are also at higher risk of experiencing cardiac events, such as arrhythmias and bradycardia. In the Canadian Myeloma 10 trial, in which quality of life was assessed, patients treated with thalidomide maintenance reported a higher incidence of dyspnea, constipation, dry mouth, leg swelling, and balance problems (Spencer et al. 2009).

PN is also the major toxicity of bortezomib treatment. It is characteristically sensory and often painful neuropathy, but rarely presents with motor signs. Similarly to thalidomide-induced PN, bortezomib-induced PN is dose-dependent, reaching a plateau at a cumulative dose between 30 and 45 mg/m^2. Side effects of bortezomib treatment other than PN mainly include fatigue and diarrhea, reported in about 10% of patients. In the HOVON-65/GSSG-HD4 trial enrolling transplant-eligible MM patients, bortezomib maintenance was better tolerated than thalidomide, with only 11% of patients discontinuing treatment due to toxicity compared to 30% in the thalidomide arm ($P < 0.001$). Newly developed PN of grade 3–4 occurred in 5% of patients on bortezomib maintenance, as compared to 8% of patients receiving thalidomide (Sonneveld et al. 2012).

The possibility to administer bortezomib subcutaneously has further improved its toxicity profile, significantly reducing the probability of developing bortezomib-induced PN (Moreau et al. 2011b).

Of the currently available drugs, lenalidomide is more promising in a maintenance setting. Lenalidomide's major side effect is myelotoxicity, mainly characterized by neutropenia and thrombocytopenia. However, despite grade 3–4 neutropenia being reported in about 25% of the patients, grade 3–4 febrile neutropenia is rare, occurring in less than 10% of cases (Dimopoulos et al. 2007; Rajkumar et al. 2010). Most importantly, lenalidomide lacks the neurologic toxicity than is the major side effect and significantly limits the use of both thalidomide and bortezomib. This favorable toxicity profile, together with the oral availability of the compound, has led to the extensive investigation of the specific role of

lenalidomide as a maintenance therapy. As expected, a higher hematological toxicity for lenalidomide-treated patients was reported in all the trials. Between 20% to approximately half of the patients receiving lenalidomide maintenance after ASCT developed grade 3–4 neutropenia, and 5–20% of patients enrolled in clinical trials had to stop treatment early due to adverse events (Attal et al. 2012; Palumbo et al. 2014a; McCarthy et al. 2012). However, the most worrying and unexpected adverse event reported in the some of the trials was an increased risk of developing SPMs in patients randomized to the lenalidomide maintenance arm compared to the control group. The rate of SPMs was increased of 2.6 and 3-folds in the CALGB100104 and in IFM 05-02 studies, respectively (Attal et al. 2012; McCarthy et al. 2012). This data were however not confirmed in the GIMEMA study, where the rate of SPMNs was low (2.8%) with no difference observed between the maintenance and the observation arm (Palumbo et al. 2014a). Interpretation of the risk of developing SPMs for patients with prolonged exposure to lenalidomide is complicated by the observation that new primary malignancies, particularly myelodysplastic syndromes (MDS) and acute myeloid leukemia (AML), occur with increased frequency even in the absence of cytotoxic/genotoxic therapy, as is the case of monoclonal gammopathy of undetermined significance (Mailankody et al. 2011). In addition to a possible intrinsic risk of second cancers in plasma cell disorders with a high genomic instability, additional drugs other than lenalidomide may predispose to secondary malignancies. In this regard, the IFM 2005-02 study identified prior exposure to the DCEP regimen including dexamethasone, cyclophosphamide, etoposide, and cisplatin as an adverse prognostic factor for the development of SPMs while on lenalidomide maintenance (Attal et al. 2012). Moreover, it is well known that exposure to melphalan is associated with an increased risk of MDS/AML (Rowley et al. 1981; Finnish Leukaemia Group 2000; Bergsagel et al. 1979).

A recent meta-analysis of more than 3000 newly diagnosed MM patients treated or not with lenalidomide identified the combination of lenalidomide and oral melphalan as the combination at a higher risk of developing SMPs. More specifically the exposure to lenalidomide plus oral melphalan significantly increased hematological second primary malignancy risk as compared to melphalan alone (HR 4.86, 95% CI 2.79–8.46, $P < 0.0001$). Exposure to lenalidomide plus cyclophosphamide (HR 1.26, 95% CI 0.30–5.38, $P = 0.75$) or lenalidomide plus dexamethasone (HR 0.86, 95% CI 0.33–2.24, $p = 0.76$) did not increase hematological second primary malignancy risk versus melphalan alone. Overall the cumulative incidences of all second primary malignancies at 5 years were 6.9% (95% CI 5.3–8.5) in patients who received lenalidomide and 4.8% (2.0–7.6) in those who did not (HR 1.55 95% CI 1.03–2.34, $P = 0.037$). There was no difference in the rate of developing solid tumors between lenalidomide treated and not treated patients, whilst the cumulative 5-year incidence of hematological second primary malignancies was 3.1% (95% CI 1.9–4.3) and 1.4% (95% CI 0.0–3.6), for lenalidomide treated and not treated patients respectively (HR 3.8, 95% CI 1.15–12.62, $P = 0.029$) (Palumbo et al. 2014b).

Although it appears that the risk of secondary cancers in newly diagnosed MM receiving prolonged therapy with lenalidomide is relatively small and is likely counterbalanced by improved clinical outcomes, both physicians and patients must carefully outweigh pros and cons of a maintenance strategy with this drug.

With the ever increasing availability of effective new drugs and their potential incorporation into the maintenance armamentarium, physicians have to take into account the issues of economic cost and impact of treatment on quality of life (QoL). Only a single trial of thalidomide maintenance evaluated the QoL (Spencer et al. 2009), while none of the studies focusing on bortezomib maintenance was designed to specifically address this important issue. Regarding lenalidomide maintenance, results on QoL are available only in the nontransplant setting, where patients receiving maintenance lenalidomide do not have a worse QoL compared to patients in the no maintenance arm (Palumbo et al. 2012). Therefore

conclusive data regarding the impact of continuous treatment on QoL are still lacking and prospective studies in the future should be specifically designed to address this important issue.

Extended PFS and OS reported with the recent introduction of the new drugs into the maintenance treatment phase have also raised major concerns about the optimal duration and economic cost of this strategy. The optimal duration of maintenance therapy is, at present, undefined, while costs of maintenance treatments are in the range of $150,000 per year (Badros 2012).

3.3.5 Which Group of Patients Benefit the Most from Maintenance Treatment?

When evaluating the choice of the best maintenance treatment for MM, it has to be taken into account that the efficacy of novel agents may be different according to the different clinical and biological characteristics of the disease, which ultimately drive clinical outcomes (Cavo et al. 2010; Brioli et al. 2013, 2014a; Barlogie et al. 2008c; Neben et al. 2012; Nair et al. 2010). The International Staging System based on the serum levels of beta-2 microglobulin (β2-m) and albumin has allowed the definition of different risk groups using readily available laboratory tests (Greipp et al. 2005). Other markers of pivotal importance in predicting the risk of MM patients are cytogenetic abnormalities (Chiecchio et al. 2006; Avet-Louseau et al. 2000; Ross et al. 2012). The combination of adverse cytogenetic lesion, identified by fluorescence in situ hybridization (FISH) with ISS stage and LDH can further refine patients' risk stratification, identifying patients with a ultrahigh risk myeloma and at higher risk of early myeloma progression related death (Boyd et al. 2012; Avet-Loiseau et al. 2013; Moreau et al. 2014). Moreover, different GEP signatures have also been shown by independent groups to be associated with different outcomes of the disease (Shaughnessy et al. 2007; Decaux et al. 2008; Dickens et al. 2010).

Although long-term results of TT2 suggested that the major benefit with thalidomide maintenance was mostly seen in patients with metaphase defined high-risk disease (Barlogie et al. 2008c), many other groups failed to confirm these data (Morgan et al. 2012; Attal et al. 2006). In the French IFM 99-02 study, thalidomide maintenance significantly improved PFS and OS of patients lacking high-risk features, including del(13q) and high β2-m (Attal et al. 2006). Similarly, in the MRC Myeloma IX trial patients with favorable FISH abnormalities and who were randomized to receive thalidomide maintenance had a significantly longer PFS compared to the control group. By the opposite, thalidomide-treated patients with adverse abnormalities, including $t(4;14)$, $t(14;16)$, $t(14;20)$, del(17p) and gain 1q had no improvement on PFS, and even a shorter OS than those assigned to observation (Morgan et al. 2012). The advantage of thalidomide maintenance on low-risk patients was confirmed also when a modified risk stratification based on the co-segregation of adverse FISH lesions was applied (Brioli et al. 2013).

The incorporation of bortezomib into the ASCT sequence has been reported to improve the adverse prognosis related to several genetic lesions, in particular $t(4;14)$ (Cavo et al. 2010; Avet-Loiseau et al. 2010). In the HOVON-65/ GMMG-HD4 trial patients, with a high-risk cytogenetic profile, including gain 1q and $t(4;14)$, benefited from prolonged exposure to bortezomib as part of induction and subsequent maintenance therapy (Mateos et al. 2012). Interestingly, in contrast with what seen by the French group, where bortezomib did not improve the outcome of patients harboring the deletion of chromosome 17 (del (17p)) (Avet-Loiseau et al. 2010), in the HOVON Study an OS benefit for patients with del(17p) was also observed (Sonneveld et al. 2015; Neben et al. 2012). In contrast with these findings, the Arkansans group failed to show any improvement with bortezomib use in GEP-defined high-risk patients (Nair et al. 2010).

In the IFM 05-02 study, the PFS benefit reported with lenalidomide maintenance in the entire patient population was retained across subgroups of patients with del(13q), del(17p) and $t(4;14)$, although their outcome was poorer compared to that of patients who were randomized to

the same maintenance arm but who lacked these unfavorable cytogenetic abnormalities (Attal et al. 2012). No data on the impact of lenalidomide maintenance on the outcome of the high-risk cytogenetic subgroup has been reported so far for both the CALGB100104 and GIMEMA trials (Palumbo et al. 2014a; McCarthy et al. 2012).

More recently, improved understanding of the biology of MM has led to the conclusion that the disease is characterized by intra-clonal heterogeneity, defined as the presence of multiple clones detectable at the same time in the same patients. Indeed, at least 4–6 different clones can be identified in MM patients at presentation (Melchor et al. 2014; Walker et al. 2012). Provided that MM is a heterogeneous disease, it is likely that a maintenance therapy should ideally aim to modifying residual disease behavior, selecting for the more indolent clones with the target of keeping the disease under control. Some concerns have been recently raised about the possibility that maintenance treatment might favor the selection of treatment resistant clones and that, in particular, prolonged exposure to lenalidomide might be associated with refractoriness to IMiD-based therapies, a finding ultimately translating into a shorter OS from first relapse (Attal et al. 2013). However, until now no study has specifically addressed the issue of maintenance impact on different disease clones, and data regarding the impact of maintenance therapy on clonal behavior are still lacking. Analyses of sequential paired patient samples will be the way forward to identify how the different maintenance treatments can modify residual disease biology, ultimately granting for a longer PFS and OS.

3.3.6 Conclusions

To date, in many countries still none of the novel agents has been approved as maintenance therapy for newly diagnosed MM patients, making it difficult to provide definite recommendation regarding maintenance treatment (Brioli et al. 2014b). NCCN 2016 guidelines list thalidomide and lenalidomide as category 1 (uniform consensus that the intervention is appropriate based upon high-level evidence) preferred maintenance regimens, whilst evidence for bortezomib maintenance places this treatment in category 2A (uniform consensus that the intervention is appropriate based upon lower-level evidence). Even lower evidence level has combination regimen such as steroid, interferon, or bortezomib plus prednisone or thalidomide (category 2B, consensus that the intervention is appropriate based upon lower-level evidence).

Thalidomide maintenance was effective in reducing the risk of relapse or death in patients with low-risk disease identified by FISH analysis, and is a possible option in this specific subgroup after either ASCT or conventional dose therapy (Morgan et al. 2012; Attal et al. 2006; Brioli et al. 2013). The toxicity profile of this drug, however, limits its applicability as maintenance therapy. Consistently with the guidelines provided by the IMWG, thalidomide should be given at the minimal effective dose (e.g., 50 mg daily) to reduce the emergence of side effects, mainly PN and constipation, and possibly for no longer than 1 year (Ludwig et al. 2012b).

Lenalidomide maintenance was associated with remarkable prolongation of PFS, while the OS benefit was variable (Attal et al. 2012; Palumbo et al. 2014a; McCarthy et al. 2012). Controversies also exist concerning the gain offered by lenalidomide maintenance in patients with different disease status before starting maintenance (e.g., CR vs less than CR) and with different cytogenetic profiles at baseline (e.g., low-risk vs. high-risk) (Attal et al. 2012; McCarthy et al. 2012). Although an increased incidence of SPMs with long-term lenalidomide exposure was reported by several groups, this finding was not consistently observed (Attal et al. 2012; Palumbo et al. 2014a, b; McCarthy et al. 2012). In addition, uncertainties also include the optimal duration of lenalidomide treatment (e.g., until relapse/progression or for a definite period of time, such as 1–3 years) and the possible selection of tumor resistant, in particular IMiD-refractory, clones induced by prolonged exposure to lenalidomide (Attal et al. 2012, 2013; McCarthy et al. 2012).

Studies available on bortezomib maintenance were designed in a way that does not allow drawing any definitive conclusion. Patients receiving bortezomib maintenance had received bortezomib during induction or a more intensified induction compared to the control group. From the available data it seems that a treatment strategy including bortezomib induction and maintenance is be able to overcome, or at least improve, the negative impact of adverse genetic lesions, such as $t(4;14)$ and even del(17p) (Sonneveld et al. 2012; Neben et al. 2012). For this reason, despite the fact that the impact of maintenance with bortezomib "per se" still has to be investigated, based on the available data it would be reasonable to offer patients with a biologically high-risk disease prolonged exposure to a proteasome inhibitor. Whether the impact of bortezomib maintenance will be different in case of the presence of a single or more than one adverse genetic lesion is an issue that still has to be addressed.

Although formally not approved in MM, the concept of maintenance treatment is becoming more and more familiar to MM experts.

The recent availability of monoclonal antibodies targeting candidate molecules expressed on the surface of MM cells, such as CS1, CD38 and CD138, might also change the maintenance treatment paradigm in MM. A currently ongoing clinical study has investigated the role of elotuzumab (a humanized anti-CS1 antibody) in association with lenalidomide and dexamethasone as first line treatment for MM patients. Elotuzumab is to be given until disease progression, with a maintenance design after the nineteenth cycle. Based on the results of a phase III study with an identical design in relapsed/refractory myeloma patients, elotuzumab was granted a fast track approval by the FDA and EMA in association with lenalidomide and dexamethasone in this category of patients (Lonial et al. 2015). Daratumumab, the anti-CD38 antibody, might also prove to be useful in a maintenance setting, and is currently being investigated in the IFM2015/HOVON131 study for newly diagnosed transplant eligible myeloma patients. After induction and consolidation with VTD plus daratumumab, the monoclonal antibody will be administered as maintenance treatment for up to 2 years.

In the recent era characterized by developments in the field of evolutionary biology and remarkable therapeutic advances, the concept of maintenance therapy is probably one of the most promising and interesting for the treatment and cure of MM. Alternating selective pressure and preventing the emergence of resistant clones might be the key for long-term disease control. Future and ongoing studies will help us to address these important questions and to balance risks and benefits in the treatment of myeloma.

3.4 Part 3: Allogeneic Stem Cell Transplantation

Whereas allogeneic hematopoietic stem cell transplantation from a HLA-matched related or unrelated donor has become a standard treatment for many patients with hematological malignancies, the role of this treatment approach in the treatment of patients with symptomatic multiple myeloma remains controversial.

Allogeneic stem cell transplantation is still the best curative approach for younger patients with MM. Allogeneic stem cell transplantation has the advantage when compared to autologous stem cell transplantation that the stem cell graft does not contain any tumor cells and that, due the transfer of a new—allogeneic—immune system to the patient, a graft versus myeloma effect can be generated and further enhanced using immunomodulatory agents like lenalidomide or interferon-@. Additional strategies to stimulate the graft-versus myeloma effect are the transfer of donor lymphocytes from the donor, especially following a lymphodepleting pretreatment.

3.4.1 Front-Line Treatment

Due to the higher median age of patients with MM allogeneic stem cell transplantation with myeloablative conditioning results in a very high transplant-related mortality ranging between 40% and 50% (Barlogie et al. 2006a; Gahrton et al. 1991) and a cure-rate of only 15–30% for patients with MM. To reduce the high transplant-related mortality the dose-reduced conditioning was increasingly administered prior to an allograft for patients with MM which resulted in significant reduction in the transplant-related mortality now being reported to be around 10–15% (Bruno et al. 2007, 2009; Giaccone et al. 2011; Moreau et al. 2008; Rotta et al. 2009).

Because of the higher relapse rate found to be associated with the reduced intensity conditioning protocols several trials used a tandem transplant approach with an autologous-allogeneic transplantation in the first line therapy for patients with multiple myeloma and additionally also for patients relapsing after a previous autograft (Bruno et al. 2007; Moreau et al. 2008; Rosiñol et al. 2008).

When tandem-autologous-RIC-allogeneic transplantation was compared to tandem or single autologous stem cell transplantation an advantage for the allogeneic stem cell transplantation did not emerge until after 2–3 years since during the first 1–2 years the allo patients did worse due to the significantly higher transplant-related mortality (10–13% vs 3–4%). Among the six trials comparing tandem-auto-allo SCT and tandem or single autologous stem cell transplantation are two showing a significant advantage of the allogeneic arm (EBMT study; (Bruno et al. 2007; El-Cheikh et al. 2013)); these are the studies with the longest follow-up. In contrast four trials showed no difference (Pethema Study (Rosiñol et al. 2008), IFM study (Moreau et al. 2008), BMT-CTN (Krishnan et al. 2011), HOVON study (Lokhorst et al. 2012)).

Especially in the very high risk patients (characterized by p53 deletion/mutation, extramedullary disease, especially plasma cell leukemia and high serum LDH levels) even induction with at least one of the novel agents and tandem high dose chemotherapy followed by autologous stem cell transplantation only offers an overall survival of less than 2 years. Thus in these patients increasingly allogeneic stem cell transplantation is used in prospective clinical trials and has shown in one in a preliminary analysis to be superior to tandem autografting, esp. in patients with p53 deletion/mutation.

3.4.2 Treatment for Relapsed Disease

Several studies of allogeneic stem cell transplantation to treat relapse following autologous SCT report long-term disease control and event free survival after allogeneic stem cell transplantation—even in patients who relapsed after an autologous SCT (Einsele et al. 2003; El-Cheikh et al. 2013). Ten years after alloSCT an OS and EFS of 32% and 24% were reported with a plateau 6 years after alloSCT (El-Cheikh et al. 2013).

In a study (Patriarca et al. 2012) patients who received novel agents for treatment of relapsing multiple myeloma after autologous stem cell transplantation the patients with a suitable donor who underwent allogeneic stem cell transplantation showed an improved progression-free survival when compared to the no donor group. An update of the study with a longer follow-up presented at the last IMWG meeting in Rome in 2015 showed also a significant improvement of overall survival for the donor group who received the allograft.

3.4.3 How to Increase the Graft-Versus Myeloma Effect After Allogeneic SCT

3.4.3.1 Donor Lymphocyte Infusions (DLI)

The efficacy of donor T cells given with donor leukocyte infusions (DLI) as treatment has been demonstrated for relapse of various hematologic malignancies after allogeneic bone marrow transplantation (BMT). In a trial 28 patients were studied of whom 24 had a complete donor T cell chimerism. The malignancies were as follows: chronic myeloid leukemia (CML) in chronic phase (CP) ($n = 9$); more advanced CML ($n = 5$); multiple myeloma (MM) ($n = 5$); acute leukemia (AL) ($n = 9$). T cell doses varied from 0.1 to 33×10^7 T cells/kg. Eight patients received two to four DLI courses because they failed to respond to one course. Thirteen of 14 patients with CML achieved complete remission (CR).

All five patients with MM responded, including three CRs. Six patients (three with CML, three with MM) responded only after two to four DLI courses. Patients with CML-CP were likely to respond to as few as 1×10^7 T cells/kg whereas patients with MM generally responded when they received > or =10×10^7 T cells/kg. The likelihood of response was strongly related to the occurrence of graft-versus-host disease (GVHD) in patients with CML and MM ($P = 0.0002$). Finally, there were no obvious differences in responses between complete donor T cell chimeras and mixed T cell chimeras (Krishnan et al. 2011; Kröger et al. 2009; Lioznov et al. 2010; Lokhorst et al. 1997). In patients relapsing with their MM post-allogeneic stem cell transplantation only a minority showed a mixed chimerism prior to the documented relapse in contrast to patients with acute or chronic leukemias (Rasche et al. ASH 2015). Thus monitoring of chimerism does not allow to predict relapses for MM patients undergoing allogeneic stem cell transplantation.

Several studies suggested that achievement of CR after high-dose chemotherapy would prolong survival. In comparison with autologous stem cell transplantation, CR rate after allogeneic stem cell transplantation is higher, and even without novel agents about 50% of patients with CR will achieve molecular remission with a high probability of long-term disease freedom. Therefore, because prior to the era of novel agents 50–60% of patients already achieved negative immunofixation after allografting with 25% even a CR on molecular level. This percentage will definitely increase following the introduction of novel agents also in protocols of allogeneic stem cell transplantation for patients with multiple myeloma.

In addition increasingly post-transplantation therapies are applied to investigate if, in patients without CR after allografting, a durable CR—if possible on molecular level—can be induced by posttransplantation therapies such as DLI with or without novel agents thalidomide, bortezomib, and lenalidomide. DLI has shown activity after allogeneic stem cell transplantation in myeloma patients, but has been investigated mainly in the setting of relapsed disease. The novel less-toxic agents offer a new possibility to treat patients after transplantation in order to upgrade or maintain remission. The immunomodulating drugs lenalidomide and thalidomide especially induce T-cell as well as natural killer cell activation. The proteasome inhibitor bortezomib has shown, in preclinical mouse models, that proteasome inhibition prevents T-cell proliferation and acute GVHD with retaining the graft-vs-tumor effect. These drugs have shown remarkable activity in patients with multiple myeloma and relapse after allogeneic stem cell transplantation, even if DLI has failed. The activity of these novel agents might be increased if they were given in combination with DLI. No severe grade III or IV toxicity of thalidomide, bortezomib, or lenalidomide was observed in our study. Thus in one trial 59% of patients achieved a CR, and this CR resulted in significantly improved progression-free survival at 5 years (58 vs 35%). CR by flow cytometry could be achieved in 63%, and this resulted in an even more favorable event-free survival at 5 years (74% vs 15%).

3.4.3.2 Lenalidomide Post-AlloSCT

The optimal salvage therapy for patients with MM relapsing after allogeneic stem cell transplantation remains to be determined. Usually such patients have been extensively pretreated and present at relapse with a relatively refractory disease. Immunomodulatory properties of lenalidomide may be beneficial by facilitating a graft-versus myeloma effect after allogeneic stem cell transplantation. However, the safety of such treatment is still under debate. In contrast a high efficacy of lenalidomide has been reported in patients with MM relapsing after allogeneic stem cell transplantation.

Lioznov et al. reported 24 MM patients relapsing after allograft who received Len/Dex (with 15 or 25 mg/day Lenalidomide d1-21 in a 4-week cycle). The reported overall response rate was 66%, the median time to progression 9.7 months and the incidence of grade 1–2 GvHD 13%. Coman et al. reported 52 patients who were diagnosed with a relapsed myeloma after allogeneic stem cell transplantation and received a Len/dex

in the classical dose scheme (25 mg d1–12, 40 mg weekly). Len was discontinued in 22% of patients due to GvHD and >50% of patients responded with a PFS and OS of 18 and 30.5 months, respectively (Coman et al. 2013; Lioznov et al. 2010)

In patients who have undergone an allogeneic stem cell transplantation residual or proliferating MM cells are specifically sensitive to lenalidomide. When patients treated with lenalidomide and dexamethasone after at two lines of prior therapy were analyzed for treatment outcome, recipients of an allogeneic stem cell graft as well as patients achieving significant tumor reduction had the best chances to achieve long-term responses as defined as at least partial responses lasting for at least 12 months (Rosiñol et al. 2008).

The role of lenalidomide as maintenance treatment is controversial. The HOVON group has investigated Len 10 mg d1–d21 of a 28-day cycle as a maintenance therapy post- alloSCT from a HLA-matched sibling donor. Due to the fact tha 37% of patients developed a GvHD grade 2 or higher which was thought to correlate with Len treatment and a drop out rate of 43% was reported Lenalidomide maintenance, especially when started eraly post-transplant did not seem to be feasible. Kroeger et al. reported that lenalidomide (median dose 5 mg/day d1–d21 of a 28 day cycle) is feasible. In this study the rate of acute GvHD grade 2–3 after lenalidomide was 28% and the drop-out rate 30% (Krishnan et al. 2011).

References

Alexanian R, Weber D, Dimopoulos M, Delasalle K, Smith TL (2000) Randomized trial of alpha-interferon or dexamethasone as maintenance treatment for multiple myeloma. Am J Hematol 65:204–209

Attal M et al (1996) A prospective, randomized trial of autologous bone marrow transplantation and chemotherapy in multiple myeloma. Intergroupe Francais du Myelome. N Engl J Med 335(2):91–97

Attal M et al (2003) Single versus double autologous stem-cell transplantation for multiple myeloma. N Engl J Med 349(26):2495–2502

Attal M et al (2006) Maintenance therapy with thalidomide improves survival in patients with multiple myeloma. Blood 108:3289–3294

Attal M et al (2012) Lenalidomide maintenance after stem-cell transplantation for multiple myeloma. N Engl J Med 366:1782–1791

Attal M et al (2013) Lenalidomide maintenance after stem-cell transplantation for multiple myeloma: follow-up analysis of the IFM 2005-02 trial. Blood 122:406–406

Attal M et al (2015) Autologous transplantation for multiple myeloma in the era of new drugs: a phase III study of the Intergroupe Francophone Du Myeloma (IFM/DFCI 2009 trial). Blood 126:391–391

Avet-Loiseau H et al (2010) Bortezomib plus dexamethasone induction improves outcome of patients with t(4;14) myeloma but not outcome of patients with del(17p). J Clin Oncol 28:4630–4634

Avet-Loiseau H et al (2013) Combining fluorescent in situ hybridization data with ISS staging improves risk assessment in myeloma: an International Myeloma Working Group collaborative project. Leukemia 27:711–717

Avet-Louseau H, Daviet A, Sauner S, Bataille R, Intergroupe Francophone du Myélome (2000) Chromosome 13 abnormalities in multiple myeloma are mostly monosomy 13. Br J Haematol 111:1116–1117

Badros AZ (2012) Lenalidomide in myeloma–a high-maintenance friend. N Engl J Med 366:1836–1838

Barlogie B et al (1987) High-dose chemoradiotherapy and autologous bone marrow transplantation for resistant multiple myeloma. Blood 70(3):869–872

Barlogie B et al (1997) Superiority of tandem autologous transplantation over standard therapy for previously untreated multiple myeloma. Blood 89:789–793

Barlogie B et al (1999) Total therapy with tandem transplants for newly diagnosed multiple myeloma. Blood 93:55–65

Barlogie B et al (2006a) Standard chemotherapy compared with high-dose chemoradiotherapy for multiple myeloma: final results of phase III US Intergroup Trial S9321. J Clin Oncol 24(6):929–936

Barlogie B et al (2006b) Thalidomide and hematopoietic-cell transplantation for multiple myeloma. N Engl J Med 354(10):1021–1030

Barlogie B et al (2006c) Total therapy 2 without thalidomide in comparison with total therapy 1: role of intensified induction and posttransplantation consolidation therapies. Blood 107:2633–2638

Barlogie B et al (2008a) Complete remission sustained 3 years from treatment initiation is a powerful surrogate for extended survival in multiple myeloma. Cancer 113:355–359

Barlogie B et al (2008b) Completion of premaintenance phases in total therapies 2 and 3 improves clinical outcomes in multiple myeloma: an important variable to be considered in clinical trial designs. Cancer 112:2720–2725

Barlogie B et al (2008c) Thalidomide arm of total therapy 2 improves complete remission duration and survival

in myeloma patients with metaphase cytogenetic abnormalities. Blood 112:3115–3121

Barlogie B et al (2010) Long-term follow-up of auto-transplantation trials for multiple myeloma: update of protocols conducted by the Intergroupe Francophone du Myeloma, Southwest Oncology Group, and University of Arkansas for Medical Sciences. J Clin Oncol 28(7):1209–1214

Belch A et al (1988) A randomized trial of maintenance versus no maintenance melphalan and prednisone in responding multiple myeloma patients. Br J Cancer 57:94–99

Benboubker L et al (2014) Lenalidomide and dexamethasone in transplant-ineligible patients with myeloma. N Engl J Med 371:906–917

Berenson JR et al (2002) Maintenance therapy with alternate-day prednisone improves survival in multiple myeloma patients. Blood 99:3163–3168

Bergsagel DE et al (1979) The chemotherapy on plasma-cell myeloma and the incidence of acute leukemia. N Engl J Med 301:743–748

Blade J et al (2005) High-dose therapy intensification compared with continued standard chemotherapy in multiple myeloma patients responding to the initial chemotherapy: long-term results from a prospective randomized trial from the Spanish cooperative group PETHEMA. Blood 106(12):3755–3759

Boyd KD et al (2012) A novel prognostic model in myeloma based on co-segregating adverse FISH lesions and the ISS: analysis of patients treated in the MRC Myeloma IX trial. Leukemia 26:349–355

Brioli A et al (2013) Biologically defined risk groups can be used to define the impact of thalidomide maintenance therapy in newly diagnosed multiple myeloma. Leuk Lymphoma 54:1975–1981

Brioli A, Melchor L, Cavo M, Morgan GJ (2014a) The impact of intra-clonal heterogeneity on the treatment of multiple myeloma. Br J Haematol 165:441–454

Brioli A, Tacchetti P, Zamagni E, Cavo M (2014b) Maintenance therapy in newly diagnosed multiple myeloma: current recommendations. Expert Rev Anticancer Ther 14:581–594

Bruno B, Rotta M, Patriarca F, Mordini N, Allione B, Carnevale-Schianca F, Giaccone L, Sorasio R, Omedè P, Baldi I, Bringhen S, Massaia M, Aglietta M, Levis A, Gallamini A, Fanin R, Palumbo A, Storb R, Ciccone G, Boccadoro M (2007) A comparison of allografting with autografting for newly diagnosed myeloma. N Engl J Med 356(11):1110–1120

Bruno B, Rotta M, Patriarca F, Mattei D, Allione B, Carnevale-Schianca F, Sorasio R, Rambaldi A, Casini M, Parma M, Bavaro P, Onida F, Busca A, Castagna L, Benedetti E, Iori AP, Giaccone L, Palumbo A, Corradini P, Fanin R, Maloney D, Storb R, Baldi I, Ricardi U, Boccadoro M (2009) Nonmyeloablative allografting for newly diagnosed multiple myeloma: the experience of the Gruppo Italiano Trapianti di Midollo. Blood 113(14):3375–3382

Cavo M et al (2005) Superiority of thalido-mide and dexamethasone over vincristine-doxorubicindexamethasone (VAD) as primary therapy in preparation for autologous transplantation for multiple myeloma. Blood 106(1):35–39

Cavo M et al (2007) Prospective, randomized study of single compared with double autologous stem-cell transplantation for multiple myeloma: Bologna 96 clinical study. J Clin Oncol 25:2434–2441

Cavo M et al (2009) Short-term thalidomide incorporated into double autologous stem-cell transplantation improves outcomes in comparison with double auto-transplantation for multiple myeloma. J Clin Oncol 27:5001–5007

Cavo M et al (2010) Bortezomib with thalidomide plus dexamethasone compared with thalidomide plus dexamethasone as induction therapy before, and consolidation therapy after, double autologous stem-cell transplantation in newly diagnosed multiple myeloma: a randomised phase 3 study. Lancet 376(9758):2075–2085

Cavo M et al (2011) International Myeloma Working Group consensus approach to the treatment of multiple myeloma patients who are candidates for autologous stem cell transplantation. Blood 117:6063–6073

Cavo M et al (2012) Bortezomib-thalidomide-dexamethasone is superior to thalidomide-dexamethasone as consolidation therapy after autologous hematopoietic stem cell transplantation in patients with newly diagnosed multiple myeloma. Blood 120:9–19

Cavo M et al (2013a) Double vs single autologous stem cell transplantation after bortezomib-based induction regimens for multiple myeloma: an integrated analysis of patient-level data from phase European III studies. Blood 122:767–767

Cavo M et al (2013b) Role of consolidation therapy in transplant eligible multiple myeloma patients. Semin Oncol 40:610–617

Cavo M et al (2015) Bortezomib-thalidomide-dexamethasone (VTD) is superior to bortezomib-cyclophosphamide-dexamethasone (VCD) as induction therapy prior to autologous stem cell transplantation in multiple myeloma. Leukemia 29(12):2429–2431

Chanan-Khan AA, Giralt S (2010) Importance of achieving a complete response in multiple myeloma, and the impact of novel agents. J Clin Oncol 28:2612–2624

Chiecchio L et al (2006) Deletion of chromosome 13 detected by conventional cytogenetics is a critical prognostic factor in myeloma. Leukemia 20:1610–1617

Child JA et al (2003) High-dose chemotherapy with hematopoietic stem-cell rescue for multiple myeloma. N Engl J Med 348(19):1875–1883

Coman T, Bachy E, Michallet M, Socié G, Uzunov M, Bourhis JH, Lapusan S, Brebion A, Vigouroux S, Maury S, François S, Huynh A, Lioure B, Yakoub-Agha I, Hermine O, Milpied N, Mohty M, Rubio MT (2013) Lenalidomide as salvage treatment for multiple myeloma relapsing after allogeneic hematopoietic stem cell transplantation: a report from the French Society of Bone Marrow and Cellular Therapy. Haematologica 98(5):776–783

Decaux O et al (2008) Prediction of survival in multiple myeloma based on gene expression profiles reveals cell cycle and chromosomal instability signatures in high-risk patients and hyperdiploid signatures in low-risk patients: a study of the Intergroupe Francophone du Myélome. J Clin Oncol 26:4798–4805

Dickens NJ et al (2010) Homozygous deletion mapping in myeloma samples identifies genes and an expression signature relevant to pathogenesis and outcome. Clin Cancer Res 16:1856–1864

Dimopoulos M et al (2007) Lenalidomide plus dexamethasone for relapsed or refractory multiple myeloma. N Engl J Med 357:2123–2132

Einsele H, Schäfer HJ, Hebart H, Bader P, Meisner C, Plasswilm L, Liebisch P, Mamberg M, Faul C, Kanz L (2003) Follow-up of patients woth progressive multiple myeloma undergoing allografts after reduced intensity conditioning. Br J Haematol 121:411–418

El-Cheikh J, Crocchiolo R, Furst S, Stoppa AM, Ladaique P, Faucher C, Calmels B, Lemarie C, De Colella JM, Granata A, Coso D, Bouabdallah R, Chabannon C, Blaise D (2013) Long-term outcome after allogeneic stem-cell transplantation with reduced-intensity conditioning in patients with multiple myeloma. Am J Hematol 88(5):370–374

Fermand JP (2005) High dose therapy supported with autologous stem cell transplantation in multiple myeloma: long term follwo-up of the prospective studies of the MAG group. Haematol. 10th Int. Myeloma Workshop Meet. Abstr. S40

Fermand JP et al (1998) High-dose therapy and autologous peripheral blood stem cell transplantation in multiple myeloma: up-front or rescue treatment? Results of a multicenter sequential randomized clinical trial. Blood 92(9):3131–3136

Fermand JP et al (2005) High-dose therapy and autologous blood stem-cell transplantation compared with conventional treatment in myeloma patients aged 55 to 65 years: long-term results of a randomized control trial from the Group Myelome-Autogreffe. J Clin Oncol 23(36):9227–9233

Ferrero S et al (2015) Long-term results of the GIMEMA VEL-03-096 trial in MM patients receiving VTD consolidation after ASCT: MRD kinetics' impact on survival. Leukemia 29:689–695

Finnish Leukaemia Group (2000) Acute leukaemia and other secondary neoplasms in patients treated with conventional chemotherapy for multiple myeloma: a Finnish Leukaemia Group study. Eur J Haematol 65:123–127

Fritz E, Ludwig H (2000) Interferon-alpha treatment in multiple myeloma: meta-analysis of 30 randomised trials among 3948 patients. Ann Oncol 11:1427–1436

Gahrton G, Tura S, Ljungman P, Belanger C, Brandt L, Cavo M, Facon T, Granena A, Gore M, Gratwohl A et al (1991) Allogeneic bone marrow transplantation in multiple myeloma. European Group for Bone Marrow Transplantation. N Engl J Med 325(18):1267–1273

Gay F et al (2015) Chemotherapy plus lenalidomide versus autologous transplantation, followed by lenalidomide plus prednisone versus lenalidomide maintenance, in patients with multiple myeloma: a randomised, multicentre, phase 3 trial. Lancet Oncol 16:1617–1629

Giaccone L, Storer B, Patriarca F, Rotta M, Sorasio R, Allione B, Carnevale-Schianca F, Festuccia M, Brunello L, Omedè P, Bringhen S, Aglietta M, Levis A, Mordini N, Gallamini A, Fanin R, Massaia M, Palumbo A, Ciccone G, Storb R, Gooley TA, Boccadoro M, Bruno B (2011) Long-term follow-up of a comparison of nonmyeloablative allografting with autografting for newly diagnosed myeloma. Blood 117(24):6721–6727

Giralt S et al (2015) American Society of Blood and Marrow Transplantation, European Society of Blood and Marrow Transplantation, Blood and Marrow Transplant Clinical Trials Network, and International Myeloma Working Group consensus conference on salvage hematopoietic cell transplantation in patients with relapsed multiple myeloma. Biol Blood Marrow Transplant 21(12):2039–2051

Goldschmidt H (2005) Single vs double high-dose therapy in multiple myeloma:second analysis of the GMMG-HD2 trial. Haematol. 10th Int. Myeloma Workshop Meet. Abstr. S38

Greipp PR et al (2005) International staging system for multiple myeloma. J Clin Oncol 23:3412–3420

Hahn-Ast C et al (2011) Improved Pregression-free and Overall survival with Thalidomide maintenance therapy after autologous stem cell transplantation in multiple myeloma: a meta-analysis of five randomized trials (16th Congress of the European Hematology Association, London, United Kingdom, 19–12 June 2011). Haematologica 96(s2):Abstract 2884

Harousseau JL, Moreau P (2009) Autologous hematopoietic stem-cell transplantation for multiple myeloma. N Engl J Med 360(25):2645–2654

Harousseau JL et al (2009) Achievement of at least very good partial response is a simple and robust prognostic factor in patients with multiple myeloma treated with high-dose therapy: long-term analysis of the IFM 99-02 and 99-04 trials. J Clin Oncol 27(34):5720–5726

Harousseau JL et al (2010) Bortezomib plus dexamethasone is superior to vincristine plus doxorubicin plus dexamethasone as induction treatment prior to autologous stem-cell transplantation in newly diagnosed multiple myeloma: results of the IFM 2005-01 phase III trial. J Clin Oncol 28(30):4621–4629

Koreth J et al (2007) High-dose therapy with single autologous transplantation versus chemotherapy for newly diagnosed multiple myeloma: a systematic review and meta-analysis of randomized controlled trials. J Am Soc Blood Marrow Transplant 13:183–196

Krishnan A et al (2011) Autologous haemopoietic stem-cell transplantation followed by allogeneic or autologous haemopoietic stem-cell transplantation in patients with multiple myeloma (BMT CTN 0102): a phase 3 biological assignment trial. Lancet Oncol 12:1195–1203

Kröger N, Badbaran A, Lioznov M, Schwarz S, Zeschke S, Hildebrand Y, Ayuk F, Atanackovic D, Schilling G, Zabelina T, Bacher U, Klyuchnikov E, Shimoni A, Nagler A, Corradini P, Fehse B, Zander A (2009) Post-transplant immunotherapy with donor-lymphocyte infusion and novel agents to upgrade partial into complete and molecular remission in allografted patients with multiple myeloma. Exp Hematol 37(7):791–798

Kumar A, Kharfan-Dabaja MA, Glasmacher A, Djulbegovic B (2009) Tandem versus single autologous hematopoietic cell transplantation for the treatment of multiple myeloma: a systematic review and meta-analysis. J Natl Cancer Inst 101:100–106

Kumar S et al (2012) Randomized, multicenter, phase 2 study (EVOLUTION) of combinations of bortezomib, dexamethasone, cyclophosphamide, and lenalidomide in previously untreated multiple myeloma. Blood 119(19):4375–4382

Ladetto M et al (2010) Major tumor shrinking and persistent molecular remissions after consolidation with bortezomib, thalidomide, and dexamethasone in patients with autografted myeloma. J Clin Oncol 28:2077–2084

Lahuerta JJ et al (2008) Influence of pre- and post-transplantation responses on outcome of patients with multiple myeloma: sequential improvement of response and achievement of complete response are associated with longer survival. J Clin Oncol 26(35):5775–5782

Lahuerta JJ et al (2010) Busulfan 12 mg/kg plus melphalan 140 mg/m^2 versus melphalan 200 mg/m^2 as conditioning regimens for autologous transplantation in newly diagnosed multiple myeloma patients included in the PETHEMA/GEM2000 study. Haematologica 95(11):1913–1920

Leleu X et al (2013) Consolidation with VTd significantly improves the complete remission rate and time to progression following VTd induction and single autologous stem cell transplantation in multiple myeloma. Leukemia 27:2242–2244

Lioznov M, El-Cheikh J Jr, Hoffmann F, Hildebrandt Y, Ayuk F, Wolschke C, Atanackovic D, Schilling G, Badbaran A, Bacher U, Fehse B, Zander AR, Blaise D, Mohty M, Kröger N (2010) Lenalidomide as salvage therapy after allo-SCT for multiple myeloma is effective and leads to an increase of activated NK (NKp44(+)) and T (HLA-DR(+)) cells. Bone Marrow Transplant 45(2):349–353

Lokhorst HM, Schattenberg A, Cornelissen JJ, Thomas LL, Verdonck LF (1997) Donor leukocyte infusions are effective in relapsed multiple myeloma after allogeneic bone marrow transplantation. Blood 90(10):4206–4211

Lokhorst HM et al (2010) A randomized phase 3 study on the effect of thalidomide combined with adriamycin, dexamethasone, and high-dose melphalan, followed by thalidomide maintenance in patients with multiple myeloma. Blood 115(6):1113–1120

Lokhorst HM, van der Holt B, Cornelissen JJ, Kersten MJ, van Oers M, Raymakers R, Minnema MC, Zweegman S, Janssen JJ, Zijlmans M, Bos G, Schaap N, Wittebol S, de Weerdt O, Ammerlaan R, Sonneveld P (2012) Donor versus no-donor comparison of newly diagnosed myeloma patients included in the HOVON-50 multiple myeloma study. Blood 119(26):6219–6225

Lokhorst HM et al (2015) Targeting CD38 with daratumumab monotherapy in multiple myeloma. N Engl J Med 373:1207–1219

Lonial S, Anderson KC (2014) Association of response endpoints with survival outcomes in multiple myeloma. Leukemia 28:258–268

Lonial S et al (2015) Elotuzumab therapy for relapsed or refractory multiple myeloma. N Engl J Med 373:621–631

Lonial S et al (2016) Daratumumab monotherapy in patients with treatment-refractory multiple myeloma (SIRIUS): an open-label, randomised, phase 2 trial. Lancet Lond Engl 387:1551–1560

Ludwig H et al (2012a) European perspective on multiple myeloma treatment strategies: update following recent congresses. Oncologist 17(5):592–606

Ludwig H et al (2012b) IMWG consensus on maintenance therapy in multiple myeloma. Blood 119:3003–3015

Ludwig H et al (2014) European perspective on multiple myeloma treatment strategies in 2014. Oncologist 19(8):829–844

Mai EK et al (2016) Single versus tandem high-dose melphalan followed by autologous blood stem cell transplantation in multiple myeloma: long-term results from the phase III GMMG-HD2 trial. Br J Haematol 173(5):731–741. https://doi.org/10.1111/bjh.13994

Mailankody S et al (2011) Risk of acute myeloid leukemia and myelodysplastic syndromes after multiple myeloma and its precursor disease (MGUS). Blood 118:4086–4092

Mateos M-V et al (2012) Maintenance therapy with bortezomib plus thalidomide or bortezomib plus prednisone in elderly multiple myeloma patients included in the GEM2005MAS65 trial. Blood 120:2581–2588

McCarthy PL et al (2012) Lenalidomide after stem-cell transplantation for multiple myeloma. N Engl J Med 366:1770–1781

McElwain TJ, Powles RL (1983) High-dose intravenous melphalan for plasma-cell leukaemia and myeloma. Lancet 2(8354):822–824

Melchor L et al (2014) Single-cell genetic analysis reveals the composition of initiating clones and phylogenetic patterns of branching and parallel evolution in myeloma. Leukemia 28:1705–1715

Mellqvist U-H et al (2013) Bortezomib consolidation after autologous stem cell transplantation in multiple myeloma: a Nordic Myeloma Study Group randomized phase 3 trial. Blood 121:4647–4654

Moreau P et al (2002) Comparison of 200 mg/m(2) melphalan and 8 Gy total body irradiation plus 140 mg/m(2) melphalan as conditioning regimens for peripheral blood stem cell transplantation in patients with newly diagnosed multiple myeloma: final analysis of the Intergroupe Francophone du Myelome 9502 randomized trial. Blood 99(3):731–735

Moreau P, Garban F, Attal M, Michallet M, Marit G, Hulin C, Benboubker L, Doyen C, Mohty M, Yakoub-Agha I, Leyvraz S, Casassus P, Avet-Loiseau H, Garderet L, Mathiot C, Harousseau JL, IFM Group (2008) Long-term follow-up results of IFM99-03 and IFM99-04 trials comparing nonmyeloablative allotransplantation with autologous transplantation in high-risk de novo multiple myeloma. Blood 112(9):3914–3915

Moreau P et al (2011a) Bortezomib plus dexamethasone versus reduced-dose bortezomib, thalidomide plus dexamethasone as induction treatment before autologous stem cell transplantation in newly diagnosed multiple myeloma. Blood 118(22):5752–5758. quiz 5982

Moreau P et al (2011b) Subcutaneous versus intravenous administration of bortezomib in patients with relapsed multiple myeloma: a randomised, phase 3, non-inferiority study. Lancet Oncol 12:431–440

Moreau P et al (2014) Combination of international scoring system 3, high lactate dehydrogenase, and t(4;14) and/or del(17p) identifies patients with multiple myeloma (MM) treated with front-line autologous stem-cell transplantation at high risk of early MM progression-related death. J Clin Oncol 32:2173–2180

Moreau P, Mary JY, Attal M (2015) Bortezomib-thalidomide-dexamethasone versus bortezomib-cyclophosphamide-dexamethasone as induction therapy prior to autologous stem cell transplantation in multiple myeloma. Br J Haematol 168(4):605–606

Morgan GJ et al (2011) Cyclophosphamide, thalidomide, and dexamethasone (CTD) as initial therapy for patients with multiple myeloma unsuitable for autologous transplantation. Blood 118(5):1231–1238

Morgan GJ et al (2012) The role of maintenance thalidomide therapy in multiple myeloma: MRC myeloma IX results and meta-analysis. Blood 119:7–15

Myeloma Trialists' Collaborative Group (2001) Interferon as therapy for multiple myeloma: an individual patient data overview of 24 randomized trials and 4012 patients. Br J Haematol 113:1020–1034

Nair B et al (2010) Superior results of Total Therapy 3 (2003-33) in gene expression profiling-defined low-risk multiple myeloma confirmed in subsequent trial 2006-66 with VRD maintenance. Blood 115:4168–4173

Neben K et al (2012) Administration of bortezomib before and after autologous stem cell transplantation improves outcome in multiple myeloma patients with deletion 17p. Blood 119:940–948

Palumbo A et al (2004) Intermediate-dose melphalan improves survival of myeloma patients aged 50 to 70: results of a randomized controlled trial. Blood 104(10):3052–3057

Palumbo A et al (2012) Continuous lenalidomide treatment for newly diagnosed multiple myeloma. N Engl J Med 366:1759–1769

Palumbo A et al (2014a) Autologous transplantation and maintenance therapy in multiple myeloma. N Engl J Med 371:895–905

Palumbo A et al (2014b) Second primary malignancies with lenalidomide therapy for newly diagnosed myeloma: a meta-analysis of individual patient data. Lancet Oncol 15:333–342

Patriarca F, Einsele H, Spina F, Bruno B, Isola M, Nozzoli C, Nozza A, Sperotto A, Morabito F, Stuhler G, Festuccia M, Bosi A, Fanin R, Corradini P (2012) Allogeneic stem cell transplantation in multiple myeloma relapsed after autograft: a multicenter retrospective study based on donor availability. Biol Blood Marrow Transplant 18:617–626

Rajkumar SV et al (2010) Lenalidomide plus high-dose dexamethasone versus lenalidomide plus low-dose dexamethasone as initial therapy for newly diagnosed multiple myeloma: an open-label randomised controlled trial. Lancet Oncol 11:29–37

Rosiñol L et al (2015) Maintenance therapy after stem-cell transplantation for multiple myeloma with bortezomib/thalidomide vs. thalidomide Vs. alfa2b-interferon: final results of a phase III pethema/GEM randomized trial. Blood 120:334–334

Rosiñol L, Pérez-Simón JA, Sureda A, de la Rubia J, de Arriba F, Lahuerta JJ, González JD, Díaz-Mediavilla J, Hernández B, García-Frade J, Carrera D, León A, Hernández M, Abellán PF, Bergua JM, San Miguel J, Bladé J (2008) Programa para el Estudio y la Terapéutica de las Hemopatías Malignas y Grupo Español de Mieloma (PETHEMA/GEM). A prospective PETHEMA study of tandem autologous transplantation versus autograft followed by reduced-intensity conditioning allogeneic transplantation in newly diagnosed multiple myeloma. Blood 112(9):3591–3593

Rosiñol L et al (2012) Superiority of bortezomib, thalidomide, and dexamethasone (VTD) as induction pretransplantation therapy in multiple myeloma: a randomized phase 3 PETHEMA/GEM study. Blood 120:1589–1596

Ross FM et al (2012) Report from the European Myeloma Network on interphase FISH in multiple myeloma and related disorders. Haematologica 97:1272–1277

Rotta M, Storer BE, Sahebi F, Shizuru JA, Bruno B, Lange T, Agura ED, McSweeney PA, Pulsipher MA, Hari P, Maziarz RT, Chauncey TR, Appelbaum FR, Sorror ML, Bensinger W, Sandmaier BM, Storb RF, Maloney DG (2009) Long-term outcome of patients with multiple myeloma after autologous hematopoietic cell transplantation and nonmyeloablative allografting. Blood 113(14):3383–3391

Roussel M et al (2010) Bortezomib and high-dose melphalan as conditioning regimen before autologous stem cell transplantation in patients with de novo multiple myeloma: a phase 2 study of the Intergroupe Francophone du Myelome (IFM). Blood 115(1):32–37

Roussel M et al (2014) Front-line transplantation program with lenalidomide, bortezomib, and dexamethasone combination as induction and consolidation followed by lenalidomide maintenance in patients with multiple myeloma: a phase II study by the Intergroupe Francophone du Myelome. J Clin Oncol 32(25):2712–2717

Rowley JD, Golomb HM, Vardiman JW (1981) Nonrandom chromosome abnormalities in acute leukemia and dysmyelopoietic syndromes in patients with previously treated malignant disease. Blood 58:759–767

Segeren CM et al (2003) Overall and event-free survival are not improved by the use of myeloablative therapy following intensified chemotherapy in previously untreated patients with multiple myeloma: a prospective randomized phase 3 study. Blood 101(6):2144–2151

Selby P et al (1988) The development of high dose melphalan and of autologous bone marrow transplantation in the treatment of multiple myeloma: Royal Marsden and St Bartholomew's Hospital studies. Hematol Oncol 6(2):173–179

Shaughnessy JD et al (2007) A validated gene expression model of high-risk multiple myeloma is defined by deregulated expression of genes mapping to chromosome 1. Blood 109:2276–2284

Shustik C et al (2007) A randomised comparison of melphalan with prednisone or dexamethasone as induction therapy and dexamethasone or observation as maintenance therapy in multiple myeloma: NCIC CTG MY.7. Br J Haematol 136:203–211

Sonneveld P et al (2012) Bortezomib induction and maintenance treatment in patients with newly diagnosed multiple myeloma: results of the randomized phase III HOVON-65/ GMMG-HD4 trial. J Clin Oncol 30(24):2946–2955

Sonneveld P et al (2013) Bortezomib induction and maintenance treatment improves survival in patients with newly diagnosed multiple myeloma: extended follow-up of the HOVON-65/GMMG-HD4 trial. Blood 122:404–404

Sonneveld P et al (2015) Bortezomib induction and maintenance in patients with newly diagnosed multiple myeloma: long-term follow-up of the HOVON-65/ GMMG-HD4 trial. Blood 126:27–27

Spencer A et al (2009) Consolidation therapy with low-dose thalidomide and prednisolone prolongs the survival of multiple myeloma patients undergoing a single autologous stem-cell transplantation procedure. J Clin Oncol 27(11):1788–1793

Stewart AK et al (2013) A randomized phase 3 trial of thalidomide and prednisone as maintenance therapy after
ASCT in patients with MM with a quality-of-life assessment: the National Cancer Institute of Canada Clinicals
Trials Group Myeloma 10 trial. Blood 121:1517–1523

Tacchetti P et al (2014a) Superior PFS2 with VTD Vs
TD for newly diagnosed, transplant eligible, multiple
myeloma (MM) patients: updated analysis of gimema
MMY-3006 study. Blood 124:196–196

Tacchetti P et al (2014b) Bortezomib- and thalidomide-
induced peripheral neuropathy in multiple myeloma:
clinical and molecular analyses of a phase 3 study. Am
J Hematol 89:1085–1091

Terpos E et al (2014) VTD consolidation, without
bisphosphonates, reduces bone resorption and is associated with a very low incidence of skeletal-related
events in myeloma patients post ASCT. Leukemia
28:928–934

Walker BA et al (2012) Intraclonal heterogeneity and
distinct molecular mechanisms characterize the
development of t(4;14) and t(11;14) myeloma. Blood
120:1077–1086

Weber DM et al (2007) Lenalidomide plus dexamethasone for relapsed multiple myeloma in North America.
N Engl J Med 357:2133–2142

Treatment of Elderly Patients with Multiple Myeloma

4

Eileen Mary Boyle, Thierry Facon,
Maria Victoria Mateos, and Antonio Palumbo

4.1 Introduction

In Europe and North America, the majority of patients diagnosed with cancer are over 65 years old. This particularly applies to myeloma that has a median age at diagnosis of 69 years old including 35% of patients diagnosed after 75 and 10% after 85 years of age, Fig. 4.1 (SEER data 2016). This is likely to increase in the years to come especially in Europe where it is foreseen that the percentage of Europeans aged over 65 will increase from 85 million (17% of the population) in 2008 to 151 million (30% of the population) in 2060 (European commission 2009).

Since both the incidence and prevalence of chronic illness increase with age and chronic ailments are a major cause of disability, these patients are more likely to harbour various psychosocial and physical co-morbidities and disabilities (SEER data 2016; Siegel et al. 2014; Smith et al. 2009) than their younger counterparts resulting in a heterogeneous group of patients.

The new elderly population, however, may be healthier than previous cohorts of elderly patients because they will have experienced a lifetime of different and better medical care. These factors will have complex effects on mortality rates, utilisation of services and treatment approaches leading to specific treatment strategies in the elderly myeloma population that we plan, based on current data, to outline hereafter.

4.2 What is Special about Myeloma in the Elderly

4.2.1 Myeloma Cytogenetics and Biology

The genetic make-up of myeloma is vastly similar in terms of cytogenetic abnormalities and mutational spectrum among the young and the elderly (Walker et al. 2015; Avet-Loiseau et al. 2013a). Interestingly, the incidence of $t(4;14)$ and del(13q) decreases with age, whereas del(17p) is remarkably stable (Avet-Loiseau et al. 2013a). From a mutational perspective, the mutational spectrum does not vary in between young and older patients, but a mutational signature related to age according to Alexandrov et al. (2013) may be found in myeloma tumour samples (Walker et al. 2015).

E. M. Boyle • T. Facon (✉)
Department of Hematology, Hopital Huriez, CHRU,
Lille, France
e-mail: thierry.facon@chru-lille.fr

M. V. Mateos
Hospital Universitario de Salamanca, Instituto
Biosanitario de Salamanca (IBSAL),
Salamanca, Spain

A. Palumbo
Takeda Italia, Rome, Italy

© Springer International Publishing Switzerland 2018
M. A. Dimopoulos et al. (eds.), *Multiple Myeloma and Other Plasma Cell Neoplasms*,
Hematologic Malignancies, https://doi.org/10.1007/978-3-319-25586-6_4

Benboubker et al. (38)	Rd	535	73	25.2	4y-OS	Any III IV: 70 vs 75%
	Rd18	541		20.7	59%	
	MPT	547		21.2	4y-OS	
					56%	
					4y-OS	
					51%	

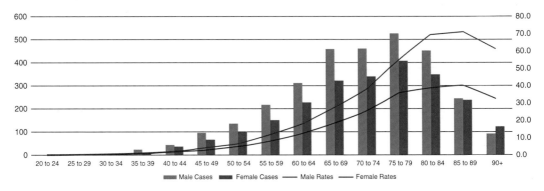

Fig. 4.1 Average number of new cases per year and age-specific incidence rates per 100,000 population, UK, 2012–2014 (ONS 2010)

4.2.2 Clinical Features

Besides these slight biological variations, clinical differences ought to be taken into consideration when treating elderly patients.

Age and the human ageing process it reflects are an essential component that cannot define by itself this population (Smith et al. 2009; Walker et al. 2015; Avet-Loiseau et al. 2013a; Alexandrov et al. 2013; Palumbo et al. 2014). In order to account for the heterogeneity of this population, age should be combined to notions such as frailty and co-morbidity that can also predict outcome.

Frailty is a distinct clinically recognized phenotype but no single sign or symptom is sufficient to define it. Usually, it requires at least three core elements among the following list: weakness, poor endurance, weight loss, low physical activity, slow gate and speed. Specific indexes have been developed (Table 4.1, adapted from Palumbo et al. 2014) to measure and compare frailty between patients and have been used to predict poor outcomes in oncology (Alexandrov et al. 2013; Palumbo et al. 2014).

The second important component we ought to take into account is the presence of co-morbidities

Table 4.1 Frailty indices

Frailty grade	Description
Very fit	Active, energetic patients, who exercise regularly or occasionally
Moderately fit	Patients not regularly active beyond routinely walking
Vulnerable	Patients who can perform limited activities but yet do not need help from other people
Mildly frail	Patients who need help for household tasks (shopping, walking several blocks, managing their finances and medications)
Moderately frail	Patients who need partial help for their personal care (dressing, bathing, toileting, eating)
Severely frail	Patients completely dependent on other people for their personal care

or treatment requiring associated diseases. Among the frequently used scales to quantify co-morbidities, the Charlson scale (Linn et al. 1968) is often perceived too complicated for routine clinical practice (Engelhardt et al. 2017) and replaced by the user friendly, well-validated, CIRS index (Linn et al. 1968).

Both age and co-morbidities can influence treatment toxicity. The human ageing processes are associated with a decrease in physiologic reserves and a change in body composure (decrease in muscle mass, increase in fat, increase in intracellular water) and age-related changes in organ function. These elements affect metabolism, distribution, pharmacokinetics and pharmacodynamics of myeloma drugs and often account for the poor tolerability of the treatment. Co-morbidity, and the subsequent polymedication, may be associated with drug interactions and modified toxicity profiles (Palumbo et al. 2014). The factors that should be taken into consideration in the choice of treatment may be summarized in Fig. 4.2. In that respect Palumbo et al. developed an easily applicable in the clinic IMWG score that stratifies patients into three groups in order to predict both mortality and toxicity (Palumbo et al. 2014). This myeloma-specific score, although it can be improved, constitutes the baseline that leaves room for improvement with more concise versions being published (Engelhardt et al. 2017).

4.3 Induction Treatment

4.3.1 When to Treat?

Like in the younger fitter patients, the diagnosis of symptomatic myeloma is based on the CRAB criteria (hypercalcaemia, renal failure, anaemia and bone lesions) and usually requires treatment (Rajkumar et al. 2014).

The diagnosis of symptomatic myeloma is sometimes less obvious in the elderly and may be mistaken for other coexisting conditions. For instance, osteoporosis should not be mistaken for myeloma bone disease. Mild kidney impairment is also very common in elderly patients. Often resulting from hypertension or diabetes, it should not be mistaken for myeloma kidney disease (Mallappallil et al. 2014). Sometimes, kidney biopsies may be required. Finally, regarding anaemia, if the degree of anaemia seems out of proportion to the disease burden, concurrent causes should be sought after. Community-based studies

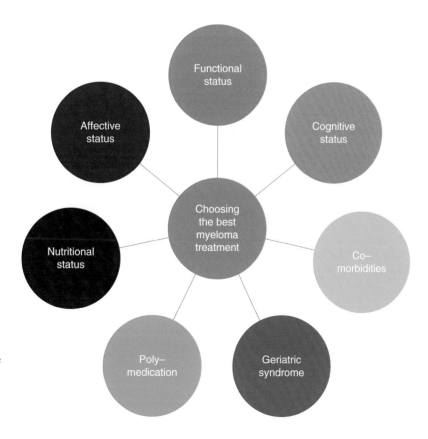

Fig. 4.2 Comprehensive assessment component prior to choosing the optimal treatment for myeloma

found that 10% and 20% of the ≥65 and ≥85, respectively, were anaemic (Patel 2008) and the most common causes of anaemia were iron deficiency, vitamin deficiency (chiefly B9 and B12), chronic inflammation, chronic kidney disease and myelodysplastic syndrome. Often more than one cause were identified per patients (Goodnough and Schrier 2014; Guralnik et al. 2004; Price et al. 2011; Pennypacker et al. 1992) suggesting that a complete anaemia workup should be performed in an elderly myeloma patient presenting with anaemia and a paraprotein without other evidence of symptomatic myeloma.

4.3.2 What to Aim for?

Achieving a complete remission (CR) is an important goal among the young patients (Rawstron et al. 2013; Davies et al. 2001; Larocca et al. 2013a; Barlogie et al. 2014). Until recently, this was not achievable in the elderly given the treatment combinations used. Evidence from recent trials suggests that the depth of response does affect outcome in the elderly (Niesvizky et al. 2008; Gay et al. 2011) although this was not confirmed in the Myeloma IX experience (Rawstron et al. 2013). Moreover, in older patients, the difference between attempting to achieve a CR at any cost and settling for a lower degree of response may be significant as treatment-related toxicities could outshine any benefit derived from the achievement of a CR. If significant toxicity is seen, obtaining good disease control whilst maintaining quality of life is reasonable. Symptom control is achieved through effective disease-specific (Larocca et al. 2013b) and supportive therapy.

4.3.3 Induction Regimens Options

For a long term, melphalan-prednisone was the only standard offered to elderly myeloma patients for many years since its first description by Alexanian et al. (1968) despite yielding low response rates and poor overall survival.

The combination of MP with thalidomide (MPT) was shown to delay disease progression in several randomized trials (Facon et al. 2007; Wijermans et al. 2010; Hulin et al. 2009; Palumbo et al. 2006, 2008; Waage et al. 2010; Beksac et al. 2011) and to improve OS in some of them (Facon et al. 2007; Wijermans et al. 2010; Hulin et al. 2009). A meta-analysis of published data from six randomized trials confirmed an improvement in progression-free survival (PFS) and OS with MPT compared with MP alone (Fayers et al. 2011). The reported median PFS and OS with MPT were 20.3 and 39.3 months, respectively. Toxicity, especially disabling neuropathy, was higher in the MPT arm (Facon et al. 2007; Hulin et al. 2009; Palumbo et al. 2008).

The addition of bortezomib to MP is now a well-established regimen. When first developed in the VISTA trial (San Miguel et al. 2008, 2013), it involved twice-weekly intravenous (I.V.) bortezomib. When first published, VMP was superior to MP across all efficacy endpoints, including response rate, CR rate, median TTP [24 months vs 16.6 months using a stringent definition of disease progression (change from immunofixation negativity to positivity)] and OS. The CR rates were approximately 30% versus 5% in the MP arm. MPV yielded better results over all cytogenetic and renal failure subgroups (San Miguel et al. 2008). Neuropathy was the major side effect of this regimen. In the final analysis of the VISTA trial after a median follow-up of 60 months, the superiority of VMP over MP in terms of median time to second-line anti-myeloma therapy (31 months vs 20.5 months) and median OS (56 months vs 43 months) was sustained (San Miguel et al. 2013).

The results of a study comparing MP and MPR induction with or without lenalidomide maintenance (MM-015, MPR-R or MPR) showed that MPR-R was associated with a PFS benefit over MPR (Falco et al. 2013). Furthermore, in the E1A06 trial that compared MPT-T versus MPR-R, there was no significant difference in terms of response and outcome in between the two arms suggesting that the potential benefit that may be acquired from lenalidomide is outshone by the toxicity profile (Stewart et al. 2014).

In the phase III trial, the FIRST study (IFM 2007-01/MM-020), involving 1623 newly diagnosed transplant-ineligible patients, continuous Rd regimen administered until disease progression or intolerance or for a fixed duration of 18 cycles (72 weeks; Rd18), was compared to MPT administered for 12 cycles (72 weeks). Continuous Rd significantly improved PFS, with an OS benefit, compared with MPT. With a median follow-up of 37 months, the median PFS was 25.5 months for Rd, compared with 20.7 months for Rd18 and 21.2 months for MPT. The 4-year estimated OS was 59% for Rd, 56% for Rd18 and 51% for MPT. In addition, Rd was superior to MPT across all other efficacy endpoints, including response rate TTP, time to treatment failure, time to second-line anti-myeloma therapy and duration of response. Of note, Rd was also generally better tolerated than MPT (Benboubker et al. 2014; Facon 2016).

Adding bortezomib to the Rd backbone showed a significant impact on both PFS (43 vs 30 months) and OS (73 vs 64 months). Nevertheless, only 42% of the patients in this large phase III trial were over 65 years of age (Durie et al. 2017) suggesting this combination may only be suitable for the fit-elderly patients. This led to the development of a customized dose scheduling of VRD, the RVD-lite combination for the elderly (O'Donnell 2015). Despite short follow-up, toxicity profiles and efficacy of the novel dose scheduling appear safe.

Recently the phase III CLARION trial evaluated an investigational regimen of carfilzomib, melphalan and prednisone (KMP) versus bortezomib, melphalan and prednisone (VMP) for 54 weeks in patients with newly diagnosed multiple myeloma who were ineligible for haematopoietic stem-cell transplant. The trial did not meet the primary endpoint of superiority in progression-free survival (PFS) (median PFS 22.3 months for KMP versus 22.1 months for VMP, HR = 0.91, 95% CI, 0.75–1.10, Hulin C et al., submitted).

4.3.4 Choice of Induction

For an elderly patient with a recent diagnosis of symptomatic myeloma, the primary objective is to determine an appropriate treatment approach on the basis of biologic age, performance status, co-morbidities and drug availability (Table 4.2).

Clinical trials may reflect more an idealized population than the daily reality where elderly patients are often clinically frail and vulnerable. Elderly and frail patients have been underrepresented in clinical trials especially those investigating new drugs (Zweegman et al. 2014). There have been a few studies that have been dedicated to patients over the age of 75 years (Larocca et al. 2013a; Hulin et al. 2009), but to date there is, to the extent of our knowledge, currently no ongoing study based on frailty in myeloma. Recruiting these patients into trials is challenging but would help us define safe tailored regimens.

The bortezomib-based VMP (or VCD or VD) or lenalidomide-based Rd or VRD regimens are the most widely used regimens (Moreau et al. 2013). When bortezomib and/or lenalidomide are available, thalidomide is no longer an attractive treatment option. Since 2013, bortezomib is usually administered subcutaneously, and weekly dosing seems to be preferred over twice-weekly infusions for frail patients. Twice-weekly dosing may still be recommended, at least at start of therapy, for patients with renal impairment or aggressive disease (Ludwig et al. 2014). In the absence of direct, prospective comparisons, it is not possible to recommend one regimen over another, although several patient- and disease-related characteristics (such as medical history of thrombosis or neuropathy) may suggest one approach over the other.

Selected patients may benefit from prednisone rather than dexamethasone (Falco et al. 2013). The key aspect of therapy is to use all available drugs and combinations appropriately. Re-challenge with any of the drugs is reasonable, provided it was effective when used previously.

4.3.5 Future Induction Regimens

Other proteasome inhibitors (i.e. ixazomib-NCT01850524), as well as monoclonal antibodies, such as anti-CD38 (daratumumab-NCT02252172),

Table 4.2 Randomized clinical trials for the elderly in myeloma using a novel agent upfront

Study	Regimen	Number	Median age (range)	PFS (months)	OS (months)	Toxicity (exp vs std)
Palumbo et al. (2006)	MPT	129	72 (60–85)	22	3y-OS 80%	Neuropathy GIII–IV: 10%
	MP	126			3y-OS 60%	
Facon et al. (2007)	MPT	125	69 (65–75)	27.5	51.6	Neuropathy III–IV: 6% vs 0%
	MP	196		17.8	33.2	Neuropathy I–II: 20% vs 9%
	Mel100	126		19.4	38.3	Neutropenia III–IC: 23 vs 20%
Hulin et al. (2009)	MPT	113	78.5 (76–91)	27.1	45.3	Neuropathy III–IV: 2% vs 0%
	MP	116		19	17.7	
Waage et al. (2010)	MPT	182	74.5 (49–92)	16	29	Neuropathy III–IV: 6% vs 1%
	MP	180		14	33	Neuropathy I–II: 21% vs 6%
Beksac et al. (2011)	MPT	62	70.6	21	26	Any III–IV: 22.4 vs 7%
	MP	60		14	28	
Wijermans et al. (2010)	MPT	168	72 (65–87)	EFS: 13	40	Any III–IV: 50 vs 29%
	MP	165	30% >75	EFS: 9	31	3% DVT
						Infection II–IV: 28 vs 18%
Morgan et al. (2011)	CTDa	426	73 (57–89)	13	30.6	DVT: 15.6 vs 5
	MP	423		12.7	33.2	Neuropathy: 23 vs 6%
						Infection: 32 vs 26%
Ludwig et al. (2009)	TD	145	73 (54–86)	21.2	45	Neuropathy I–II: 65 vs 32%
	MP	143	10% >80%	29.1	58	Leukopenia: 3 vs 20%
						Infection: 13 vs 8%
San Miguel et al. (2008)	VMP	334	71 (30% >75%)	24	NR	Neutropenia 40 vs 38%
	MP	338		16.6	43.1	Neuropathy III–IC: 13 vs 0%
Mateos et al. (2010)	VMP	125		32	63	Neuropathy: 9% vs 7%
	VTP	128		23	43	Infection: 7% vs 1%
Stewart et al. (2014)	MPR	306		47.7	2y-72%	Any grade III–IV: 58 vs 73%
	MPT			52.6	2y 78%	

anti-CS1/SLAMF7 (elotuzumab-NCT01891643), and anti-PD1 (pembrolizumab-NCT02880228) are currently under investigation in the upfront setting.

4.3.6 ASCT in Elderly Patients

Although age does not affect the outcome of ASCT (Siegel et al. 1999), biological features are powerful determinants of prognosis. The 65-year-old cut-off is commonly used to determine ASCT eligibility in patients with myeloma, even if the feasibility of ASCT is well-established in fit patients up to the age of 70 (Gertz and Dingli 2014). Evidence from the IFM 99-06 trial did not suggest any benefit of ASCT in this population, but the transplant arm did not incorporate any novel agents (the induction regimen was VAD) (Facon et al. 2007). Early ASCT may nevertheless be appropriate in selected patients between 65 and 75 years of age. However this may need to be established in the context of a clinical trial in the era of three and potentially four drug induction and consolidation regimens incorporating new agents. Lower doses (100–140 mg/m^2) may be used for older patients (Zweegman et al. 2014). ASCT in elderly patients with significantly compromised renal function should be avoided.

4.3.7 Maintenance

Several studies have recently evaluated the role of maintenance or continuous therapy. These approaches include bortezomib, melphalan, prednisone, thalidomide (VMPT) followed by bortezomib, thalidomide (VT) maintenance (Palumbo et al. 2010; Mateos et al. 2010), VMP or bortezomib, thalidomide, prednisone (VTP) followed by VT or bortezomib, prednisone (VP) maintenance (Mateos et al. 2012), lenalidomide maintenance after MPR (Falco et al. 2013) or continuous Rd (Benboubker et al. 2014). Taken together, these studies support the role of continuous therapy, at least in terms of PFS and time to second-line anti-myeloma therapy. Only lenalidomide has so far a satisfactory long-term safety profile, but second-generation proteasome inhibitors and monoclonal antibodies represent potential effective drugs for maintenance and are currently actively investigated.

4.3.8 Impact of Cytogenetics in Elderly Patients

With the exception of the NCRI trials (Myeloma IX and XI) and the registration studies (Facon et al. 2007; Benboubker et al. 2014; Boyd et al. 2012), most of the cytogenetic data collected in the past few years have come from younger, transplant-eligible newly diagnosed patients. The Intergroupe Francophone du Myélome (IFM) group recently reported on a series of 1890 elderly patients (median age 72 years; 651 patients >75 years of age), including 1095 patients with updated data on treatment modalities and survival (Avet-Loiseau et al. 2013a). Regardless of treatment, both $t(4;14)$ and del(17p) were associated with a worse clinical outcome. The median PFS in patients with $t(4;14)$ and del(17p) was 14 and 11 months, respectively, compared with 24 months for patients lacking both abnormalities. Similarly, the median OS was 32 and 19 months, respectively, compared with 50 months.

When considering treatment, the use of VMP did not improve the outcome of high-risk patients over MP (San Miguel et al. 2013). Similarly, the Rd arms did not offer a substantial benefit over MPT in the FIRST trial (Avet-Loiseau et al.

2013b). By extension to the data seen in the younger fitter patients and in the relapsed setting, the combination of a proteasome inhibitor and an IMID may improve this. Evidence supporting this hypothesis should be available from the combination trials such as the IRD trial (NCT01850524). Finally the outcome of high-risk and ultra-high-risk patients is always dismal.

4.4 Supportive Care and Management of Co-morbidities

Co-morbidities are frequent in the elderly patients, and several co-morbidities may be present in a given patient. As they may be aggravated by the myeloma drugs, some ought to be taken into account before a treatment decision in made. The most common are hereafter summarized.

4.4.1 Thromboembolic Events

Age, cancer and impaired mobility are well known risk factors of deep vein thrombosis (Lee et al. 2003). This risk is increased by IMIDs such as thalidomide or lenalidomide especially when combined to conventional chemotherapy agents (including steroids). Thromboprophylaxis using low-molecular weight heparin is an effective preventive measure (Larocca et al. 2012) but for patients unable to tolerate them or with a past medical history of thrombosis whilst on prophylaxis, alternative approaches may be preferable. The risk of thrombosis is nevertheless limited when these drugs are used alone, option worth exploring in selected cases (Boyle et al. 2012).

4.4.2 Renal Failure

The use of fast-acting combinations is important to minimize tumour burden and maximize the chance of restoring a near-to-normal renal function in patients with myeloma-related kidney failure. The dose of lenalidomide must be adjusted to renal function. Thalidomide and bortezomib can be used at full doses in patients with renal dysfunction including in patients requiring haemodialysis (Kastritis et al. 2013). Cyclophosphamide is also easier to manage than melphalan in case of renal failure. Compared with thalidomide, bortezomib exerts faster and deeper responses, which could result in a greater chance of reversal of renal failure. Bisphosphonates should be used with caution with renal dysfunction as they may increase tubular necrosis (Hirschberg 2012). Of note there was no differential impact on renal failure of clodronate or zoledronic acid (Jackson et al. 2014). Finally, as age and renal dysfunction both increase morbidity and mortality of transplant, ASCT should therefore not be performed in older patients regardless of the aetiology of the renal failure (Harousseau and Attal 2002).

4.4.3 Cardiovascular Disease

Steroids are associated with multiple side effects, the most common being cardiovascular such as hypertension, heart failure, fluid retention, making regimens such as Rd, with reduced steroids appealing. Thalidomide (and to a lesser extent, lenalidomide) may cause bradycardia (Fahdi et al. 2004). The concomitant use of these drugs with a beta-blocker may increase that risk (Yamaguchi 2008). Furthermore, lenalidomide may increase levels of digoxine; they should therefore be monitored closely upon treatment initiation (Chen et al. 2014). Finally, maintaining adequate haemoglobin is important in patients with cardiovascular disease to minimize the risk of ischemic episodes and heart failure (Azad and Lemay 2014).

4.4.4 Diabetes

Diabetes and diabetes-related end-organ damage are common in elderly patients. Monitoring and adjusting the glycaemia control regimen whilst on steroids are essential. A recent review of 1240 patients with diabetes and myeloma suggested its adverse prognosis, especially when steroid-induced (Wu et al. 2014). Furthermore, as diabetic patients are also at risk of peripheral neuropathy, a clear evaluation of baseline diabetes-related complications is required prior to introducing drugs such as thalidomide and bortezomib and should therefore influence treatment.

4.4.5 QOL

The current treatment aims in myeloma are to control the disease, to improve overall survival and to increase the quality of life. Despite improvements in overall survival, novel agents are associated with adverse events that may, in conjunction with persistent myeloma-related symptoms, impair quality of life (Sonneveld et al. 2013). The QOL scores improved among responders in bortezomib (Fayers et al. 2011; Chen et al. 2014; Azad and Lemay 2014) and lenalidomide (Delforge et al. 2015). As some treatment options have prolonged survival in myeloma patients, and owing to the impact of treatment-related toxicity on QOL, this data have become increasingly relevant. In the absence of differences in treatment efficacy, the choice of initial treatment should be based on QOL indicators, among other patient-related factors.

Conclusion

The clinical management of elderly patients with myeloma remains challenging. Not only does it require an up-to-date knowledge of tumour biology and clinical trials, day-to-day practice requires an accurate assessment of many clinical and social parameters. Novel agents, including thalidomide-lenalidomide and bortezomib have participated to the improvement of outcome of elderly myeloma patients with median OS in elderly NDMM patients increasing from roughly 30 to 60 months. The way forward lies within future development of second- and third-generation immunomodulatory drugs and proteasome inhibitors, new drug families such as monoclonal antibodies and histone deacetylase inhibitors and better tools to develop more effective treatment strategies and clinical trials tailored to the specific needs of these patients.

References

Alexandrov LB, Nik-Zainal S, Wedge DC, Aparicio SAJR, Behjati S, Biankin AV et al (2013) Signatures of mutational processes in human cancer. Nature 500(7463):415–421

Alexanian R, Bergsagel DE, Migliore J, Vaughn WK, Howe CD (1968) Melphalan therapy for plasma cell myeloma. Blood 31(1):1–10

Avet-Loiseau H, Hulin C, Campion L, Rodon P, Marit G, Attal M et al (2013a) Chromosomal abnormalities are major prognostic factors in elderly patients with multiple myeloma: the intergroupe francophone du myélome experience. J Clin Oncol Off J Am Soc Clin Oncol 31(22):2806–2809

Avet-Loiseau H, Hulin C, Campion L, Rodon P, Marit G, Attal M et al (2013b) Chromosomal abnormalities are major prognostic factors in elderly patients with multiple myeloma: the intergroupe Francophone du Myélome experience. J Clin Oncol 31(22):2806–2809

Azad N, Lemay G (2014) Management of chronic heart failure in the older population. J Geriatr Cardiol JGC 11(4):329–337

Barlogie B, Mitchell A, van Rhee F, Epstein J, Morgan GJ, Crowley J (2014) Curing myeloma at last: defining criteria and providing the evidence. Blood 124(20):3043–3051

Beksac M, Haznedar R, Firatli-Tuglular T, Ozdogu H, Aydogdu I, Konuk N et al (2011) Addition of thalidomide to oral melphalan/prednisone in patients with multiple myeloma not eligible for transplantation: results of a randomized trial from the Turkish myeloma study group. Eur J Haematol 86(1):16–22

Benboubker L, Dimopoulos MA, Dispenzieri A, Catalano J, Belch AR, Cavo M et al (2014) Lenalidomide and dexamethasone in transplant-ineligible patients with myeloma. N Engl J Med 371(10):906–917

Boyd KD, Ross FM, Chiecchio L, Dagrada GP, Konn ZJ, Tapper WJ et al (2012) A novel prognostic model in myeloma based on co-segregating adverse FISH lesions and the ISS: analysis of patients treated in the MRC myeloma IX trial. Leukemia 26(2):349–355

Boyle EM, Fouquet G, Manier S, Gauthier J, Noel MP, Borie C et al (2012) Immunomodulator drug-based therapy in myeloma and the occurrence of thrombosis. Expert Rev Hematol 5(6):617–626. quiz 627

Chen N, Weiss D, Reyes J, Liu L, Kasserra C, Wang X et al (2014) No clinically significant drug interactions between lenalidomide and P-glycoprotein substrates and inhibitors: results from controlled phase I studies in healthy volunteers. Cancer Chemother Pharmacol 73(5):1031–1039

Davies FE, Forsyth PD, Rawstron AC, Owen RG, Pratt G, Evans PA et al (2001) The impact of attaining a minimal disease state after high-dose melphalan and autologous transplantation for multiple myeloma. Br J Haematol 112(3):814–819

Delforge M, Minuk L, Eisenmann JC, Arnulf B, Canepa L, Fragasso A et al (2015) Health-related quality-of-life in patients with newly diagnosed multiple myeloma in the FIRST trial: lenalidomide plus low-dose dexamethasone versus melphalan, prednisone, thalidomide. Haematologica 100(6):826–833

Durie BGM, Hoering A, Abidi MH, Rajkumar SV, Epstein J, Kahanic SP et al (2017) Bortezomib with lenalidomide and dexamethasone versus lenalidomide and dexamethasone alone in patients with newly diagnosed myeloma without intent for immediate autologous stem-cell transplant (SWOG S0777): a randomised, open-label, phase 3 trial. Lancet Lond Engl 389(10068):519–527

Engelhardt M, Domm A-S, Dold SM, Ihorst G, Reinhardt H, Zober A et al (2017) A concise revised myeloma comorbidity index as a valid prognostic instrument in a large cohort of 801 multiple myeloma patients. Haematologica 102(5):910–921. https://doi.org/10.3324/haematol.2016.162693

European commission (2009) Ageing report: economic and budgetary projections for the EU-27 Member States (2008–2060)

Facon T (2016) Paper: final analysis of overall survival from the first trial [Internet]. [cited 2017 Apr 3]. Available from: https://ash.confex.com/ash/2016/webprogram/Paper91328.html

Facon T, Mary JY, Hulin C, Benboubker L, Attal M, Pegourie B et al (2007) Melphalan and prednisone plus thalidomide versus melphalan and prednisone alone or reduced-intensity autologous stem cell transplantation in elderly patients with multiple myeloma (IFM 99-06): a randomised trial. Lancet 370(9594):1209–1218

Fahdi IE, Gaddam V, Saucedo JF, Kishan CV, Vyas K, Deneke MG et al (2004) Bradycardia during therapy for multiple myeloma with thalidomide. Am J Cardiol 93(8):1052–1055

Falco P, Cavallo F, Larocca A, Rossi D, Guglielmelli T, Rocci A et al (2013) Lenalidomide-prednisone induction followed by lenalidomide-melphalan-prednisone consolidation and lenalidomide-prednisone maintenance in newly diagnosed elderly unfit myeloma patients. Leukemia 27(3):695–701

Fayers PM, Palumbo A, Hulin C, Waage A, Wijermans P, Beksaç M et al (2011) Thalidomide for previously untreated elderly patients with multiple myeloma: meta-analysis of 1685 individual patient data from 6 randomized clinical trials. Blood 118(5):1239–1247

Gay F, Larocca A, Wijermans P, Cavallo F, Rossi D, Schaafsma R et al (2011) Complete response correlates with long-term progression-free and overall survival in elderly myeloma treated with novel agents: analysis of 1175 patients. Blood 117(11):3025–3031

Gertz MA, Dingli D (2014) How we manage autologous stem cell transplantation for patients with multiple myeloma. Blood 124(6):882–890

Goodnough LT, Schrier SL (2014) Evaluation and management of anemia in the elderly. Am J Hematol 89(1):88–96

Guralnik JM, Eisenstaedt RS, Ferrucci L, Klein HG, Woodman RC (2004) Prevalence of anemia in persons 65 years and older in the United States: evidence for a high rate of unexplained anemia. Blood 104(8):2263–2268

Harousseau J-L, Attal M (2002) The role of stem cell transplantation in multiple myeloma. Blood Rev 16(4):245–253

Hirschberg R (2012) Renal complications from bisphosphonate treatment. Curr Opin Support Palliat Care 6(3):342–347

Hulin C, Facon T, Rodon P, Pegourie B, Benboubker L, Doyen C et al (2009) Efficacy of melphalan and prednisone plus thalidomide in patients older than 75 years with newly diagnosed multiple myeloma: IFM 01/01 trial. J Clin Oncol Off J Am Soc Clin Oncol 27(22):3664–3670

Jackson GH, Morgan GJ, Davies FE, Wu P, Gregory WM, Bell SE et al (2014) Osteonecrosis of the jaw and renal safety in patients with newly diagnosed multiple myeloma: Medical Research Council myeloma IX study results. Br J Haematol 166(1):109–117

Kastritis E, Terpos E, Dimopoulos MA (2013) Current treatments for renal failure due to multiple myeloma. Expert Opin Pharmacother 14(11):1477–1495

Larocca A, Cavallo F, Bringhen S, Di Raimondo F, Falanga A, Evangelista A et al (2012) Aspirin or enoxaparin thromboprophylaxis for patients with newly diagnosed multiple myeloma treated with lenalidomide. Blood 119(4):933–939. quiz 1093

Larocca A, Cavallo F, Magarotto V, Palumbo A (2013a) Reduced dose-intensity subcutaneous bortezomib plus prednisone (VP) or plus cyclophosfamide (VCP) or plus melphalan (VMP) for newly diagnosed multiple myeloma patients older than 75 years of age. Blood 122:539

Larocca A, Child JA, Cook G, Jackson GH, Russell N, Szubert A et al (2013b) The impact of response on bone-directed therapy in patients with multiple myeloma. Blood 122(17):2974–2977

Lee AYY, Levine MN, Baker RI, Bowden C, Kakkar AK, Prins M et al (2003) Low-molecular-weight heparin versus a coumarin for the prevention of recurrent venous thromboembolism in patients with cancer. N Engl J Med 349(2):146–153

Linn BS, Linn MW, Gurel L (1968) Cumulative illness rating scale. J Am Geriatr Soc 16(5):622–626

Ludwig H, Hajek R, Tóthová E, Drach J, Adam Z, Labar B et al (2009) Thalidomide-dexamethasone compared with melphalan-prednisolone in elderly patients with multiple myeloma. Blood 113(15):3435–3442

Ludwig H, Sonneveld P, Davies F, Bladé J, Boccadoro M, Cavo M et al (2014) European perspective on multiple myeloma treatment strategies in 2014. Oncologist 19(8):829–844

Mallappallil M, Friedman EA, Delano BG, McFarlane SI, Salifu MO (2014) Chronic kidney disease in the elderly: evaluation and management. Clin Pract Lond Engl 11(5):525–535

Mateos M-V, Oriol A, Martínez-López J, Gutiérrez N, Teruel A-I, de Paz R et al (2010) Bortezomib, melphalan, and prednisone versus bortezomib, thalidomide, and prednisone as induction therapy followed by maintenance treatment with bortezomib and thalidomide versus bortezomib and prednisone in elderly patients with untreated multiple myeloma: a randomised trial. Lancet Oncol 11(10):934–941

Mateos M-V, Oriol A, Martínez-López J, Gutiérrez N, Teruel A-I, López de la Guía A et al (2012) Maintenance therapy with bortezomib plus thalidomide or bortezomib plus prednisone in elderly multiple myeloma patients included in the GEM2005MAS65 trial. Blood 120(13):2581–2588

Moreau P, San Miguel J, Ludwig H, Schouten H, Mohty M, Dimopoulos M et al (2013) Multiple myeloma: ESMO clinical practice guidelines for diagnosis, treatment and follow-up. Ann Oncol Off J Eur Soc Med Oncol 24(Suppl 6):vi133–vi137

Morgan GJ, Davies FE, Gregory WM, Russell NH, Bell SE, Szubert AJ et al (2011) Cyclophosphamide, thalidomide, and dexamethasone (CTD) as initial therapy for patients with multiple myeloma unsuitable for autologous transplantation. Blood 118(5):1231–1238

Niesvizky R, Richardson PG, Rajkumar SV, Coleman M, Rosiñol L, Sonneveld P et al (2008) The relationship between quality of response and clinical benefit for patients treated on the bortezomib arm of the international, randomized, phase 3 APEX trial in relapsed multiple myeloma. Br J Haematol 143(1):46–53

O'Donnell EK (2015) Paper: a phase II study of modified lenalidomide, bortezomib, and dexamethasone (RVD-lite) for transplant-ineligible patients with newly diagnosed multiple myeloma [Internet]. [cited 2017 Apr 3]. Available from: https://ash.confex.com/ash/2015/webprogramscheduler/Paper80503.html

ONS (2010) Office for National Statistics (ONS) [Internet]. Office for National Statistics [cited 2015 Jan 4]. Available from: http://www.ons.gov.uk/ons/index.html

Palumbo A, Bringhen S, Caravita T, Merla E, Capparella V, Callea V et al (2006) Oral melphalan and prednisone chemotherapy plus thalidomide compared with melphalan and prednisone alone in elderly patients with multiple myeloma: randomised controlled trial. Lancet 367(9513):825–831

Palumbo A, Bringhen S, Liberati AM, Caravita T, Falcone A, Callea V et al (2008) Oral melphalan, prednisone, and thalidomide in elderly patients with multiple myeloma: updated results of a randomized controlled trial. Blood 112(8):3107–3114

Palumbo A, Bringhen S, Rossi D, Cavalli M, Larocca A, Ria R et al (2010) Bortezomib-melphalan-prednisone-thalidomide followed by maintenance with bortezomib-thalidomide compared with bortezomib-melphalan-prednisone for initial treatment of multiple myeloma: a randomized controlled trial. J Clin Oncol Off J Am Soc Clin Oncol 28(34):5101–5109

Palumbo A, Rajkumar SV, San Miguel JF, Larocca A, Niesvizky R, Morgan G et al (2014) International myeloma working group consensus statement for the management, treatment, and supportive care of patients with myeloma not eligible for standard autologous stem-cell transplantation. J Clin Oncol Off J Am Soc Clin Oncol 32(6):587–600

Patel KV (2008) Epidemiology of anemia in older adults. Semin Hematol 45(4):210–217

Pennypacker LC, Allen RH, Kelly JP, Matthews LM, Grigsby J, Kaye K et al (1992) High prevalence of cobalamin deficiency in elderly outpatients. J Am Geriatr Soc 40(12):1197–1204

Price EA, Mehra R, Holmes TH, Schrier SL (2011) Anemia in older persons: etiology and evaluation. Blood Cells Mol Dis 46(2):159–165

Rajkumar SV, Dimopoulos MA, Palumbo A, Blade J, Merlini G, Mateos M-V et al (2014) International myeloma working group updated criteria for the diagnosis of multiple myeloma. Lancet Oncol 15(12):e538–e548

Rawstron AC, Child JA, de Tute RM, Davies FE, Gregory WM, Bell SE et al (2013) Minimal residual disease assessed by multiparameter flow cytometry in multiple myeloma: impact on outcome in the Medical Research Council myeloma IX study. J Clin Oncol Off J Am Soc Clin Oncol 31(20):2540–2547

San Miguel JF, Schlag R, Khuageva NK, Dimopoulos MA, Shpilberg O, Kropff M et al (2008) Bortezomib plus melphalan and prednisone for initial treatment of multiple myeloma. N Engl J Med 359(9):906–917

San Miguel JF, Schlag R, Khuageva NK, Dimopoulos MA, Shpilberg O, Kropff M et al (2013) Persistent overall survival benefit and no increased risk of second malignancies with bortezomib-melphalan-prednisone versus melphalan-prednisone in patients with previously untreated multiple myeloma. J Clin Oncol Off J Am Soc Clin Oncol 31(4):448–455

SEER data (2016) US Population data 1969–2012-SEER Datasets [Internet]. [cited 2015 Jan 4]. Available from: http://seer.cancer.gov/data/citation.html

Siegel DS, Desikan KR, Mehta J, Singhal S, Fassas A, Munshi N et al (1999) Age is not a prognostic variable with autotransplants for multiple myeloma. Blood 93(1):51–54

Siegel R, Ma J, Zou Z, Jemal A (2014) Cancer statistics, 2014. CA Cancer J Clin 64(1):9–29

Smith BD, Smith GL, Hurria A, Hortobagyi GN, Buchholz TA (2009) Future of cancer incidence in the United States: burdens upon an aging, changing nation. J Clin Oncol Off J Am Soc Clin Oncol 27(17):2758–2765

Sonneveld P, Verelst SG, Lewis P, Gray-Schopfer V, Hutchings A, Nixon A et al (2013) Review of health-related quality of life data in multiple myeloma patients treated with novel agents. Leukemia 27(10):1959–1969

Stewart AK, Jacobus SJ, Fonseca R, Weiss M, Callander NS, Chanan-Khan AAA et al (2014) E1A06: a phase III trial comparing melphalan, prednisone, and thalidomide (MPT) versus melphalan, prednisone, and lenalidomide (MPR) in newly diagnosed multiple myeloma (MM). J Clin Oncol 32(5s):8511. Available from: http://meetinglibrary.asco.org/content/131886-144

Waage A, Gimsing P, Fayers P, Abildgaard N, Ahlberg L, Björkstrand B et al (2010) Melphalan and prednisone plus thalidomide or placebo in elderly patients with multiple myeloma. Blood 116(9):1405–1412

Walker BA, Boyle EM, Wardell CP, Murison A, Begum DB, Dahir NM et al (2015) Mutational spectrum, copy number changes, and outcome: results of a sequencing study of patients with newly diagnosed myeloma. J Clin Oncol Off J Am Soc Clin Oncol 33(33):3911–3920

Wijermans P, Schaafsma M, Termorshuizen F, Ammerlaan R, Wittebol S, Sinnige H et al (2010) Phase III study of the value of thalidomide added to melphalan plus prednisone in elderly patients with newly diagnosed multiple myeloma: the HOVON 49 study. J Clin Oncol Off J Am Soc Clin Oncol 28(19):3160–3166

Wu W, Merriman K, Nabaah A, Seval N, Seval D, Lin H et al (2014) The association of diabetes and anti-diabetic medications with clinical outcomes in multiple myeloma. Br J Cancer 111(3):628–636

Yamaguchi T (2008) Syncope and sinus bradycardia from combined use of thalidomide and beta-blocker. Pharmacoepidemiol Drug Saf 17(10):1033–1035

Zweegman S, Palumbo A, Bringhen S, Sonneveld P (2014) Age and aging in blood disorders: multiple myeloma. Haematologica 99(7):1133–1137

Treatment of Relapsed/Refractory Patients with Multiple Myeloma

5

Jacob P. Laubach, Philippe Moreau,
Meletios A. Dimopoulos, and Paul G. Richardson

5.1 Introduction

Twenty years ago, this subject would not have warranted a separate chapter. Clinicians had only a limited number of chemotherapy options with which to attempt to manage their relapsed/refractory multiple myeloma (RRMM) patients, and this was reflected in the poor outcomes for patients with multiple myeloma (MM) overall, for whom median overall survival was only 3 years (Kyle et al. 2003). However, the past two decades have witnessed an unprecedented increase in the number and variety of therapeutic options for MM (Larsen and Kumar 2015), including the emergence of four novel classes of agents with distinct mechanisms of action (Boudreault et al. 2017) and the approval of ten new individual agents.

These developments have been made possible through our significantly increased understanding of the biology and genetics of the disease (Manier et al. 2017), enabling the identification of rational targets for anti-myeloma agents (Egan et al. 2016). Furthermore, insights into clonal evolution of MM and the consequent clonal heterogeneity of the disease (Manier et al. 2017; Bianchi and Ghobrial 2014), particularly as it progresses through its course, are shaping our understanding of the management of MM across the disease course and highlighting the importance of treatment selection and sequencing in the RRMM setting (Yee and Raje 2016).

Indeed, treatment selection and sequencing are emerging as important new issues for consideration by clinicians when planning for the longer-term (and, in some cases, chronic) management of their MM patients (Sonneveld and Broijl 2016), for whom survival times are increasingly likely to exceed 10 years (National Cancer Institute 2016; Kumar et al. 2014; Pulte et al. 2014). Additionally, the emerging treatment paradigms of triplet versus doublet therapy (Boudreault et al. 2017; Anderson 2016; Sun et al. 2017; Moreau and de Wit 2017) and the use of treat-to-progression and/or maintenance approaches (Musto and Montefusco 2016) are influencing the treatment of RRMM, and, with the availability of numerous novel agents and regimens, the affordability of treating MM as a chronic disease is also an increasingly relevant consideration (Fonseca et al. 2017; Rajkumar and Harousseau 2016).

J. P. Laubach • P. G. Richardson (✉)
Medical Oncology, Dana-Farber Cancer Institute,
Boston, MA, USA
e-mail: paul_richardson@dfci.harvard.edu

P. Moreau
Department of Hematology, University Hospital
Hôtel Dieu, Nantes, France

M. A. Dimopoulos
National and Kapodistrian University of Athens,
School of Medicine, Athens, Greece

© Springer International Publishing Switzerland 2018
M. A. Dimopoulos et al. (eds.), *Multiple Myeloma and Other Plasma Cell Neoplasms*,
Hematologic Malignancies, https://doi.org/10.1007/978-3-319-25586-6_5

Despite remarkable improvements in outcome for patients with MM (National Cancer Institute 2016; Kumar et al. 2014; Pulte et al. 2014) and frontline therapy becoming increasingly effective, with prolonged disease control, MM remains incurable and relapse remains an inevitability for the majority of patients (Dimopoulos et al. 2015a). Therefore, with the wealth of therapeutic options becoming available to us, it is important to try to establish recommended treatment options for RRMM patients to guide selection of subsequent therapies based on key factors of importance. Furthermore, the development of new agents with unique mechanisms of anti-myeloma activity remains a very high priority in the field. For example, the recent availability of the monoclonal antibodies daratumumab and elotuzumab has changed the treatment paradigm considerably and has expanded treatment options for patients through this novel mechanism of action (Laubach et al. 2017). Additionally, new approaches to MM management, including immunotherapies such as chimeric antigen receptor (CAR) T-cell therapies (Kumar and Anderson 2016), Bcl-2 inhibition with venetoclax (Terpos and International Myeloma Society 2017), and novel monoclonal antibodies with unique targets (Touzeau et al. 2017) are likely to further change the treatment paradigm in the coming years.

This chapter aims to provide a succinct overview of the issues affecting the treatment of RRMM patients, including a summary of important recent data on each of the available treatment options, and recommendations for treatment approaches in different patient subgroups and in different disease settings. It also aims to provide a longer-term perspective, examining how treatment of RRMM patients may evolve in parallel with the evolution of frontline therapy and with the emergence of additional novel agents in the future.

5.2 Currently Approved Treatment Options for RRMM

The approval of multiple new therapeutic agents over the past two decades has led to a large and growing number of treatment options for RRMM patients. While there are a number of single-agent options, many of these new options are two-, three-, and even four-drug regimens that incorporate multiple mechanisms of action. Inevitably, given this wealth of options, there is limited head-to-head evidence from randomized studies between all the different regimens. However, a substantial number of large, randomized and, in some cases, placebo-controlled phase 3 studies have been conducted, and our use of regimens for RRMM is guided in many cases by the evidence from such randomized studies demonstrating improved efficacy— category 1 level evidence in the United States National Comprehensive Cancer Network (NCCN) guidelines (National Comprehensive Cancer Network 2016). Tables 5.1 and 5.2 summarize the single-agent/doublet and triplet regimens, respectively, available for RRMM for which such category 1 level evidence exists, and here we summarize some of the key information and data on each regimen.

5.2.1 Single-Agent/Doublet Regimens

The only single-agent therapy for which phase 3 study data are available in RRMM is bortezomib, which was compared with single-agent dexamethasone in the APEX trial in patients who had received 1–3 prior lines of therapy (Richardson et al. 2007, 2005). An overall response rate (ORR) of 43% was reported with bortezomib after prolonged follow-up, compared to only 18% with dexamethasone, including 15% vs 2% complete/near-complete responses (CR/nCR), along with superior time to progression (TTP; median 6.2 vs 3.5 months, hazard ratio [HR] 0.55) (Richardson et al. 2005) and overall survival (OS; median 29.8 vs 23.7 months, HR 0.77) (Richardson et al. 2007). However, increased rates of certain toxicities were reported with bortezomib, notably peripheral neuropathy (PN) (Richardson et al. 2009), gastrointestinal toxicities (Richardson et al. 2005), thrombocytopenia (Lonial et al. 2008), and herpes zoster reactivation (Chanan-Khan et al. 2008).

Table 5.1 Single-agent/doublet regimens evaluated in phase 3 studies for the treatment of RRMM

Trial	Regimen	N	Prior lines	≥MR, %	≥PR, %	≥VGPR, %	≥CR, %	TTP, mos	PFS, mos	OS, mos
APEX (Richardson et al. 2005, 2007)	Bortezomib	333	2	NR	43	NR	15[a]	6.2	NR	29.8
	Dex	336	2	NR	18	NR	2[a]	3.5	NR	23.7
MMY-3021 (Arnulf et al. 2012; Moreau et al. 2011)	SC V ± d	148	1	NR	52	27	23[a]	9.7	9.3	28.7
	IV V ± d	74	1	NR	52	25	22[a]	9.6	8.4	NE
MMY-3001 (Orlowski et al. 2007, 2016)	Bortezomib + PLD	324	66% ≥2	NR	44	27	13[a]	9.3	9.0	33.0
	Bortezomib	322	66% ≥2	NR	41	19	10[a]	6.5	6.5	30.8
MM-009 (US, Canada) (Weber et al. 2007)	Rd	177	62% ≥2	NR	61	NR	24[a]	11.1	NR	Combined (Dimopoulos et al. 2009) 38.0 vs 31.6
	Dex	176	62% ≥2	NR	20	NR	2[a]	4.7	NR	
MM-010 (ex-N America) (Dimopoulos et al. 2007)	Rd	176	2	NR	60	NR	24[a]	11.3	NR	
	Dex	175	2	NR	24	NR	5[a]	4.7	NR	
NIMBUS (San Miguel et al. 2013)	Pom-dex	302	5	39	31	6	1	4.7	4.0	12.7
	Dex	153	5	16	10	<1	0	2.1	1.9	8.1
ENDEAVOR (Dimopoulos et al. 2016a; Siegel et al. 2017)	Kd	464	2	82	77	54	13	NR	18.7	47.6
	Vd	465	2	74	63	29	6	NR	9.4	40.0

Prior lines, TTP, PFS, OS data shown as medians except where indicated

CR complete response, *Dex* dexamethasone, *IV* intravenous, *Kd* carfilzomib-dexamethasone, *MR* minimal response, *nCR* near-complete response, *NR* not reported, *OS* overall survival, *PFS* progression-free survival, *PLD* pegylated liposomal doxorubicin, *Pom-dex* pomalidomide-dexamethasone, *PR* partial response, *Rd* lenalidomide-dexamethasone, *SC* subcutaneous, *TTP* time to progression, *Vd* bortezomib-dexamethasone, *VGPR* very good partial response

[a]CR/nCR

Table 5.2 Triplet regimens evaluated in phase 3 studies for the treatment of RRMM

Trial	Regimen	N	Prior lines	≥MR, %	≥PR, %	≥VGPR, %	≥CR, %	TTP, mos	PFS, mos	OS, mos
ASPIRE (Stewart et al. 2015; Amgen 2017)	Carfilzomib-Rd	396	2	91	87	70	32	31.4	26.3	48.3
	Rd	396	2	76	67	40	9	19.4	17.6	40.4
TOURMALINE-MM1 (Moreau et al. 2016a)	Ixazomib-Rd	360	1	NR	78	48	12	21.4	20.6	NR
	Placebo-Rd	362	1	NR	72	39	7	15.7	14.7	NR
ELOQUENT-2 (Lonial et al. 2015; Dimopoulos et al. 2017a)	Elotuzumab-Rd	321	2	86	79	33	4	NR	19.4	48.0
	Rd	325	2	76	66	28	7	NR	14.9	40.0
POLLUX (Dimopoulos et al. 2016c)	Daratumumab-Rd	286	1	95	93	76	43	NR	NE	NE
	Rd	283	1	86	76	44	19	NR	18.4	NE
CASTOR (Palumbo et al. 2016)	Daratumumab-Vd	251	2	87	83	59	19	NE	NE	NE
	Vd	247	2	72	63	29	9	7.3	7.2	NE
PANORAMA1 (San-Miguel et al. 2014, 2016)	Panobinostat-Vd	387	1	67	61	NR	28[a]	12.7	12.0	40.3
	Placebo-Vd	381	1	66	55	NR	16[a]	8.5	8.1	35.8

Prior lines, TTP, PFS, OS data shown as medians except where indicated

CR complete response, MR minimal response, NE not estimable, NR not reported, OS overall survival, PFS progression-free survival, PR partial response, Rd lenalidomide-dexamethasone, TTP time to progression, Vd bortezomib-dexamethasone, VGPR very good partial response

[a]CR/near-CR rate

The NCCN guidelines give category 1 recommendation to bortezomib plus dexamethasone, rather than single-agent bortezomib, because although no phase 3 study has demonstrated superiority of this doublet over an older regimen, a number of studies and analyses in RRMM have shown that addition of dexamethasone to bortezomib can augment efficacy and improve patient responses and outcomes (Jagannath et al. 2006; Mikhael et al. 2009; Dimopoulos et al. 2015b). Indeed, in the phase 3 study of subcutaneous (SC) versus intravenous (IV) bortezomib, with or without added dexamethasone, in patients with RRMM after 1–3 prior lines of therapy, 56% versus 53% of patients had dexamethasone added after four cycles of single-agent bortezomib, resulting in 13% of patients improving response from partial response (PR) to CR, and 30% improving response from <PR to PR, on each arm (Moreau et al. 2011). This study also demonstrated the benefit of SC versus IV bortezomib in terms of significantly reduced rates of PN (Moreau et al. 2011). In another phase 3 study in RRMM patients after 1–3 prior lines of therapy, improved outcomes were also reported with the doublet regimen comprising pegylated liposomal doxorubicin plus bortezomib, compared to bortezomib alone (Orlowski et al. 2007, 2016). TTP (median 9.3 vs 6.5 months, HR 1.82) and duration of response (median 10.2 vs 7.0 months) were improved with this steroid-free doublet versus single-agent bortezomib, but there was no significant improvement in OS (median 33 vs 30.8 months, HR 1.047), and the combination resulted in increased rates of some toxicities, including neutropenia, thrombocytopenia, diarrhea, and hand-foot syndrome (Orlowski et al. 2007, 2016).

The second-generation proteasome inhibitor carfilzomib is approved for the treatment of RRMM as a doublet regimen with dexamethasone, having demonstrated improved efficacy versus bortezomib-dexamethasone in the ENDEAVOR phase 3 study in patients with RRMM after 1–3 prior therapies (Dimopoulos et al. 2016a). The primary endpoint of progression-free survival (PFS) was significantly improved with carfilzomib-dexamethasone (median 18.7 vs 9.4 months, HR 0.53), as were ORR (77% vs 63%) and rates of very good partial response or better (≥VGPR; 54% vs 29%) and ≥CR (13% vs 6%) (Dimopoulos et al. 2016a).

Notably, these findings were similar in subgroup analyses according to patients' prior treatment status (Moreau et al. 2017a), cytogenetic status (Chng et al. 2017), and age (Ludwig et al. 2017). A follow-up analysis also demonstrated prolonged OS with carfilzomib-dexamethasone (median 47.6 vs 40.0 months, HR 0.79) (Siegel et al. 2017). Reflecting the safety profile seen in earlier-phase carfilzomib studies, the rate of PN was significantly lower with carfilzomib-dexamethasone (grade $\geq$ 2 PN: 6% vs 32%, odds ratio [OR] 0.14). Conversely, carfilzomib was associated with higher rates of some adverse events (AEs), including anemia, dyspnea, hypertension, acute renal failure, and cardiac failure (Dimopoulos et al. 2016a).

The two immunomodulatory drugs lenalidomide and pomalidomide have likewise demonstrated efficacy benefits in doublet combination regimens with dexamethasone in phase 3 studies in RRMM. Two parallel phase 3 studies of lenalidomide-dexamethasone versus placebo-dexamethasone in RRMM patients following 1–3 prior therapies were conducted in North America (Weber et al. 2007) and the rest of the world (Dimopoulos et al. 2007), and both demonstrated superior ORRs (61% vs 20%; 60% vs 24%), rates of CR (14% vs 1%; 16% vs 3%), and TTP (median 11.1 vs 4.7 months; median 11.3 vs 4.7 months). A combined long-term analysis showed a superior OS with lenalidomide-dexamethasone (median 38.0 vs 31.6 months) (Dimopoulos et al. 2009), and subsequent analyses indicated that both higher quality of response to lenalidomide-dexamethasone (Harousseau et al. 2010) and longer duration of treatment (San-Miguel et al. 2011) were associated with better outcomes in these treat-to-progression protocols. Notable toxicities that occurred more frequently with the doublet regimen included neutropenia, thrombocytopenia, and venous thromboembolism, although an analysis demonstrated that the latter did not adversely affect survival (Zangari et al. 2010). In addition, the risk of second primary malignancies (SPMs) in RRMM patients treated with lenalidomide-dexamethasone appeared to be increased compared with those receiving pla-cebo-dexamethasone (incidence rate, per 100 patient-years, 3.98 vs 1.38) (Dimopoulos et al. 2012).

The efficacy and safety of pomalidomide-dexamethasone has also been demonstrated in a phase 3 randomized study of pomalidomide-dexamethasone versus high-dose dexamethasone alone. Patients in the NIMBUS (MM-003) study had relapsed and refractory disease and had to have failed at least two prior treatments including bortezomib and lenalidomide (San Miguel et al. 2013). In this hard-to-treat population, who have poor prognosis (Kumar et al. 2012), pomalidomide-dexamethasone demonstrated superior PFS (median 4.0 vs 1.9 months, HR 0.48) and OS (median 12.7 vs 8.1 months, HR 0.74), with a generally consistent benefit seen in patients who were refractory to both lenalidomide and bortezomib, intolerant to prior bortezomib, or who had received lenalidomide or bortezomib in their last prior regimen (San Miguel et al. 2013). A benefit was also seen in patients with high-risk cytogenetics, with specific benefit with pomalidomide-dexamethasone reported in RRMM patients with del(17p) (Dimopoulos et al. 2015c; Leleu et al. 2015). Overall, these findings showed the potential for pomalidomide-dexamethasone in this later setting in the RRMM treatment algorithm. Additionally, the phase 3b STRATUS study confirmed these findings with pomalidomide plus low-dose dexamethasone in a heavily pretreated patient population that was mostly refractory to both lenalidomide and bortezomib; the ORR was 33%, and median PFS and OS were 4.6 and 11.9 months, respectively (Dimopoulos et al. 2016b). Common toxicities across both MM-003 and STRATUS were neutropenia, anemia, thrombocytopenia, and pneumonia (San Miguel et al. 2013; Dimopoulos et al. 2016b; Moreau et al. 2017b). Notably, as with lenalidomide-dexamethasone, an analysis of another study of pomalidomide-dexamethasone showed that patients who remained on therapy longer (>1 vs <1 year) in the treat-to-progression protocol had significantly better PFS and OS than those receiving shorter duration of therapy (Fouquet et al. 2016).

5.2.2 Triplet Regimens

Doublets based on a proteasome inhibitor or an immunomodulatory drug combined with dexamethasone have become standards of care in RRMM based on the results outlined above. Consequently, these regimens have been used as the backbone to which novel agents have been added to develop multiple triplet regimens, and these more extensive therapies have been demonstrating superior activity and outcomes compared with doublets in RRMM patients (Sun et al. 2017). For example, four recent phase 3 studies in RRMM have utilized the lenalidomide-dexamethasone backbone, adding the IV proteasome inhibitor carfilzomib (Stewart et al. 2015), SLAMF7-directed monoclonal antibody elotuzumab (Lonial et al. 2015), the oral proteasome inhibitor ixazomib (Moreau et al. 2016a), and the CD38-directed monoclonal antibody daratumumab (Dimopoulos et al. 2016c), to create highly active novel triplet regimens.

Phase 3 studies have demonstrated that addition of either of the proteasome inhibitors carfilzomib or ixazomib to lenalidomide-dexamethasone in patients with RRMM after 1–3 prior therapies results in improvements in activity and outcomes. In the open-label ASPIRE (Stewart et al. 2015) and placebo-controlled TOURMALINE-MM1 (Moreau et al. 2016a) studies, PFS was significantly increased (median 26.3 vs 17.6 months, HR 0.69; and median 20.6 vs 14.7 months, HR 0.74, respectively) after a median follow-up of ~32 months and ~15 months, respectively, and ORRs (87% vs 67%; and 78% vs 72%, respectively), $\geq$VGPR rates (70% vs 40%; and 48% vs 39%), and $\geq$CR rates (32% vs 9%; and 12% vs 7%) were also significantly higher with the triplet regimens versus lenalidomide-dexamethasone alone. Subgroup analyses showed that both triplets provided benefit across the RRMM patient population, regardless of prior therapy exposure or cytogenetic risk (Stewart et al. 2015; Moreau et al. 2016a; Avet-Loiseau et al. 2016a, b; Dimopoulos et al. 2017b, c; Mateos et al. 2016a). Notably, PFS in patients with high-risk cytogenetics treated with ixazomib-lenalidomide-dexamethasone appeared similar to that in standard-risk patients, suggesting that this regimen might partially overcome the poor prognosis associated with some high-risk features (Moreau et al. 2016a; Avet-Loiseau et al. 2016b). Both triplet regimens appeared well tolerated over a lengthy duration of treatment, with only limited increases in rates of toxicity seen versus the doublet arm. Of note, neither proteasome inhibitor-based regimen was associated with a substantially higher rate of PN than lenalidomide-dexamethasone, indicating that this key AE of bortezomib is not a major complication of either carfilzomib or ixazomib. However, in ASPIRE (Stewart et al. 2015), higher rates of diarrhea, cough, hypokalemia, dyspnea, and hypertension were seen in the carfilzomib arm, while in TOURMALINE-MM1 ixazomib-lenalidomide-dexamethasone was associated with higher rates of thrombocytopenia, gastrointestinal toxicities, and rash, compared to lenalidomide-dexamethasone alone (Moreau et al. 2016a).

In the ELOQUENT-2 phase 3 trial, addition of the monoclonal antibody elotuzumab to lenalidomide-dexamethasone for the treatment of RRMM patients after 1–3 prior therapies demonstrated superior PFS (median 19.4 vs 14.9 months, HR 0.70) after a median follow-up of 24.5 months, as well as a higher ORR (79% vs 66%) (Lonial et al. 2015). A lower rate of CR was reported in the elotuzumab arm, but this may have been due to false-positive M-protein spikes arising from the monoclonal antibody (Murata et al. 2016). The PFS benefit with the triplet was seen across patient subgroups, and treatment was well tolerated, with lymphocytopenia reported more commonly in the elotuzumab arm. Elotuzumab also resulted in a higher rate of infusion reactions, with the majority being grade 1 or 2 and occurring during the first infusion (Lonial et al. 2015).

A second monoclonal antibody-lenalidomide-dexamethasone combination has demonstrated superiority to lenalidomide-dexamethasone alone. In the POLLUX phase 3 study, RRMM patients who had received a median of 1 prior line of therapy (range 1–11) were randomized to daratumumab plus lenalidomide-dexamethasone or lenalidomide-dexamethasone alone, with treatment continuing until progression or unacceptable toxicity (Dimopoulos et al. 2016c). The triplet resulted in highly superior PFS (median not reached vs 18.4 months, HR 0.37) after a median follow-up of 13.5 months, as well as a significantly higher ORR (93% vs 76%), ≥VGPR rate (76% vs 44%), and ≥CR rate (43% vs 19%). As reported with elotuzumab, the PFS benefit was seen across patient subgroups, regardless of prior lenalidomide or proteasome inhibitor exposure, or number of prior lines of therapy, as well as in patients with high-risk cytogenetic features (Moreau et al. 2016b). Notably, treatment appeared very well tolerated, with limited additional toxicity reported; higher rates of neutropenia, diarrhea, upper respiratory tract infection, and cough were seen with the triplet regimen. Additionally, as reported with elotuzumab, daratumumab resulted in a higher rate of infusion reactions, which were mostly grade 1 or 2 and occurred primarily during the first infusion. The rate of infusion reactions appeared somewhat higher with daratumumab compared to elotuzumab. There was no increase in the rate of discontinuations with the triplet versus doublet regimen (Dimopoulos et al. 2016c).

Two phase 3 studies have utilized bortezomib-dexamethasone as a backbone regimen. In the CASTOR phase 3 study, RRMM patients who had received a median of 2 prior lines of therapy (range 1–10) were randomized to daratumumab plus bortezomib-dexamethasone or bortezomib-dexamethasone alone, with treatment comprising eight cycles of the triplet/doublet followed by single-agent daratumumab until progression or unacceptable toxicity (Palumbo et al. 2016). As in POLLUX, the triplet regimen resulted in highly superior PFS (median not reached vs 7.2 months, HR 0.39) after a median follow-up of 7.4 months, a benefit that was seen across patient subgroups defined by prior treatment exposure, as well as a significantly higher ORR (83% vs 63%), ≥VGPR rate (59% vs 29%), and ≥CR rate (19% vs 9%). The triplet was associated with somewhat higher rates of toxicities than bortezomib-dexamethasone alone, with thrombocytopenia, neutropenia, lymphopenia, diarrhea,

upper respiratory tract infection, cough, dyspnea, and peripheral edema more common in the daratumumab arm and the rate of PN also slightly higher. Infusion-related reactions with daratumumab were similar to those reported in POLLUX and, as in POLLUX, the rate of discontinuations was not higher in the triplet versus doublet arm (Palumbo et al. 2016).

Bortezomib-dexamethasone has also been studied in combination with the histone deacetylase inhibitor panobinostat in the placebo-controlled PANORAMA1 phase 3 trial in RRMM patients after 1–3 prior lines of therapy (San-Miguel et al. 2014). Panobinostat-bortezomib-dexamethasone resulted in a significantly longer PFS than bortezomib-dexamethasone alone (median 11.99 vs 8.08 months, HR 0.63), as well as a higher CR/near-CR rate (28% vs 16%), but the ORRs were similar (61% vs 55%). Particular benefit was noted in the subgroups of relapsed and refractory patients, and patients previously exposed to bortezomib and immunomodulatory drugs, and a specific analysis was conducted in patients with at least 2 prior regimens including bortezomib and an immunomodulatory drug (Richardson et al. 2016). An enhanced PFS benefit was seen in this population (median 12.5 vs 4.78 months, HR 0.47), and these data led to the approval of panobinostat in this indication. An updated analysis of the study showed a modest OS benefit with the triplet regimen (median 40.3 vs 35.8 months, HR 0.94) that appeared similar in the subgroup of patients who had received at least 2 prior regimens including bortezomib and an immunomodulatory drug (median 25.5 vs 19.5 months, HR 1.01). The efficacy benefit of the triplet regimen was accompanied by increased toxicity, including gastrointestinal and hematologic AEs, and a higher rate of on-treatment deaths (San-Miguel et al. 2014; Richardson et al. 2016).

5.2.3 Other Regimens Not Supported by Phase 3 Study Data

A number of treatment regimens that have not been evaluated in a phase 3 study in RRMM are nevertheless widely used in this setting, and Table 5.3 provides a summary of those for which the strongest evidence is available, for example from large phase 2 studies. Of note, single-agent daratumumab is used in this setting, particular for patients with multiple prior lines of therapy or relapsed and refractory disease following treatment with a proteasome inhibitor and lenalidomide, as this is the setting in which daratumumab was initially approved in the United States (Raedler 2016). Approval was based on the results from two phase 2 studies, GEN-501 (Lokhorst et al. 2015) and SIRIUS (Lonial et al. 2016). In the former, an ORR of 36% and a median PFS of 5.6 months were reported in 42 RRMM patients treated at the approved dose of 16 mg/kg who had received a median of 4 prior therapies, of whom approximately three-quarters were refractory to bortezomib and lenalidomide (Lokhorst et al. 2015). Similarly, in SIRIUS, which included RRMM patients who were more heavily pretreated (median 5 prior lines) and were more frequently refractory to proteasome inhibitors and immunomodulatory drugs than in GEN-501, an ORR of 29% and a median PFS of 3.7 months were reported (Lonial et al. 2016). In both studies, single-agent daratumumab demonstrated good tolerability and was shown to have a relative limited toxicity profile, with mostly mild AEs, including infusion-related AEs.

Numerous other regimens with a less-than-category 1 level of evidence are also utilized for the treatment of RRMM. Similarly to daratumumab, single-agent carfilzomib was initially approved in the United States for heavily pretreated RRMM patients (Kortuem and Stewart 2013), although its use has now expanded to earlier in the treatment algorithm based upon the results from ENDEAVOR and ASPIRE. The doublet regimen of ixazomib-dexamethasone has been studied in relapsed MM patients who were not refractory to bortezomib (Kumar et al. 2015a, 2016), demonstrating an ORR of 31% at a 4 mg dose and 54% at a 5.5 mg dose, and a median event-free survival of 5.7 months in bortezomib-exposed patients and 11.0 months in bortezomib-naïve patients. The higher dose of ixazomib was associated with more toxicity than the 4.0 mg dose.

Reflecting the emerging paradigm, multiple additional triplet regimens are frequently used for the treatment of RRMM, demonstrating notable activity in this setting. Combinations that have been investigated in phase 2 studies and have a category 2A recommendation in the NCCN guidelines (Network 2016) include bortezomib-lenalidomide-dexamethasone (Richardson et al. 2014), bortezomib (de Waal et al. 2015), lenalidomide (Schey et al. 2010), or pomalidomide (Baz et al. 2016) in combination with cyclophosphamide-dexamethasone, elotuzumab-bortezomib-dexamethasone (Jakubowiak et al. 2016), and bortezomib (Ludwig et al. 2014) or lenalidomide (Kumar et al. 2015b) plus bendamustine-dexamethasone. Another noteworthy regimen that is frequently considered in the United States for patients with high-risk disease is carfilzomib-pomalidomide-dexamethasone (Shah et al. 2015), which has demonstrated an ORR of 64%, including 26% ≥ VGPR, and a median PFS of 9.2 months in a phase 1/2 multicenter study in RRMM patients after 1–3 prior lines of therapy (Bringhen et al. 2017a). Key data on all these regimens are summarized in Table 5.3.

5.3 Factors to Consider when Selecting Therapy in RRMM

The availability of the large and growing number of treatment regimens for RRMM raises important questions pertaining to clinical practice, regarding how to make an appropriate choice of treatment at each relapse and how to plan to sequence the available regimens in an individual patient. As well as having a large number of different treatment options, MM is a highly heterogeneous disease (Manier et al. 2017) for which therapy must be individualized based on a range of factors. While there is currently limited information on optimized sequencing of available therapies (Yee and Raje 2016; Mohty et al. 2012), it is widely acknowledged that multiple considerations related to a patient's characteristics, their disease characteristics, their personal circumstances and goals and preferences for treatment, and their previous treatment history must all be taken into account when selecting a treatment for

Table 5.3 Regimens evaluated in earlier-phase studies for the treatment of RRMM

Regimen/trial	Phase	N	Prior lines	≥MR, %	≥PR, %	≥VGPR, %	≥CR, %	PFS, mos	OS, mos
Single-agent regimens									
Carfilzomib (PX-171-003-A1) (Siegel et al. 2012)	2	266	5	37	24	6	<1	3.7	15.6
Carfilzomib (PX-171-004) (Vij et al. 2012a)	2	70 (cohort 2)	2 Btz-naive	64	52	28	2	NE	NE
Daratumumab (GEN-501) (Lokhorst et al. 2015)	2	42 (MTD)	4	NR	36	10	5	5.6	NE
Daratumumab (SIRIUS) (Lonial et al. 2016)	2	106	5	34	29	12	3	3.7	NE
Doublet regimens									
Ixazomib-dex (Kumar et al. 2015a, 2016)	2	35 (4 mg)	4	46	31	23	3	8.4	NE
		35 (5.5 mg)	4	57	54	31	3	7.8	NE
Triplet regimens									
VRD (Richardson et al. 2014)	2	64	2	80	64	28	25[a]	9.5	30
VCD (de Waal et al. 2015)	NR	59	1	72	66	33	7	18.4	28.1
RCD (Schey et al. 2010)	1/2	31	3	84	81	36	29	NE	NE
Pom-CD (Baz et al. 2016)	2	34	4	80	65	12	3	9.5	NE
EVD (Jakubowiak et al. 2016)	2	77	1	71	66	37	4	9.7	NR
Benda-Vd (Ludwig et al. 2014)	2	79	2	76	61	36	15	9.7	25.6
Benda-Rd (Kumar et al. 2015b)	1/2	71	3	55	49	29	NR	11.8	NE
V-Pom-dex (Paludo et al. 2017)	1/2	50	2	NR	86	50	22	13.7	NR
K-Pom-dex (Shah et al. 2015)	1	32	6	66	50	16	0	7.2	20.6
K-Pom-dex (Bringhen et al. 2017a)	1/2	48 (RP2D)	NR	NR	64	26	6[a]	9.2	NE

Prior lines, TTP, PFS, OS data shown as medians except where indicated

Benda-Vd/Rd bendamustine plus bortezomib-dexamethasone/lenalidomide-dexamethasone, *CR* complete response, *EVD* elotuzumab, bortezomib, dexamethasone, *K-Pom-dex* carfilzomib, pomalidomide, dexamethasone, *MTD* maximum tolerated dose, *NE* not estimable, *NR* not reported, *OS* overall survival, *PFS* progression-free survival, *Pom-CD* pomalidomide, cyclophosphamide, dexamethasone, *PR* partial response, *RCD* lenalidomide, cyclophosphamide, dexamethasone, *Rd* lenalidomide-dexamethasone, *VCD* bortezomib, cyclophosphamide, dexamethasone, *Vd* bortezomib-dexamethasone, *VGPR* very good partial response, *V-Pom-dex* bortezomib, pomalidomide, dexamethasone, *VRD* bortezomib, lenalidomide, dexamethasone

[a]CR/near-CR rate

RRMM, as well as the efficacy and safety of the various treatment options being considered.

5.3.1 Disease Characteristics

A key question to consider with regards to RRMM disease characteristics is: what constitutes relapse? The definition of RRMM encompasses a number of different patient scenarios (Rajkumar et al. 2011), which can have an impact on prognosis (Kumar et al. 2012; Majithia et al. 2015), and thus warrant differentiation. Patients with RRMM may be classified as having relapsed disease, relapsed and refractory disease, or primary refractory disease. Per the International Myeloma Working Group (IMWG) consensus guidelines (Rajkumar et al. 2011), relapsed MM comprises previously responding disease (minimal response [MR] or better) that has subsequently progressed (Rajkumar et al. 2011). Disease defined as 'refractory' is associated with poorer prognosis than relapsed MM, as refractoriness is indicative of lower sensitivity of the MM clone to treatment. Refractory disease comprises two classifications: relapsed and refractory disease includes MM that has progressed during or within 60 days of completing previous treatment in patients who have achieved at least a MR to any prior line of therapy, whereas primary refractory disease is MM that has not responded (MR or better) to any prior therapy (Laubach et al. 2016).

In addition to considering the above issue when a patient relapses or progresses, a full diagnostic evaluation is also needed—including patient history, clinical exam, laboratory testing (comprehensive metabolic panel, complete blood count), protein electrophoresis with immunofixation, radiography, and bone marrow evaluation if necessary—in order to characterize the nature of the disease at relapse (Laubach et al. 2016). MM patients may experience different types of relapse as they progress through their disease course, which may be associated with different outcomes and may warrant consideration when selecting subsequent treatment options. A primary distinction can be made between indolent or aggressive progression. Indolent progression may be characterized solely by biochemical progression (i.e.

Table 5.4 Characteristics defining high-risk relapsed disease (Laubach et al. 2016)

Disease characteristics	Notes
Adverse cytogenetic abnormalities	Hypodiploidy, $t(4;14)$, del(17p), amp(1q21)
Advanced-stage disease	High (>5.5 mg/L) β_2-microglobulin or low (<3.5 mg/dL) albumin
Extramedullary disease	There are no notes associated with these disease characteristics
Short duration of response to prior therapy	Or progression while on current therapy
Aggressive clinical features	Rapid symptomatic onset
	Extensive disease at relapse
	MM-related organ dysfunction (renal failure, hypercalcemia, skeletal events)
High lactate dehydrogenase levels	There are no notes associated with these disease characteristics
Isotype transformation	Light chain escape
	Development of hyposecretory disease
Circulating plasma cells	There are no notes associated with these disease characteristics

reappearance of M-protein) in the absence of any other disease symptoms or associated end-organ dysfunction, and unless this increase in the M-protein spike is rapid (e.g. doubling within 3 months) these patients may not necessarily need immediate treatment (Laubach et al. 2016). By contrast, aggressive progression may be associated with a rapid return and development of disease, including marked symptomatology and organ involvement, for example renal failure and appearance of plasmacytomas. Such aggressive clinical features represent one of the characteristics of high-risk relapsed disease, as defined in the IMWG recommendations on the management of relapsed MM (Laubach et al. 2016)—these characteristics are summarized in Table 5.4.

5.3.2 Patient Characteristics

A number of patient characteristics are important considerations when selecting subsequent therapy for RRMM (Sonneveld and Broijl 2016;

Moreau and de Wit 2017; Dimopoulos et al. 2015a, d; Laubach et al. 2016; Malard et al. 2017), including age, performance status, and comorbidities, as well as the goals for the patient's care and the patient's preferences with respect to treatment and its impact on their quality of life. One obvious example is the consideration of a patient's age and performance status when determining if they are eligible for receiving salvage autologous stem cell transplantation (ASCT), with only younger and fitter patients typically able to undergo a repeat ASCT (if received as part of frontline therapy, with lengthy PFS) or a first ASCT in the RRMM setting. However, beyond this, a patient's age and fitness/frailty, as determined by the presence of comorbidities and cognitive/physical functioning (Palumbo et al. 2015), is of relevance for determining feasible treatment options, as elderly or frail patients are not able to tolerate more intensive therapy as well as younger, fitter patients, and may consequently require less dose-intense options or attenuated therapies (Dimopoulos et al. 2015d; Rosko et al. 2017; Willan et al. 2016; Larocca and Palumbo 2015). Similarly, the presence of specific comorbidities, which may be more frequent in elderly patients, may preclude the use of particular treatment approaches in these patients, or may make the patients more susceptible to the known toxicities of a particular regimen (Dimopoulos et al. 2015a; Palumbo et al. 2015). For example, the presence of pre-existing peripheral neuropathy, either associated with MM itself or with previous treatment, may result in a recommendation not to utilize a bortezomib-based or a thalidomide-based regimen, whereas in patients with elevated venous thromboembolic risk, lenalidomide and thalidomide may not be recommended (Dimopoulos et al. 2015a).

A patient's age may have an impact on the treatment goals for that patient, which can independently affect treatment decisions. For example, in older patients the primary goal of treatment may be to prolong survival while maintaining quality of life (Mateos and San Miguel 2013), rather than achieve as deep a response as possible using intensive therapy that

may be associated with substantial toxicity. Other patient preferences may also influence the goals of treatment and the treatment options (Postmus et al. 2016); analyses have identified a number of factors associated with treatment that can affect the quality of life of MM patients, such as the mode of treatment administration and the impact of clinic visits (Baz et al. 2015). Other aspects of treatment burden, such as the inconvenience and the financial impact, have also been shown to affect quality of life, along with symptomatic burden, AEs associated with treatment, and comorbidities (Baz et al. 2015; Osborne et al. 2014; Osborne et al. 2015), and these various considerations may thus affect patients' preferences when selecting a treatment option. Such aspects are of direct clinical relevance, as better quality of life has been shown to be associated with prolonged survival (Viala et al. 2007; Montazeri 2009).

5.3.3 History of Prior Therapies

Patients with RRMM may be recorded as having a certain number of prior lines of therapy, with prognosis generally becoming poorer and duration of therapy becoming shorter with increasing numbers of prior lines (Kumar et al. 2004, 2015c; Yong et al. 2016b; Jagannath et al. 2016). However, definitions of what constitutes a prior line of therapy have varied, and have not always required disease relapse between 'lines' of therapy; therefore, in 2015, Rajkumar et al. published a short paper containing recommendations to provide a clear definition of what constitutes a line of therapy in MM, in order to provide a uniform methodology for defining this metric (Rajkumar et al. 2015a). The number of prior lines of therapy is important because the extent of prior treatment can affect patients' frailty and their ability to tolerate treatment, for example due to a limited bone marrow reserve, with such effects becoming increasingly marked with increasing number of prior lines (Dimopoulos et al. 2015a, d; Song et al. 2016). Similarly, various comorbidities and toxicities have been shown to become increasingly common through the disease course, including renal impairment and cardiovascular complications (Yong et al. 2016a, b).

The types of prior therapies received, as well as the duration of these therapies, the duration of response/PFS, and the toxicities associated with prior therapies, are also very important factors to consider when selecting RRMM treatment options. For example, if a patient has not yet been treated with a particular agent (or class of agents), then a treatment option incorporating this agent may be a good choice (Laubach et al. 2016). Subsequently, an alternating approach may be considered, with key drug classes being switched between lines of therapy, as outlined in guidelines from the European Myeloma Network (Sonneveld and Broijl 2016). This is a rational approach in the context of the known clonal heterogeneity of MM and the clonal evolution that can occur over the course of the disease (Morgan et al. 2012; Bahlis 2012). For example, a dominant clone that is sensitive to a particular class of agents may be eradicated by treatment containing such an agent, but then at relapse a different clone may drive the reappearance of the disease, a process known as clonal tiding (Keats et al. 2012; Binder et al. 2016; Egan et al. 2012), this clone, which could be a pre-existing minor clone, an ancestral clone, or a newly evolved clone, may have different characteristics and so may be sensitive to a different class of agents (having not been eliminated by the previous therapy) (Bahlis 2012).

However, relapse may also occur through the recovery of the same clone, and thus in patients who have achieved a good response to a prior treatment, with a duration of response of at least 6–9 months, retreatment with this agent—either within the same regimen or as part of a different regimen—can also be considered (Sonneveld and Broijl 2016; Laubach et al. 2016). Immediate and delayed retreatment has been shown to be feasible and effective in RRMM with bortezomib (Petrucci et al. 2013; Knopf et al. 2014), lenalidomide (Madan et al. 2011), pomalidomide (Nooka et al. 2016), and daratumumab (Nooka et al. 2016). Similarly, repeating ASCT in the salvage setting, following frontline use, has been

shown to be feasible, with patients considered eligible if they achieved a PFS after their first ASCT of at least 18–24 months (Laubach et al. 2016). It is important to note, however, that repeating an agent or a specific treatment option may become less feasible with the widespread adoption of treat-to-progression or maintenance paradigms in the frontline and relapsed settings. Continued use of a therapy until disease progression may give rise to disease refractory to that therapy, thus potentially limiting its utility in subsequent lines of therapy.

As discussed earlier, the issue of sequencing has not been thoroughly explored in RRMM. However, with multiple different agents available within the two main classes—proteasome inhibitors and immunomodulatory drugs—the issue of whether prior therapy with one drug in a particular class affects efficacy with another drug in the same class has been investigated in a number of studies. For the proteasome inhibitors, there is evidence to suggest that previous exposure to another proteasome inhibitor may reduce somewhat the activity of the subsequent agent, just as bortezomib retreatment in responding patients did not result in a second response in all those treated (Petrucci et al. 2013). For example, early-phase studies of carfilzomib alone or in combination with dexamethasone indicated that response rates and outcomes were poorer in RRMM patients who had received or were refractory to prior bortezomib (Vij et al. 2012a; Lendvai et al. 2014; Vij et al. 2012b). In the phase 3 ENDEAVOR study of carfilzomib-dexamethasone versus bortezomib-dexamethasone, median PFS appeared somewhat shorter in both arms among patients with prior bortezomib exposure compared to bortezomib-naïve patients, although the magnitude of the benefit of carfilzomib-dexamethasone versus bortezomib-dexamethasone was similar in both groups (Moreau et al. 2017a). Similar findings were seen in analyses by prior treatment exposure of the phase 3 ASPIRE study of carfilzomib-lenalidomide-dexamethasone versus lenalidomide-dexamethasone (Dimopoulos et al. 2017c), and the phase 3 TOURMALINE-MM1 study of ixazomib-lenalidomide-dexamethasone versus placebo-lenalidomide-dexamethasone (Mateos et al. 2016a). For the immunomodulatory drugs, an analysis of two phase 3 studies of lenalidomide-dexamethasone in RRMM showed that exposure to prior thalidomide resulted in a significantly lower response rate and shorter TTP and PFS, but did not affect OS (Wang et al. 2008). By contrast, an analysis by prior therapy exposure of the phase 3 MM-003 study of pomalidomide-dexamethasone versus dexamethasone in patients who had all received prior lenalidomide showed similar response rates and outcomes regardless of prior thalidomide exposure or lenalidomide-refractory status (San Miguel et al. 2015). No clinical data on pomalidomide in lenalidomide-naïve patients have been reported.

A final important consideration regarding prior therapies is that of residual or ongoing toxicity, which may influence treatment options in RRMM. As noted earlier, the presence of ongoing peripheral neuropathy from a previous line of treatment may result in a recommendation not to utilize a bortezomib-based or a thalidomide-based regimen, and the presence of ongoing renal toxicity or cardiac events might preclude the selection of specific regimens (Dimopoulos et al. 2015a). With the improvements in median OS for MM patients, this issue of ongoing toxicity and of late and long-term consequences of treatment is becoming increasingly important, as outlined in a paper by Snowden et al. for the UK Myeloma Forum and British Society for Haematology (Snowden et al. 2017). With survival times increasingly likely to exceed 10 years (National Cancer Institute 2016; Kumar et al. 2014; Pulte et al. 2014), the cumulative effects of multiple lines of therapy must be considered when selecting treatment options for RRMM and when developing a long-term management plan for MM patients. For example, as summarized by Snowden et al., long-term consequences of treatment might include progressive immunosuppression and thus increased susceptibility to infections, increased renal impairment, ongoing neurologic complications, increasing cardiovascular and respiratory complications, ongoing gastrointestinal complications, increasing fatigue, and diminishing bone marrow capacity (Snowden et al. 2017).

5.3.4 Strength of Clinical Trial Evidence

As summarized in Tables 5.1, 5.2, and 5.3, there is an abundance of data from high-quality phase 3 clinical trials in RRMM, as well as from important earlier-phase trials, to help guide treatment selection in this setting. Indeed, anticipated efficacy of treatment is a primary consideration for therapy selection, and strength of clinical trial evidence supporting this efficacy should also be borne in mind, with data from phase 3 trials regarded as the gold standard. It is important to note, however, that cross-trial comparisons between phase 3 trials should be avoided or approached with caution, as differences between studies in various aspects of study design, eligibility criteria, and other factors may affect absolute values of response and outcomes data. For example, exclusion of a poor prognosis subgroup of patients from one study but not another may result in a higher median PFS in the former versus the latter study, despite the 'true' effects of the treatments being similar.

A more stringent and valid approach for evaluating the multiple different treatment options in the RRMM setting is to use a network meta-analysis to compare the relative efficacy of each treatment option versus a common comparator, utilizing a common endpoint such as PFS. Such a network meta-analysis for RRMM has been recently published (van Beurden-Tan et al. 2017); a systematic literature review was used to identify all available evidence from relevant phase 3 randomized controlled trials, and the data in the form of HRs for PFS (or TTP where PFS was not available) from individual studies were compiled into a network that enabled the generation of HRs for PFS for each different treatment option versus the common comparator of dexamethasone. The analysis determined that the five 'best' regimens in terms of HR compared to dexamethasone were all recently approved triplet regimens, with daratumumab-lenalidomide-dexamethasone demonstrating the greatest relative efficacy (HR 0.13), followed by carfilzomib-lenalidomide-dexamethasone (HR 0.24), elotuzumab-lenalidomide-dexamethasone (HR 0.25), ixazomib-lenalidomide-dexamethasone

(HR 0.26), and daratumumab-bortezomib-dexamethasone (HR 0.27) (van Beurden-Tan et al. 2017). These findings reflect the results from the individual studies and also support the treatment paradigm of utilizing triplet regimens for RRMM where feasible and available, on the basis of efficacy improvement.

The network meta-analysis only utilized PFS or TTP data. However, other aspects of the clinical trial evidence should also be considered when making treatment choices. Depth of response is an important parameter, and high rates of quality responses (CR and VGPR), such as those seen in several of the recent phase 3 trials including POLLUX (Dimopoulos et al. 2016c), CASTOR (Palumbo et al. 2016), and ASPIRE (Stewart et al. 2015), are associated with improved outcomes (van de Velde et al. 2007, 2017; Lonial and Anderson 2014). Furthermore, elimination of minimal residual disease (MRD) has been shown to be prognostic for significantly improved outcomes (Anderson et al. 2017), with sustained MRD-negative status being a prerequisite for "operational cure" of MM (Lahuerta et al. 2017; Harousseau and Avet-Loiseau 2017). Clinical study data demonstrating high rates of MRD-negative responses would be an important efficacy consideration when selecting RRMM treatment, such as those findings reported from POLLUX and CASTOR with the daratumumab-based triplet regimens (Dimopoulos et al. 2016c; Mateos et al. 2016b). In tandem with considering the overall rates of quality responses, it is important to determine if activity is maintained in high-risk subgroups such as those with high-risk cytogenetic features. Consistent benefits in these patient subgroups have been reported with the majority of the new doublet and triplet regimens, including in the TOURMALINE-MM1 (Avet-Loiseau et al. 2016b), ASPIRE (Avet-Loiseau et al. 2016a), ENDEAVOR (Chng et al. 2017), ELOQUENT (Lonial et al. 2015), CASTOR (Mateos et al. 2016b), and POLLUX (Moreau et al. 2016b) studies. Finally, from an efficacy perspective, consideration should be given to those regimens for RRMM that demonstrate an OS benefit versus a comparator, as such a benefit is becoming increasingly difficult to demonstrate in the modern era of multiple active salvage treatment options. Notably, an OS benefit has been seen with carfilzomib-dexamethasone versus bortezomib-dexamethasone in ENDEAVOR (Siegel et al. 2017).

Any toxicity concerns arising from high-quality phase 3 trial data should be a significant consideration for RRMM treatment selection. Additionally, if data are available on patients' perspectives of treatment, in the form of quality-of-life findings, these are also valuable to consider, particularly in the context of different patient preferences for treatment and different goals of treatment. Many of the recent phase 3 studies in RRMM have reported quality-of-life endpoint data, demonstrating no detrimental impact—and in some cases a positive effect—on patient-reported outcomes following the addition of a second or third agent to a single-agent or doublet backbone, for example, with pomalidomide-dexamethasone (Weisel et al. 2015), ixazomib-lenalidomide-dexamethasone (Moreau et al. 2016a), and carfilzomib-lenalidomide-dexamethasone (Stewart et al. 2016).

5.4 Recommendations Regarding Management of RRMM

A number of important guidelines are available providing recommendations on the treatment and management of RRMM, including from the IMWG (Laubach et al. 2016), the European Society for Medical Oncology (Moreau et al. 2017c), the Mayo Clinic (Dingli et al. 2017), and the NCCN (Network 2016; Kumar et al. 2017). With the rapidly changing nature of the RRMM treatment armamentarium and the availability of regularly updated recommendations and guidelines, this chapter is not the forum for providing a detailed regimen-by-regimen or setting-by-setting consolidated summary of current recommendations. However, a number of important general principles may be derived from recent publications and the latest available data.

5.4.1 Focused Clinical Assessment of Relapse

Patients should be thoroughly evaluated at relapse to determine the nature of their relapse and the returning disease. Specifically, an aggressive relapse requires immediate treatment with highly active triplet regimens (if tolerable) in order to achieve as deep a response as possible (Laubach et al. 2016); given the likelihood of subsequent progression with aggressive disease, the treatment should be given continuously if tolerated, rather than for a finite duration (Laubach et al. 2016). Additional options for aggressive relapse include consolidation with (repeat) ASCT or consideration for allogeneic stem cell transplant (Laubach et al. 2016). In contrast, patients with indolent relapse could potentially be carefully observed for a period of time or could be considered for treatment with a less intensive treatment option such as a doublet or even single-agent therapy, particularly if not previously exposed to that regimen or if previously responsive (Laubach et al. 2016). Patients should also undergo a frailty or geriatric assessment to determine the extent of comorbidities and cognitive/physical functioning (Palumbo et al. 2015; Engelhardt et al. 2016, 2017), as this will be important for determining whether more intensive treatment options might be feasible or whether patients require attenuated therapy to balance activity and tolerability (Dimopoulos et al. 2015d; Rosko et al. 2017; Willan et al. 2016; Larocca and Palumbo 2015). A number of such approaches have been evaluated in clinical trials in MM (Tuchman et al. 2017; Quach et al. 2017; Larocca et al. 2016).

5.4.2 Use of Triplet Versus Doublet Regimens

There is now a wealth of high-quality data from phase 3 clinical trials supporting the benefit of using triplet versus doublet regimens in RRMM, if tolerable for the patient (Sun et al. 2017; Stewart et al. 2015; Moreau et al. 2016a; Lonial et al. 2015; Dimopoulos et al. 2016c; Palumbo et al. 2016; Garderet et al. 2012). As noted above,

the use of triplet therapy is particularly recommended in patients with high-risk disease, such as those with high-risk cytogenetics (Laubach et al. 2016), which aligns with the specific IMWG recommendation to treat patients with high-risk cytogenetics with a triplet combination comprising a proteasome inhibitor, lenalidomide or pomalidomide, and dexamethasone (Sonneveld et al. 2016). However, it should be noted that this recommendation was published prior to the availability of data from CASTOR and POLLUX. For those patients in whom a doublet regimen is required due to frailty or tolerability issues, it is suggested to preferentially employ a regimen containing an agent to which the patient has not been previously exposed.

5.4.3 Use of Feasible Treatment Options Offering Greatest Degree of Impact Demonstrated in Clinical Trials

It is becoming increasingly well established that early (or, indeed, upfront) use of the most active drugs is important for achieving as deep and as durable a remission as possible (Mohty et al. 2012), including MRD-negative status. Multiple studies have demonstrated better response rates and outcomes with specific regimens in earlier versus later lines of therapy (Moreau et al. 2016a, 2017a; Dimopoulos et al. 2016c, 2017c; Palumbo et al. 2016), and thus, to optimize chances of the best clinical outcome, it is recommended to use the most active regimen, based on clinical trial data, that is feasible and available for an individual RRMM patient. In this context, and in the absence of head-to-head clinical trial data, approaches such as the previously described network meta-analysis (van Beurden-Tan et al. 2017) can provide important information for clinicians selecting a treatment regimen. A counterargument to such an approach—of utilizing complex treatment regimens incorporating several classes of agent—is that it can "burn up" multiple agents early in a patient's disease course, to the detriment of subsequent treatment options; however, as noted above, data suggest the feasibility of retreatment with a number of agents, and with the increasing availability of novel treatment options, this may become less of a consideration.

It is important to acknowledge that subsequent developments in frontline therapy based on the above philosophy will obviously affect the feasibility and availability of treatment options for RRMM. For example, daratumumab-lenalidomide-dexamethasone currently appears the most active option based upon network meta-analysis of available phase 3 studies in RRMM, followed by four other triplet regimens (van Beurden-Tan et al. 2017); however, if frontline therapy were to evolve based on the findings from currently ongoing phase 3 studies of daratumumab (Cassiopeia, NCT02541383; Alcyone, NCT02195479; Maia, NCT02252172), elotuzumab (ELOQUENT-1 NCT01335399), carfilzomib (ECOG E1A11, NCT01863550), or ixazomib (TOURMALINE-MM2, NCT01850524), for example, to incorporate widespread use of these agents, then subsequent therapy selection for RRMM would be affected. Similarly, while the current consensus is to not treat patients with smoldering MM, except for those with very high risk of progression to active MM who are now reclassified as having MM and requiring therapy (Rajkumar et al. 2015b; Korde 2016), more widespread use of treatment for smoldering MM in the future may also affect the feasibility of subsequent treatment options for MM in general.

5.4.4 Consideration of Patient Preferences, Impact on Lifestyle, and Potential Long-Term Effects

In tandem with the above considerations, it is important to remember that treatment choice is not necessarily all about efficacy. Patient preferences regarding choice of therapy, route of administration, and other factors affecting lifestyle and quality of life should be taken into consideration (Baz et al. 2015; Osborne et al. 2014; Tariman et al. 2014; Lassalle et al. 2016;

Muhlbacher et al. 2008), and physicians should also consider the burden of relapse on the patient and on the caregiver, including the psychosocial impact, when making subsequent management decisions (Hulin et al. 2017; Kurtin 2017). Furthermore, the potential long-term effects of treatment, and the potential impact of the long-term effects of previous therapies, must also be taken into account given the increasing length of survival in RRMM. Specifically, as recommended in a recent paper by Snowden et al., management of RRMM patients must include consideration of the long-term physical consequences of treatment, patient frailty and evolving comorbidities, psychosocial aspects such as psychologic well-being, and the impact on a patient's work ability (Snowden et al. 2017). Additionally, the potential for side-effects based on a patient's medical background and the toxicity profile of a given regimen will require consideration (Colson 2015; Bringhen et al. 2017b), as may the financial impacts of treatment and the management of associated complications, in order to avoid "financial toxicity" from long-term therapy (Baz et al. 2015; Goodwin et al. 2013; Huntington et al. 2015).

5.5 Future Directions

As noted at the beginning of this chapter, the management of RRMM patients has changed remarkably over the past two decades, with the introduction of multiple classes of agents and numerous treatment options (Moreau and de Wit 2017). Nevertheless, however, much progress in drug development has already occurred; the RRMM treatment algorithm is likely to undergo further changes in the years ahead as novel agents and regimens currently in the pipeline progress through clinical development. A number of new agents with novel mechanisms of action are currently in phase 3 clinical trials in RRMM, as summarized in Table 5.5.

Beyond these agents there are additional promising compounds and approaches in earlier-phase development (Gonsalves et al. 2017). For example, building on the approval of the

Table 5.5 Novel agents currently in phase 3 clinical trials in RRMM (registered on ClinicalTrials.gov, July 4, 2017; phase 3 studies in RRMM not yet recruiting, open, or ongoing)

Agent	Mechanism of action	Study name	NCT
Pembrolizumab	Anti-PD-1 monoclonal antibody	KEYNOTE-183 (Shah et al. 2016)	NCT02576977
Nivolumab	Anti-PD-1 monoclonal antibody	CheckMate 602 (Lonial et al. 2017)	NCT02726581
Isatuximab	Anti-CD38 monoclonal antibody	ICARIA-MM (Richardson et al. 2017)	NCT02990338
Venetoclax	Bcl-2 inhibitor	–	NCT02755597
Selinexor	Selective inhibitor of nuclear export compound	BOSTON	NCT03110562
Plitidepsin	Cyclic depsipeptide	ADMYRE	NCT01102426
Melflufen	Peptidase potentiated alkylator	OCEAN	NCT03151811

pan-histone deacetylase inhibitor panobinostat, the histone deacetylase-6-specific inhibitors ricolinostat (Vogl et al. 2017) and ACY-241 (Niesvizky et al. 2016) have shown promising results in phase 1/2 studies in RRMM. Additionally, there is great excitement about the use of chimeric antigen receptor-engineered T-cell (CAR-T) therapy in MM, including approaches targeting the B-cell maturation antigen (BCMA) (Berdeja et al. 2017; Fan et al. 2017) and CD19 (Kochenderfer 2016), which have shown substantial activity, including durable, deep responses. Reflecting the success of antibody-drug conjugates in other malignancies, a compound targeting BCMA is also in development in RRMM (Cohen et al. 2016).

As these treatment options potentially come "online" in the future, clinicians will have an increasing range of novel regimens and different mechanisms of action with which to treat RRMM. As noted earlier, this may result in further substantial changes to the treatment algorithm, particularly if commonly used agents for RRMM move into the frontline setting. The availability of additional novel agents may also increase the cost pressures in RRMM (Fonseca et al. 2017; Rajkumar and Harousseau 2016), although this may be less of an issue in this setting compared to first-line therapy, which may evolve to encompass a four-drug induction regimen comprising at least two novel agents, possibly with stem cell transplantation, consolidation, and maintenance therapy. Nevertheless, the financial issues associated with long-term survivorship in MM will need to be considered

as part of patient management, alongside the clinical challenges of selecting the optimal therapy, choosing appropriate combination regimens and treatment sequences for individual patients, and managing toxicities from treatment over a lengthy period of time (Snowden et al. 2017).

Conclusions

The management of patients with RRMM has undergone a revolution over the past two decades, with improvements in treatment and supportive care resulting in prolonged survival and better quality of life. This has been a period of substantial positive change for both patients and clinicians, with further exciting developments on the horizon. However, patients with RRMM still have important unmet needs across the increasing duration of their disease course, and the hope is that newly available agents and emerging therapies and approaches may address these in the longer term, transforming MM into a chronic disease. In the immediate future, the wealth of novel and emerging treatment options, and increasing life expectancy of patients, are presenting their own challenges to clinicians, including determining the optimal treatment and sequence of therapies, as well as managing long-term effects and toxicities. Nevertheless, this is a positive set of problems to have, and as our MM knowledge expands further, we will move into an era of increasingly tailored, personalized therapy for patients with RRMM, with the best regimens and mechanisms of action selected based on individual patients and disease characteristics—an incredible advance on the generally bleak outlook for RRMM patients that existed just two decades ago.

References

Amgen (2017) Second phase 3 study shows KYPROLIS® (Carfilzomib) regimen significantly improves overall survival in patients with relapsed multiple myeloma, Amgen. http://www.amgen.com/en-gb/media/news-releases/2017/07/second-phase-3-study-shows-kyprolis-carfilzomib-regimen-significantly-improves-overall-survival-in-patients-with-relapsed-multiple-myeloma/

Anderson KC (2016) Progress and Paradigms in Multiple Myeloma. Clin Cancer Res 22:5419–5427

Anderson KC, Auclair D, Kelloff GJ et al (2017) The role of minimal residual disease testing in myeloma treatment selection and drug development: current value and future applications. Clin Cancer Res 23(15):3980–3993

Arnulf B, Pylypenko H, Grosicki S et al (2012) Updated survival analysis of a randomized phase III study of subcutaneous versus intravenous bortezomib in patients with relapsed multiple myeloma. Haematologica 97:1925–1928

Avet-Loiseau H, Fonseca R, Siegel D et al (2016a) Carfilzomib significantly improves the progression-free survival of high-risk patients in multiple myeloma. Blood 128:1174–1180

Avet-Loiseau J, Bahlis N, Chng WJ et al (2016b) Impact of cytogenetic risk status on efficacy and safety of ixaozmib-lenalidomide-dexamethasone (IRd) vs placebo-Rd in relapsed/refractory multiple myeloma patients in the global TOURMALINE-MM1 study. Haematologica 101:80

Bahlis NJ (2012) Darwinian evolution and tiding clones in multiple myeloma. Blood 120:927–928

Baz R, Lin HM, Hui AM et al (2015) Development of a conceptual model to illustrate the impact of multiple myeloma and its treatment on health-related quality of life. Support Care Cancer 23:2789–2797

Baz RC, Martin TG 3rd, Lin HY et al (2016) Randomized multicenter phase 2 study of pomalidomide, cyclophosphamide, and dexamethasone in relapsed refractory myeloma. Blood 127:2561–2568

Berdeja JG, Lin Y, Raje NS et al (2017) First-in-human multicenter study of bb2121 anti-BCMA CAR T-cell therapy for relapsed/refractory multiple myeloma: updated results. J Clin Oncol 35:3010

Bianchi G, Ghobrial IM (2014) Biological and clinical implications of clonal heterogeneity and clonal evolution in multiple myeloma. Curr Cancer Ther Rev 10:70–79

Binder M, Rajkumar SV, Ketterling RP et al (2016) Occurrence and prognostic significance of cytogenetic evolution in patients with multiple myeloma. Blood Cancer J 6:e401

Boudreault JS, Touzeau C, Moreau P (2017) Triplet combinations in relapsed/refractory myeloma: update on recent phase 3 trials. Expert Rev Hematol 10:207–215

Bringhen S, Oliva S, Liberati AM et al (2017a) Carfilzomib, pomalidomide and dexamethasone in relapsed and/or refractory multiple myeloma patients: a multicenter, open-label, phase 1/2 study. Clin Lymphoma Myeloma Leuk 17:e59

Bringhen S, De Wit E, Dimopoulos MA (2017b) New agents in multiple myeloma: an examination of safety profiles. Clin Lymphoma Myeloma Leuk 17(7):391–407

Chanan-Khan A, Sonneveld P, Schuster MW et al (2008) Analysis of herpes zoster events among bortezomib-treated patients in the phase III APEX study. J Clin Oncol 26:4784–4790

Chng WJ, Goldschmidt H, Dimopoulos MA et al (2017) Carfilzomib-dexamethasone vs bortezomib-dexamethasone in relapsed or refractory multiple myeloma by cytogenetic risk in the phase 3 study ENDEAVOR. Leukemia 31:1368–1374

Cohen AD, Popat R, Trudel S et al (2016) First in human study with GSK2857916, an antibody drug conjugated to microtubule-disrupting agent directed against B-cell maturation antigen (BCMA) in patients with relapsed/refractory multiple myeloma (MM): results from study BMA117159 part 1 dose escalation. Blood 128:1148

Colson K (2015) Treatment-related symptom management in patients with multiple myeloma: a review. Support Care Cancer 23:1431–1445

de Waal EG, de Munck L, Hoogendoorn M et al (2015) Combination therapy with bortezomib, continuous low-dose cyclophosphamide and dexamethasone followed by one year of maintenance treatment for relapsed multiple myeloma patients. Br J Haematol 171(5):720–725

Dimopoulos M, Spencer A, Attal M et al (2007) Lenalidomide plus dexamethasone for relapsed or refractory multiple myeloma. N Engl J Med 357:2123–2132

Dimopoulos MA, Chen C, Spencer A et al (2009) Long-term follow-up on overall survival from the MM-009 and MM-010 phase III trials of lenalidomide plus dexamethasone in patients with relapsed or refractory multiple myeloma. Leukemia 23:2147–2152

Dimopoulos MA, Richardson PG, Brandenburg N et al (2012) A review of second primary malignancy in patients with relapsed or refractory multiple myeloma treated with lenalidomide. Blood 119:2764–2767

Dimopoulos MA, Richardson PG, Moreau P, Anderson KC (2015a) Current treatment landscape for relapsed and/or refractory multiple myeloma. Nat Rev Clin Oncol 12:42–54

Dimopoulos MA, Orlowski RZ, Facon T et al (2015b) Retrospective matched-pairs analysis of bortezomib plus dexamethasone versus bortezomib monotherapy in relapsed multiple myeloma. Haematologica 100:100–106

Dimopoulos MA, Weisel KC, Song KW et al (2015c) Cytogenetics and long-term survival of patients with refractory or relapsed and refractory multiple myeloma treated with pomalidomide and low-dose dexamethasone. Haematologica 100:1327–1333

Dimopoulos MA, Terpos E, Niesvizky R, Palumbo A (2015d) Clinical characteristics of patients with relapsed multiple myeloma. Cancer Treat Rev 41:827–835

Dimopoulos MA, Moreau P, Palumbo A et al (2016a) Carfilzomib and dexamethasone versus bortezomib and dexamethasone for patients with relapsed or refractory multiple myeloma (ENDEAVOR): a randomised, phase 3, open-label, multicentre study. Lancet Oncol 17:27–38

Dimopoulos MA, Palumbo A, Corradini P et al (2016b) Safety and efficacy of pomalidomide plus low-dose dexamethasone in STRATUS (MM-010): a phase 3b study in refractory multiple myeloma. Blood 128:497–503

Dimopoulos MA, Oriol A, Nahi H et al (2016c) Daratumumab, lenalidomide, and dexamethasone for multiple myeloma. N Engl J Med 375:1319–1331

Dimopoulos MA, Lonial S, White D et al (2017a) Phase 3 ELOQUENT-2 study: extended 4-year follow-up of elotuzumab plus lenalidomide/dexamethasone vs lenalidomide/dexamethasone in relapsed/refractory multiple myeloma. Haematologica 102:167–168

Dimopoulos MA, Stewart AK, Masszi T et al (2017b) Carfilzomib, lenalidomide, and dexamethasone in patients with relapsed multiple myeloma categorised by age: secondary analysis from the phase 3 ASPIRE study. Br J Haematol 177:404–413

Dimopoulos MA, Stewart AK, Masszi T et al (2017c) Carfilzomib-lenalidomide-dexamethasone vs lenalidomide-dexamethasone in relapsed multiple myeloma by previous treatment. Blood Cancer J 7:e554

Dingli D, Ailawadhi S, Bergsagel PL et al (2017) Therapy for relapsed multiple myeloma: guidelines from the mayo stratification for myeloma and risk-adapted therapy. Mayo Clin Proc 92:578–598

Egan JB, Shi CX, Tembe W et al (2012) Whole-genome sequencing of multiple myeloma from diagnosis to plasma cell leukemia reveals genomic initiating events, evolution, and clonal tides. Blood 120:1060–1066

Egan P, Drain S, Conway C, Bjourson AJ, Alexander HD (2016) Towards stratified medicine in plasma cell myeloma. Int J Mol Sci 17:pii: E1760

Engelhardt M, Dold SM, Ihorst G et al (2016) Geriatric assessment in multiple myeloma patients: validation of the International Myeloma Working Group (IMWG) score and comparison with other common comorbidity scores. Haematologica 101(9):1110–1119

Engelhardt M, Domm AS, Dold SM et al (2017) A concise revised Myeloma Comorbidity Index as a valid

prognostic instrument in a large cohort of 801 multiple myeloma patients. Haematologica 102:910–921

Fan F, Zhao W, Liu J et al (2017) Durable remissions with BCMA-specific chimeric antigen receptor (CAR)-modified T cells in patients with refractory/relapsed multiple myeloma. J Clin Oncol 35:LBA3001

Fonseca R, Abouzaid S, Bonafede M et al (2017) Trends in overall survival and costs of multiple myeloma, 2000–2014. Leukemia 31(9):1915–1921

Fouquet G, Pegourie B, Macro M et al (2016) Safe and prolonged survival with long-term exposure to pomalidomide in relapsed/refractory myeloma. Ann Oncol 27:902–907

Garderet L, Iacobelli S, Moreau P et al (2012) Superiority of the triple combination of bortezomib-thalidomide-dexamethasone over the dual combination of thalidomide-dexamethasone in patients with multiple myeloma progressing or relapsing after autologous transplantation: the MMVAR/IFM 2005-04 Randomized Phase III Trial from the Chronic Leukemia Working Party of the European Group for Blood and Marrow Transplantation. J Clin Oncol 30:2475–2482

Gonsalves WI, Milani P, Derudas D, Buadi FK (2017) The next generation of novel therapies for the management of relapsed multiple myeloma. Future Oncol 13:63–75

Goodwin JA, Coleman EA, Sullivan E et al (2013) Personal financial effects of multiple myeloma and its treatment. Cancer Nurs 36:301–308

Harousseau JL, Avet-Loiseau H (2017) Minimal residual disease negativity is a new end point of myeloma therapy. J Clin Oncol 35(25):2863–2865

Harousseau JL, Dimopoulos MA, Wang M et al (2010) Better quality of response to lenalidomide plus dexamethasone is associated with improved clinical outcomes in patients with relapsed or refractory myeloma. Haematologica 95:1738–1744

Hulin C, Hansen T, Heron L et al (2017) Living with the burden of relapse in multiple myeloma from the patient and physician perspective. Leuk Res 59:75–84

Huntington SF, Weiss BM, Vogl DT et al (2015) Financial toxicity in insured patients with multiple myeloma: a cross-sectional pilot study. Lancet Haematol 2:e408–e416

Jagannath S, Richardson PG, Barlogie B et al (2006) Bortezomib in combination with dexamethasone for the treatment of patients with relapsed and/or refractory multiple myeloma with less than optimal response to bortezomib alone. Haematologica 91:929–934

Jagannath S, Roy A, Kish J et al (2016) Real-world treatment patterns and associated progression-free survival in relapsed/refractory multiple myeloma among US community oncology practices. Expert Rev Hematol 9:707–717

Jakubowiak A, Offidani M, Pegourie B et al (2016) Randomized phase 2 study: elotuzumab plus bortezomib/dexamethasone vs bortezomib/dexamethasone for relapsed/refractory MM. Blood 127:2833–2840

Keats JJ, Chesi M, Egan JB et al (2012) Clonal competition with alternating dominance in multiple myeloma. Blood 120:1067–1076

Knopf KB, Duh MS, Lafeuille MH et al (2014) Meta-analysis of the efficacy and safety of bortezomib re-treatment in patients with multiple myeloma. Clin Lymphoma Myeloma Leuk 14:380–388

Kochenderfer JN (2016) Blood Chimeric Antigen receptors/genetically modified T-cells. Blood 128: SCI-37

Korde N (2016) Treatment of high-risk smoldering myeloma. Semin Oncol 43:695–696

Kortuem KM, Stewart AK (2013) Carfilzomib. Blood 121:893–897

Kumar SK, Anderson KC (2016) Immune therapies in multiple myeloma. Clin Cancer Res 22:5453–5460

Kumar SK, Therneau TM, Gertz MA et al (2004) Clinical course of patients with relapsed multiple myeloma. Mayo Clin Proc 79:867–874

Kumar SK, Lee JH, Lahuerta JJ et al (2012) Risk of pro-gression and survival in multiple myeloma relapsing after therapy with IMiDs and bortezomib: a multi-center international myeloma working group study. Leukemia 26:149–157

Kumar SK, Dispenzieri A, Lacy MQ et al (2014) Continued improvement in survival in multiple myeloma: changes in early mortality and outcomes in older patients. Leukemia 28:1122–1128

Kumar SK, LaPlant B, Roy V et al (2015a) Phase 2 trial of ixazomib in patients with relapsed multiple myeloma not refractory to bortezomib. Blood Cancer J 5:e338

Kumar SK, Krishnan A, LaPlant B et al (2015b) Bendamustine, lenalidomide, and dexamethasone (BRD) is highly effective with durable responses in relapsed multiple myeloma. Am J Hematol 90:1106–1110

Kumar SK, Lee JH, Dimopoulos MA et al (2015c) Outcomes after initial relapse of multiple myeloma: an International Myeloma Working Group Study. Blood 126:4201

Kumar SK, LaPlant BR, Reeder CB et al (2016) Randomized phase 2 trial of ixazomib and dexametha-sone in relapsed multiple myeloma not refractory to bortezomib. Blood 128:2415–2422

Kumar SK, Callander NS, Alsina M et al (2017) Multiple myeloma, version 3.2017, NCCN clinical practice guidelines in oncology. J Natl Compr Cancer Netw 15:230–269

Kurtin S (2017) Living with multiple myeloma: a continuum-based approach to cancer survivorship. Semin Oncol Nurs 33(3):348–361

Kyle RA, Gertz MA, Witzig TE et al (2003) Review of 1027 patients with newly diagnosed multiple myeloma. Mayo Clin Proc 78:21–33

Lahuerta JJ, Paiva B, Vidriales MB et al (2017) Depth of response in multiple myeloma: a pooled analysis of three PETHEMA/GEM clinical trials. J Clin Oncol 35(25):2900–2910

Larocca A, Palumbo A (2015) How I treat fragile myeloma patients. Blood 126:2179–2185

Larocca A, Bringhen S, Petrucci MT et al (2016) A phase 2 study of three low-dose intensity subcutaneous bortezomib regimens in elderly frail patients with untreated multiple myeloma. Leukemia 30(6):1320

Larsen JT, Kumar S (2015) Evolving paradigms in the management of multiple myeloma: novel agents and targeted therapies. Rare Cancers Ther 3:47–68

Lassalle A, Thomare P, Fronteau C et al (2016) Home administration of bortezomib in multiple myeloma is cost-effective and is preferred by patients compared with hospital administration: results of a prospective single-center study. Ann Oncol 27:314–318

Laubach J, Garderet L, Mahindra A et al (2016) Management of relapsed multiple myeloma: recom-mendations of the International Myeloma Working Group. Leukemia 30:1005–1017

Laubach JP, Paba Prada CE, Richardson PG, Longo DL (2017) Daratumumab, elotuzumab, and the develop-ment of therapeutic monoclonal antibodies in multiple myeloma. Clin Pharmacol Ther 101:81–88

Leleu X, Karlin L, Macro M et al (2015) Pomalidomide plus low-dose dexamethasone in multiple myeloma with deletion 17p and/or translocation (4;14): IFM 2010-02 trial results. Blood 125:1411–1417

Lendvai N, Hilden P, Devlin S et al (2014) A phase 2 single-center study of carfilzomib 56 mg/m2 with or without low-dose dexamethasone in relapsed multiple myeloma. Blood 124:899–906

Lokhorst HM, Plesner T, Laubach JP et al (2015) Targeting CD38 with Daratumumab Monotherapy in Multiple Myeloma. N Engl J Med 373:1207–1219

Lonial S, Anderson KC (2014) Association of response endpoints with survival outcomes in multiple myeloma. Leukemia 28:258–268

Lonial S, Richardson PG, San Miguel J et al (2008) Characterisation of haematological profiles and low risk of thromboembolic events with bortezomib in patients with relapsed multiple myeloma. Br J Haematol 143:222–229

Lonial S, Dimopoulos M, Palumbo A et al (2015) Elotuzumab therapy for relapsed or refractory mul-tiple myeloma. N Engl J Med 373:621–631

Lonial S, Weiss BM, Usmani SZ et al (2016) Daratumumab monotherapy in patients with treatment-refractory multiple myeloma (SIRIUS): an open-label, ran-domised, phase 2 trial. Lancet 387:1551–1560

Lonial S, Richardson PG, Reece DE, Mohamed H, Shelat S, San Miguel S (2017) CheckMate 602: an open-label, randomized, phase 3 trial of combinations of nivolumab, elotuzumab, pomalidomide and dexa-methasone in relapsed/refractory multiple myeloma. J Clin Oncol 35:TPS8052

Ludwig H, Kasparu H, Leitgeb C et al (2014) Bendamustine-bortezomib-dexamethasone is an active and well-tolerated regimen in patients with relapsed or refractory multiple myeloma. Blood 123:985–991

Ludwig H, Dimopoulos MA, Moreau P et al (2017) Carfilzomib and dexamethasone vs bortezomib and dexamethasone in patients with relapsed multiple myeloma: results of the phase 3 study ENDEAVOR (NCT01568866) according to age subgroup. Leuk Lymphoma 58(10):2501–2504

Madan S, Lacy MQ, Dispenzieri A et al (2011) Efficacy of retreatment with immunomodulatory drugs (IMiDs) in patients receiving IMiDs for initial therapy of newly diagnosed multiple myeloma. Blood 118:1763–1765

Majithia N, Vincent Rajkumar S, Lacy MQ et al (2015) Outcomes of primary refractory multiple myeloma and the impact of novel therapies. Am J Hematol 90:981–985

Malard F, Harousseau JL, Mohty M (2017) Multiple myeloma treatment at relapse after autologous stem cell transplantation: a practical analysis. Cancer Treat Rev 52:41–47

Manier S, Salem KZ, Park J, Landau DA, Getz G, Ghobrial IM (2017) Genomic complexity of multiple myeloma and its clinical implications. Nat Rev Clin Oncol 14:100–113

Mateos MV, San Miguel JF (2013) How should we treat newly diagnosed multiple myeloma patients? Hematology Am Soc Hematol Educ Program 2013:488–495

Mateos MV, Masszi T, Grzasko N et al (2016a) Efficacy and safety of oral ixazomib-lenalidomide-dexamethasone (IRd) vs placebo-Rd in relapsed/refractory multiple myeloma patients: impact of prior therapy in the phase 3 TOURMALINE-MM1 study. Haematologica 101:527

Mateos M-V, Estell J, Barreto W et al (2016b) Efficacy of daratumumab, bortezomib, and dexamethasone versus bortezomib and dexamethasone in relapsed or refractory myeloma based on prior lines of therapy: updated analysis of castor. Blood 128:1150

Mikhael JR, Belch AR, Prince HM et al (2009) High response rate to bortezomib with or without dexamethasone in patients with relapsed or refractory multiple myeloma: results of a global phase 3b expanded access program. Br J Haematol 144:169–175

Mohty B, El-Cheikh J, Yakoub-Agha I, Avet-Loiseau H, Moreau P, Mohty M (2012) Treatment strategies in relapsed and refractory multiple myeloma: a focus on drug sequencing and 'retreatment' approaches in the era of novel agents. Leukemia 26:73–85

Montazeri A (2009) Quality of life data as prognostic indicators of survival in cancer patients: an overview of the literature from 1982 to 2008. Health Qual Life Outcomes 7:102

Moreau P, de Wit E (2017) Recent progress in relapsed multiple myeloma therapy: implications for treatment decisions. Br J Haematol 179(2):198–218

Moreau P, Pylypenko H, Grosicki S et al (2011) Subcutaneous versus intravenous administration of bortezomib in patients with relapsed multiple myeloma: a randomised, phase 3, non-inferiority study. Lancet Oncol 12:431–440

Moreau P, Masszi T, Grzasko N et al (2016a) Oral ixazomib, lenalidomide, and dexamethasone for multiple myeloma. N Engl J Med 374:1621–1634

Moreau P, Kaufman JL, Sutherland HJ et al (2016b) Efficacy of daratumumab, lenalidomide and dexamethasone versus lenalidomide and dexamethasone alone for relapsed or refractory multiple myeloma

among patients with 1 to 3 prior lines of therapy based on previous treatment exposure: updated analysis of pollux. Blood 128:489

Moreau P, Joshua D, Chng WJ et al (2017a) Impact of prior treatment on patients with relapsed multiple myeloma treated with carfilzomib and dexamethasone vs bortezomib and dexamethasone in the phase 3 ENDEAVOR study. Leukemia 31:115–122

Moreau P, Dimopoulos MA, Richardson PG et al (2017b) Adverse event management in patients with relapsed and refractory multiple myeloma taking pomalidomide plus low-dose dexamethasone: a pooled analysis. Eur J Haematol 99(3):199–206

Moreau P, San Miguel J, Sonneveld P et al (2017c) Multiple myeloma: ESMO Clinical Practice Guidelines for diagnosis, treatment and follow-updagger. Ann Oncol 28(Suppl_4):iv52–iv61

Morgan GJ, Walker BA, Davies FE (2012) The genetic architecture of multiple myeloma. Nat Rev Cancer 12:335–348

Muhlbacher AC, Lincke HJ, Nubling M (2008) Evaluating patients' preferences for multiple myeloma therapy, a Discrete-Choice-Experiment. Psychosoc Med 5:Doc10

Murata K, McCash SI, Carroll B et al (2016) Treatment of multiple myeloma with monoclonal antibodies and the dilemma of false positive M-spikes in peripheral blood. Clin Biochem. https://doi.org/10.1016/j.clinbiochem.2016.09.015. [Epub ahead of print]

Musto P, Montefusco V (2016) Are maintenance and continuous therapies indicated for every patient with multiple myeloma? Expert Rev Hematol 9:743–751

National Cancer Institute (2016) SEER Cancer Statistics Review, 1975–2014, based on November 2016 SEER data submission, posted to the SEER web site, April 2017. Table 18.9, Myeloma, SEER Relative Survival (Percent) By Year of Diagnosis, All Races, Males and Females 2017. National Cancer Institute, Bethesda, MD. https://seer.cancer.gov/csr/1975_2014/

National Comprehensive Cancer Network (2016) NCCN clinical practice guidelines in oncology (NCCN Guidelines). National Comprehensive Cancer Network, NCCNorg. www.nccn.org

Niesvizky R, Richardson PG, Yee AJ et al (2016) Selective HDAC6 inhibitor acy-241, an oral tablet, combined with pomalidomide and dexamethasone: safety and efficacy of escalation and expansion cohorts in patients with relapsed or relapsed-and-refractory multiple myeloma (ACE-MM-200 study). Blood 128:3307

Nooka AK, Joseph N, Boise LH, Gleason C, Kaufman JL, Lonial S (2016) Clinical efficacy of daratumumab, pomalidomide and dexamethasone in relapsed, refractory myeloma patients: utility of retreatment with daratumumab among refractory patients. Blood 128:492

Orlowski RZ, Nagler A, Sonneveld P et al (2007) Randomized phase III study of pegylated liposomal doxorubicin plus bortezomib compared with bortezomib alone in relapsed or refractory multiple myeloma:

combination therapy improves time to progression. J Clin Oncol 25:3892–3901

Orlowski RZ, Nagler A, Sonneveld P et al (2016) Final overall survival results of a randomized trial comparing bortezomib plus pegylated liposomal doxorubicin with bortezomib alone in patients with relapsed or refractory multiple myeloma. Cancer 122:2050–2056

Osborne TR, Ramsenthaler C, de Wolf-Linder S et al (2014) Understanding what matters most to people with multiple myeloma: a qualitative study of views on quality of life. BMC Cancer 14:496

Osborne TR, Ramsenthaler C, Schey SA, Siegert RJ, Edmonds PM, Higginson IJ (2015) Improving the assessment of quality of life in the clinical care of myeloma patients: the development and validation of the Myeloma Patient Outcome Scale (MyPOS). BMC Cancer 15:280

Paludo J, Mikhael JR, LaPlant BR et al (2017) Pomalidomide, bortezomib and dexamethasone (pvd) for patients with relapsed, lenalidomide refractory multiple myeloma. Blood 130:1198–1204

Palumbo A, Bringhen S, Mateos MV et al (2015) Geriatric assessment predicts survival and toxicities in elderly myeloma patients: an International Myeloma Working Group report. Blood 125:2068–2074

Palumbo A, Chanan-Khan A, Weisel K et al (2016) Daratumumab, bortezomib, and dexamethasone for multiple myeloma. N Engl J Med 375:754–766

Petrucci MT, Giraldo P, Corradini P et al (2013) A prospective, international phase 2 study of bortezomib retreatment in patients with relapsed multiple myeloma. Br J Haematol 160:649–659

Postmus D, Mavris M, Hillege HL et al (2016) Incorporating patient preferences into drug development and regulatory decision making: results from a quantitative pilot study with cancer patients, carers, and regulators. Clin Pharmacol Ther 99:548–554

Pulte D, Redaniel MT, Brenner H, Jansen L, Jeffreys M (2014) Recent improvement in survival of patients with multiple myeloma: variation by ethnicity. Leuk Lymphoma 55:1083–1089

Quach H, Fernyhough L, Henderson R et al (2017) Upfront lower dose lenalidomide is less toxic and does not compromise efficacy for vulnerable patients with relapsed refractory multiple myeloma: final analysis of the phase II RevLite study. Br J Haematol 177:441–448

Raedler LA (2016) Darzalex (Daratumumab): first anti-CD38 monoclonal antibody approved for patients with relapsed multiple myeloma. Am Health Drug Benefits 9:70–73

Rajkumar SV, Harousseau JL (2016) Next-generation multiple myeloma treatment: a pharmacoeconomic perspective. Blood 128:2757–2764

Rajkumar SV, Harousseau JL, Durie B et al (2011) Consensus recommendations for the uniform reporting of clinical trials: report of the International Myeloma Workshop Consensus Panel 1. Blood 117:4691–4695

Rajkumar SV, Richardson P, San Miguel JF (2015a) Guidelines for determination of the number of prior lines of therapy in multiple myeloma. Blood 126:921–922

Rajkumar SV, Landgren O, Mateos MV (2015b) Smoldering multiple myeloma. Blood 125:3069–3075

Richardson PG, Sonneveld P, Schuster MW et al (2005) Bortezomib or high-dose dexamethasone for relapsed multiple myeloma. N Engl J Med 352:2487–2498

Richardson PG, Sonneveld P, Schuster M et al (2007) Extended follow-up of a phase 3 trial in relapsed multiple myeloma: final time-to-event results of the APEX trial. Blood 110:3557–3560

Richardson PG, Sonneveld P, Schuster MW et al (2009) Reversibility of symptomatic peripheral neuropathy with bortezomib in the phase III APEX trial in relapsed multiple myeloma: impact of a dose-modification guideline. Br J Haematol 144:895–903

Richardson PG, Xie W, Jagannath S et al (2014) A phase 2 trial of lenalidomide, bortezomib, and dexamethasone in patients with relapsed and relapsed/refractory myeloma. Blood 123:1461–1469

Richardson PG, Hungria VT, Yoon SS et al (2016) Panobinostat plus bortezomib and dexamethasone in previously treated multiple myeloma: outcomes by prior treatment. Blood 127:713–721

Richardson PG, Attal M, San Miguel S et al (2017) A phase III, randomized, open-label study of isatuximab (SAR650984) plus pomalidomide (Pom) and dexamethasone (Dex) versus Pom and Dex in relapsed/refractory multiple myeloma. J Clin Oncol 35:TPS8057

Rosko A, Giralt S, Mateos MV, Dispenzieri A (2017) Myeloma in elderly patients: when less is more and more is more. Am Soc Clin Oncol Educ Book 37:575–585

San Miguel J, Weisel K, Moreau P et al (2013) Pomalidomide plus low-dose dexamethasone versus high-dose dexamethasone alone for patients with relapsed and refractory multiple myeloma (MM-003): a randomised, open-label, phase 3 trial. Lancet Oncol 14:1055–1066

San Miguel JF, Weisel KC, Song KW et al (2015) Impact of prior treatment and depth of response on survival in MM-003, a randomized phase 3 study comparing pomalidomide plus low-dose dexamethasone versus high-dose dexamethasone in relapsed/refractory multiple myeloma. Haematologica 100:1334–1339

San-Miguel JF, Dimopoulos MA, Stadtmauer EA et al (2011) Effects of lenalidomide and dexamethasone treatment duration on survival in patients with relapsed or refractory multiple myeloma treated with lenalidomide and dexamethasone. Clin Lymphoma Myeloma Leuk 11:38–43

San-Miguel JF, Hungria VT, Yoon SS et al (2014) Panobinostat plus bortezomib and dexamethasone versus placebo plus bortezomib and dexamethasone in patients with relapsed or relapsed and refractory multiple myeloma: a multicentre, randomised, double-blind phase 3 trial. Lancet Oncol 15:1195–1206

San-Miguel JF, Hungria VT, Yoon SS et al (2016) Overall survival of patients with relapsed multiple myeloma treated with panobinostat or placebo plus bortezomib and dexamethasone (the PANORAMA 1 trial): a randomised, placebo-controlled, phase 3 trial. Lancet Haematol 3:e506–ee15

Schey SA, Morgan GJ, Ramasamy K et al (2010) The addition of cyclophosphamide to lenalidomide and dexamethasone in multiply relapsed/refractory myeloma patients; a phase I/II study. Br J Haematol 150:326–333

Shah JJ, Stadtmauer EA, Abonour R et al (2015) Carfilzomib, pomalidomide, and dexamethasone for relapsed or refractory myeloma. Blood 126:2284–2290

Shah JJ, Jagannath S, Mateos M-V et al (2016) KEYNOTE-183: a randomized, open-label phase 3 study of pembrolizumab in combination with pomalidomide and low-dose dexamethasone in refractory or relapsed and refractory multiple myeloma (rrMM). J Clin Oncol 34:TPS8070

Siegel DS, Martin T, Wang M et al (2012) A phase 2 study of single-agent carfilzomib (PX-171-003-A1) in patients with relapsed and refractory multiple myeloma. Blood 120:2817–2825

Siegel DS, Oriol A, Rajnics P, et al (2017) Updated Results from ASPIRE and ENDEAVOR, Randomized, Open-Label, Multicenter Phase 3 Studies of Carfilzomib in Patients (Pts) with Relapsed/Refractory Multiple Myeloma (RRMM). In: Proceedings of the 2017 International Myeloma Workshop (IMW),16th IMW:e211-e2

Snowden JA, Greenfield DM, Bird JM et al (2017) Guidelines for screening and management of late and long-term consequences of myeloma and its treatment. Br J Haematol 176:888–907

Song X, Cong Z, Wilson K (2016) Real-world treatment patterns, comorbidities, and disease-related complications in patients with multiple myeloma in the United States. Curr Med Res Opin 32:95–103

Sonneveld P, Broijl A (2016) Treatment of relapsed and refractory multiple myeloma. Haematologica 101:396–406

Sonneveld P, Avet-Loiseau H, Lonial S et al (2016) Treatment of multiple myeloma with high-risk cytogenetics: a consensus of the International Myeloma Working Group. Blood 127:2955–2962

Stewart AK, Rajkumar SV, Dimopoulos MA et al (2015) Carfilzomib, lenalidomide, and dexamethasone for relapsed multiple myeloma. N Engl J Med 372:142–152

Stewart AK, Dimopoulos MA, Masszi T et al (2016) Health-related quality of life results from the open-label, randomized, phase III ASPIRE trial evaluating carfilzomib, lenalidomide, and dexamethasone versus lenalidomide and dexamethasone in patients with relapsed multiple myeloma. J Clin Oncol

Sun Z, Zheng F, Wu S, Liu Y, Guo H, Liu Y (2017) Triplet versus doublet combination regimens for the treatment of relapsed or refractory multiple myeloma: a meta-analysis of phase III randomized controlled trials. Crit Rev Oncol Hematol 113:249–255

Tariman JD, Doorenbos A, Schepp KG, Singhal S, Berry DL (2014) Older adults newly diagnosed with symptomatic myeloma and treatment decision making. Oncol Nurs Forum 41:411–419

Terpos E, International Myeloma Society (2017) Multiple Myeloma: clinical updates from the American Society of Hematology Annual Meeting 2016. Clin Lymphoma Myeloma Leuk 17:329–339

Touzeau C, Moreau P, Dumontet C (2017) Monoclonal antibody therapy in multiple myeloma. Leukemia 31:1039–1047

Tuchman SA, Moore JO, DeCastro CD et al (2017) Phase II study of dose-attenuated bortezomib, cyclophosphamide and dexamethasone ("VCD-Lite") in very old or otherwise toxicity-vulnerable adults with newly diagnosed multiple myeloma. J Geriatr Oncol 8:165–169

van Beurden-Tan CHY, Franken MG, Blommestein HM, Uyl-de Groot CA, Sonneveld P (2017) Systematic literature review and network meta-analysis of treatment outcomes in relapsed and/or refractory multiple myeloma. J Clin Oncol 35:1312–1319

van de Velde H, Londhe A, Ataman O et al (2017) Association between complete response and outcomes in transplant-eligible myeloma patients in the era of novel agents. Eur J Haematol 98:269–279

van de Velde HJ, Liu X, Chen G, Cakana A, Deraedt W, Bayssas M (2007) Complete response correlates with long-term survival and progression-free survival in high-dose therapy in multiple myeloma. Haematologica 92:1399–1406

Viala M, Bhakar AL, de la Loge C et al (2007) Patient-reported outcomes helped predict survival in multiple myeloma using partial least squares analysis. J Clin Epidemiol 60:670–679

Vij R, Wang M, Kaufman JL et al (2012a) An open-label, single-arm, phase 2 (PX-171-004) study of single-agent carfilzomib in bortezomib-naive patients with relapsed and/or refractory multiple myeloma. Blood 119:5661–5670

Vij R, Siegel DS, Jagannath S et al (2012b) An open-label, single-arm, phase 2 study of single-agent carfilzomib in patients with relapsed and/or refractory multiple myeloma who have been previously treated with bortezomib. Br J Haematol 158:739–748

Vogl DT, Raje N, Jagannath S et al (2017) Ricolinostat, the first selective histone deacetylase 6 inhibitor, in combination with bortezomib and dexamethasone for relapsed or refractory multiple myeloma. Clin Cancer Res 23(13):3307–3315

Wang M, Dimopoulos MA, Chen C et al (2008) Lenalidomide plus dexamethasone is more effective than dexamethasone alone in patients with relapsed or refractory multiple myeloma regardless of prior thalidomide exposure. Blood 112:4445–4451

Weber DM, Chen C, Niesvizky R et al (2007) Lenalidomide plus dexamethasone for relapsed multiple myeloma in North America. N Engl J Med 357:2133–2142

Weisel K, Dimopoulos M, Song KW et al (2015) Pomalidomide and low-dose dexamethasone improves health-related quality of life and prolongs time to worsening in relapsed/refractory patients with multiple myeloma enrolled in the MM-003 randomized phase III Trial. Clin Lymphoma Myeloma Leuk 15:519–530

Willan J, Eyre TA, Sharpley F, Watson C, King AJ, Ramasamy K (2016) Multiple myeloma in the very elderly patient: challenges and solutions. Clin Interv Aging 11:423–435

Yee AJ, Raje NS (2016) Sequencing of nontransplant treatments in multiple myeloma patients with active disease. Hematology Am Soc Hematol Educ Program 2016:495–503

Yong C, Seal B, Farrelly E et al (2016a) Practice patterns and outcomes in U.S. patients (pts) with relapsed/refractory multiple myeloma (RRMM) and comorbid renal dysfunction (RD) and/or cardiovascular disease (CVD). Haematologica 101:528

Yong K, Delforge M, Driessen C et al (2016b) Multiple myeloma: patient outcomes in real-world practice. Br J Haematol 175:252–264

Zangari M, Tricot G, Polavaram L et al (2010) Survival effect of venous thromboembolism in patients with multiple myeloma treated with lenalidomide and high-dose dexamethasone. J Clin Oncol 28:132–135

Minimal Residual Disease in Multiple Myeloma

Noemi Puig, Carmela Palladino, Bruno Paiva, and Marco Ladetto

6.1 Introduction

The number of drugs approved for the treatment of multiple myeloma (MM) in the last 10 years has significantly increased, and several agents with novel mechanisms of action and promising efficacy are in the pipeline (Ocio et al. 2014). The remarkable therapeutic advances achieved with the use of these drugs resulted in improved complete remission (CR) rates and significantly prolonged progression-free (PFS) and overall survival (OS) (Mateos and San Miguel 2013; McCarthy and Hahn 2013; Kumar et al. 2014). Unfortunately, most patients with MM continue to relapse despite achieving such optimal responses, thus reflecting the persistence of residual disease undetected with the currently used methods for response assessment.

Response assessment in MM has been mainly based in the measurement of the serum paraprotein and/or urinary light chain excretion. In response to improved treatment efficacy, the International Myeloma Working Group introduced in 2006 the normalization of serum-free light-chains ratio (sFLC) and the absence of bone marrow clonal plasma cells by immunohistochemistry or immunofluorescence as additional requirements to CR, in order to define a more stringent CR (Durie et al. 2006). However, immunohistochemistry cannot reliably be used to characterize small numbers of clonal plasma cells given that the regeneration of normal polyclonal plasma cells after therapy normalizes kappa/lambda ratios. Also, whereas the added prognostic value of the stringent over conventional CR criteria has been demonstrated by Kapoor et al. (2013), others have failed to show additional prognostic value of sFLC assessment among CR patients (de Larrea et al. 2009; Giarin et al. 2009; Paiva et al. 2011).

Therefore, to adapt to the rapidly evolving treatment landscape in MM, techniques that are more sensitive and more directly linked to the actual tumor burden are needed to monitor minimal residual disease (MRD). Furthermore categories of response should be updated accordingly (Rajkumar et al. 2011). Acknowledging this unmet need, the IMWG has recently published

N. Puig
Hospital Universitario de Salamanca, Instituto de Investigación Biomedica de Salamanca (IBSAL), Centro de Investigación del Cancer (IBMCC-USAL, CSIS), CIBERONC, Salamanca, Spain

C. Palladino • M. Ladetto (✉)
Divisione di Ematologia, Azienda Ospedaliera Santi Antonio e Biagio e Cesare Arrigo, Alessandria, Italy
e-mail: marco.ladetto@unito.it

B. Paiva
Clinica Universidad de Navarra, centro de Investigación Medica Aplicadas (CIMA), Instituto de Investigación Sanitaria de Navarra (IDISNA), CIBERONC, Pamplona, Spain

© Springer International Publishing Switzerland 2018
M. A. Dimopoulos et al. (eds.), *Multiple Myeloma and Other Plasma Cell Neoplasms*,
Hematologic Malignancies, https://doi.org/10.1007/978-3-319-25586-6_6

consensus criteria for MRD assessment in MM, aiming to identify better definitions of CR than those traditionally defined by conventional methods (Kumar et al. 2016). With the use of flow cytometry or gene sequencing for the identification of residual tumor cells in the bone marrow and sensitive imaging techniques to detect the presence of extramedullary residual disease, the IMWG has defined new response categories that will hopefully contribute to the uniform reporting within and outside clinical trials, to a better evaluation of treatment efficacy and also to help optimizing patient treatment according to the risk of relapse, particularly during consolidation or maintenance phases of therapy (Kumar et al. 2016).

6.2   Historic Perspective

The hypothesis that maximal cytoreduction could have a major impact on outcome is not a novel one and is accepted over the most disparate fields of onco-hematology (Harousseau et al. 2009; Abola et al. 2014). Most of the preliminary studies in this field date back to the last decade end of the previous millennium (Knulst et al. 1993; Dongen et al. 1998; van der Velden et al. 2003; Gribben et al. 1991). As a general rule, the factors which most critically impact the therapeutic relevance of MRD are the availability of effective treatment and the applicability of the method employed. For several years, both these factors acted against a rapid development of MRD detection in MM compared to other neoplasms such as acute lymphoblastic leukemia, acute promyelocytic leukemia and chronic myelogenous leukemia. Until the last decade, MM was consistently regarded as a chronic illness with limited chances of effective control and potentially "curative"; treatments such as allogeneic transplantation were considered as experimental approaches limited to highly selected groups of patients (Dhakal et al. 2016; Figueiredo et al. 2016). From the methodological point of view, both molecular and flow cytometry-based MRD approaches were in their infancy (Voena et al. 1997; Almeida et al. 1999). They were considerably labor-

intensive and had major limitations such as the nonquantitative nature of molecular MRD detection. Moreover issues of poor reproducibility and lack of standardization were consistently raised as major limitations. Finally some specific MM-related technical issues such as those related to somatic hypermutation made such evaluations definitely more complex in MM compared to other diseases. The technical scenario started to change at the turn of the century. Quantitative molecular MRD detection became a reality, and flow cytometry became increasingly feasible and reliable (Ladetto et al. 2000) In addition novel approaches became more reproducible and broadly used, while standardization efforts started in the context of other neoplasms provided the basis for method implementation in MM (van der Velden et al. 2007).

The most recent years witnessed further development in MRD detection in MM, including the development of the next-generation flow cytometry, digital droplets PCR next-generation sequencing (Martinez-Lopez et al. 2014; Lahuerta et al. 2017; Drandi et al. 2015; Ladetto et al. 2014; Flores-Montero et al. 2017). This led to the current phase in which MM should be considered one of the entities where MRD has reached one of the highest standards in terms of reliability, reproducibility, and uniform reporting compared to other mature B-cell disorders (Kumar et al. 2016).

6.3   Methodology

6.3.1   Flow

Multiparameter flow cytometry (MFC) is a method of analysis that allows the rapid study of certain physical and chemical characteristics of cells or other biological particles. The principle on which it is based is simple: the cells or biological particles to be analyzed are suspended in an isotonic fluid flow and are forced to pass, aligned, one by one and at a high speed (up to thousands of cells/second), in front of a light beam. The impact of each cell with the light beam, usually a laser of a given wavelength, produces individual signals corresponding to the different parameters of each individual cell, which are subsequently collected by detectors capable of measuring different individual physical and/or chemical characteristics. These detectors convert the signals into electronic pulses that are finally digitalized to allow the simultaneous measurement of several parameters in the same cell or particle.

MFC is particularly well-suited to study biological samples containing PCs, because it allows (1) simultaneous identification of normal vs. tumors cells at the single-cell level, (2) fast evaluation of a very high number of cells (in a few hours), (3) quantitative assessment of both normal and tumor cells and their corresponding antigen expression levels (e.g., for antibody-based therapy), (4) combined detection of cell surface and intracellular antigens (e.g., for confirmation of clonality within phenotypically aberrant cells) (Paiva et al. 2010).

Simultaneous assessment of CD38 and CD138 represents the best marker combination for specific identification of PC (Almeida et al. 1999; García-Sanz et al. 1999; Lin et al. 2004; Rawstron et al. 2001). In the event of anti-CD38 and/or anti-CD138 therapies, simultaneous surface plus intracellular staining with polyclonal anti-CD38 and/or anti-CD138 conjugates should be performed. Phenotypically aberrant clonal PCs typically show (1) underexpression of CD19, CD27, CD38, and/or CD45, (2) overexpression of CD56, and (3) asynchronous expression of CD117 (Dahl et al. 2002; Davies et al. 2001; Mateo Manzanera et al. 2005; Nowakowski et al. 2005; Pérez-Andrés et al. 2005; Rawstron et al. 2002; Robillard et al. 2005; San Miguel et al. 2002, 2006; Moreau et al. 2006). Although no single parameter reliably distinguishes clonal from normal PCs, a multiparameter approach that evaluates all markers used in a single tube can readily identify phenotypically aberrant PCs, provided enough cellular events are evaluated in the flow cytometer (Paiva et al. 2010).

The sensitivity of MFC has recently increased due to simultaneous assessment of >8 markers and evaluation of greater numbers of cells than what was previously feasible with analogical (four-color) instruments (Paiva et al. 2015). Thus, the availability of >8-color digital flow cytometers coupled to novel sample preparation procedures that allow fast and cost-effective evaluation of >5 million nucleated cells has boosted the sensitivity of modern MFC-based MRD monitoring into that achieved on molecular grounds ($\leq 10^{-5}$). It should be noted that current sensitivity of MFC is at least 1-log superior than that of previous MFC analyses (10^{-4}); therefore, ongoing MFC-based MRD monitoring should result in improved patient' risk stratification vs. 4- or 6-color analyses. Analysis of larger number of cells (i.e., >5 million events) allows visualization of previously undetectable normal PC subsets with more heterogeneous phenotypes, which implies the need for simultaneous evaluation of at least 8 parameters to improve specificity (and thereby sensitivity). Using validated and standardized 8-color panels, clonal PCs are readily and accurately distinguishable from normal PCs according to aberrant phenotypes (Paiva et al. 2015) and their clonality further confirmed by light chain restriction. Because such analyses rely on the recognition of aberrant antigenic patterns (i.e., different from normal), flow-MRD is applicable in virtually every MM patient without requiring for patient-specific diagnostic phenotypic profiles (although these are certainly useful). Equally important, the flow-MRD method incorporates a sample quality check of BM cellularity via simultaneous detection of B-cell precursors, erythroblasts, myeloid precursors, and/or mast cells. This information is critical to ensure sample quality and to identify hemodiluted BM aspirates that may lead to false-negative results.

A potential limitation of MFC is that current strategies could miss hypothetical MM cancer stem cells with more immature phenotypes. However, recent investigations conducted with sensitive ASO-PCR assessment of clonal Ig genes among FACS-sorted peripheral blood B-cell subsets revealed that such clonotypic cells are either absent or present below highly sensitive limits of detection (Thiago et al. 2014). The need for extensive expertise to analyze flow cytometric data, together with the lack of well-standardized flow-MRD methods have been pointed out as additional and perhaps the main limitations of conventional MFC immunophenotyping (Flanders et al. 2013). Furthermore, conventional visualization of flow cytometric data in bivariate (2D) dot plots becomes increasingly complex with increasing numbers of parameters. In recent years new multivariate computational tools and visualization plots (e.g., principal component analysis and canonical analysis) have been developed and integrated into innovative software packages for improved multidimensional identification and classification of different clusters of cells coexisting in a sample. These tools, together with the use of normal and malignant reference databases, further pave the way for automated detection and tracking of aberrant cell populations that deviate from the normal/reactive phenotypic profiles (Pedreira et al. 2013). Such innovative flow-MRD strategies are currently being developed by the EuroFlow Consortium under the Black Swan Research Initiative promoted by the International Myeloma Foundation (IMF), and it is likely to become the method of choice for accurate, high-sensitive, and automated flow-MRD monitoring in MM (i.e., "next-generation flow"). Regarding the potential impact of genetic heterogeneity and clonal tiding after treatment on the feasibility of MFC to detect MRD, it should be highlighted that the multidimensional approach of current flow cytometry immunophenotyping not only allows to detect clonal heterogeneity in approximately 30% of newly diagnosed patients but also to monitor all different phenotypic subclones throughout patients' treatment, thereby assessing potential (phenotypical) clonal selection upon therapy. Nevertheless, it should be noted that according to the experience of the Medical Research Council (MRC) and the Grupo Español de Mieloma (GEM) groups based on large patient cohorts, there are no major antigenic shifts for consensus markers (e.g.: CD19, CD38, CD45, or CD56) used to monitor MRD (*unpublished data*). Accordingly, potential clonal evolution throughout the course of treatment does not influence the efficacy of MFC-based MRD assessment. Additionally, discrimination between normal and myeloma PCs is still feasible in the (rare) event of phenotypic shifts from diagnostic to posttreatment MRD samples.

6.3.2 Molecular

MRD detection by molecular tools is a reliable approach which has a high degree of complementarity with respect to MFC. The technical principle is simple and based on the identification of clonotypic sequences, i.e., sequences that ideally are present exclusively on myeloma plasma cells and absent on other cells and particularly on nonmalignant plasma cells (Ferrero et al. 2011). There are several genetic sequences that fulfill these characteristics and the development of high-throughput approaches might potentially allow the detection and the monitoring of multiple targets including both universal targets representing the whole tumor burden, as well as subclonal genetic lesions which might allow monitoring of specific potentially more aggressive clones (Kotrova et al. 2017). Despite potential interest of multi-target approaches, the bulk of current knowledge on molecular evaluation of MRD was obtained using the immunoglobulin heavy and (to a lesser extent) light chain rearrangements (Ferrero et al. 2011). The immunoglobulin heavy chain rearrangement is a highly reliable target for MRD detection in MM: it is stable, contains long N insertions, and is heavily hypermutated. Therefore MRD detection is highly sensitive and specific. On the other hand, its identification was often extremely difficult especially as long as target identification relied on PCR amplification with primers derived from the framework regions followed by Sanger sequencing. Indeed this approach could be hampered by somatic mutations located in conserved regions used for consensus PCR amplification of the IgH rearrangement (Ferrero et al. 2011). Due to this limitation, DJ rearrangements and light chain rearrangements were frequently employed for patients failing IgH sequencing allowing to increase the number of molecularly evaluable patients (Puig et al. 2014). Current NGS-based approaches have basically overcome this limitation and currently ensure effective clonotype sequencing in the vast majority of patients (Ladetto et al. 2014). The subsequent step of MRD analysis following identification of a clonotypic sequence is the detection and quantification of these targets in follow-up samples. This was originally performed by nonquantitative approaches such as nested PCR (Voena et al. 1997), and further developed using real-time quantitative PCR (RQ-PCR) (Ladetto et al. 2000) and most recently digital droplet PCR (dd-PCR) (Drandi et al. 2015). Both RQ-PCR and dd-PCR ensure optimal quantification of MRD and their use allowed obtaining useful information on MRD dynamics in a number of clinical settings. More recently an NGS-based approach has been developed for MRD quantification. This method has been compared to RQ-PCR resulting in comparable sensitivity and proved highly valuable for outcome prediction (Martinez-Lopez et al. 2014; Ladetto et al. 2014). However it is usually provided as commercial service by one single company. However alternative methods are under development both at single academic institutions and within the Euro-MRD and Euro-clonality consortia (Martinez-Lopez et al. 2017; Wren et al. 2014; Brüggemann et al. 2010).

Currently both MFC and molecular MRD detection have been included in the MM consensus criteria for response, and minimal residual disease assessment in multiple myeloma has been recently developed which include the definition of "flow-MRD negative," "sequencing-MRD negative," and "sustained MRD negative," which are now routinely adopted in clinical trials addressing MRD as a secondary endpoint (Kumar et al. 2016). One potential added value of molecular MRD detection that still deserve to be addressed in detail is the use of plasma-derived cell-free DNA which seems to be of potential interest in other B-cell neoplasms.

6.3.3 Imaging

Currently, MRD assessment is mainly based on the analysis of the tumor burden in a single bone marrow aspirate. However, bone marrow infiltration in patients with MM is characteristically heterogeneous and the presence of extramedullary disease at diagnosis or during the disease is estimated in approximately 10% of MM patients (Bladé et al. 2012; Usmani et al. 2012; Short et al. 2011; Varettoni et al. 2010; Sheth et al. 2009; Dores et al. 2009). This feature is likely higher in the current era of extended OS in MM with the novel treatment options and could be even higher using sensitive imaging methods. Considering this, it becomes clear that MRD assessment in MM and the definition of high-quality responses cannot be merely based on the analysis of a single bone marrow sample but must include the analysis of the presence of extramedullary disease.

Two imaging techniques have been applied to the identification of extramedullary disease at diagnosis and to assess the presence of residual disease posttreatment: PET and MRI. 18F-fluorodeoxyglucose PET assesses tumor metabolic activity, and the low-dose CT usually performed for localization is also useful for the assessment of MM-associated bone disease. Overall, the detection of PET-positive lesions has prognostic value in MM patients at diagnosis and at the time of relapse (Zamagni et al. 2011; Usmani et al. 2013; Bartel et al. 2009; van Lammeren-Venema et al. 2012; Elliott et al. 2011). However, PET-based MRD monitoring is mainly based on the FDG uptake (rather than in the identification of bone lesions), and both false-negative and false-positive results due to coexisting infectious or inflammatory processes may be seen (Caers et al. 2014). Various studies have shown the prognostic value of MRD assessment with PET/CT at different time points within the treatment scheme of MM patients undergoing ASCT. Among them, the Italian group has shown that, among patients achieving conventional CR post-ASCT, those associating negative PET scans presented with an improved PFS and OS (Zamagni et al. 2011). Most importantly, data from the IFM2009 trial showed that among the 86 patients with PET and MRD by MFC available for analysis, PFS was significantly higher in the 41 patients presenting with negative PET scans as compared with those patients with positive results using either or both methods.

MRI is the most sensitive imaging technique to detect focal lesions in the spine (Dimopoulos et al. 2009; Hillengass and Landgren 2013). It also provides information on the extent of soft tissue disease and the pattern of marrow infiltration (normal, focal, heterogeneous, or diffuse). However, MRI responses can be significantly delayed as marrow signal abnormalities can persist a long time after therapy in both responding and non-responding patients (Elliott et al. 2011; Derlin et al. 2013; Walker et al. 2012). MRI also has a low specificity in the differentiation of viable disease from bone remodeling (Derlin et al. 2012; Shortt et al. 2009). Thus, the usefulness of MRI for the MRD assessment posttreatment warrants further investigations to be elucidated.

A recent comparison between WB-MRI and PET/CT in transplant-eligible patients showed that, against conventional response criteria, PET/CT had lower sensitivity (50% vs 80%) but higher specificity (85% vs 38%) than WB-MRI (Hillengass et al. 2011). While the utility of other MRI-based techniques is still under investigation (e.g., dynamic contrast-enhanced MRI) (Hillengass et al. 2011), the current perception is that PET/CT represents the most promising imaging tool to monitor MRD in MM. New imaging technologies are currently under development, such as PET/MRI, in which the PET detects avid focal lesions, while the MRI shows the location of the lesions and informs on myeloma cell infiltration of the bone marrow (Fraioli and Punwani 2014). Also, a small study comparing PET/CT and functional WB-MRI (diffusion-weighted imaging) showed that the latter is superior in detecting focal and diffuse infiltration of the bone marrow (Pawlyn et al. 2016). However, standardization of PET-CT (including response criteria) and comparison with other sensitive BM-based MRD methods are still needed to define which imaging technique or combination gives the higher clinical benefit for patients with MM, both at diagnosis and for response assessment (Kumar et al. 2016).

6.4 Clinical Application

6.4.1 Transplant Setting

Patients undergoing autologous or allogeneic transplantation have always been considered ideal candidates for MRD evaluation, given the heavy cytoreduction, the high rate of CR and the potential existence of ongoing graft vs myeloma effect (for allogeneic transplantation). Early reports from the 1990s showed that autologous transplantation was unable to induce MRD negativity by nested PCR in MM as opposed to allogeneic transplantation that allowed a proportion of patients to enter molecular remission and become long-term MRD-free survivors (Corradini et al. 1996; Tarella et al. 1999).

The substantial impact of the introduction of novel agents in MM on tumor clearance was clearly demonstrated by studies indicating that non-chemotherapeutic-based combinations were able to further decrease tumor burden after autologous transplantation allowing a proportion of patients to enter molecular remission (Ladetto et al. 2010). Currently a large number of reports have proven the prognostic value of MRD evaluated by both molecular and flow cytometry-based approaches on multiple survival parameters (Kumar et al. 2016) and in the context of different therapeutic programs. Moreover MRD acted as an independent prognosticator in several large trials, and its impact was independent from other important prognosticators such as cytogenetics (Paiva et al. 2011, 2008, 2012; Sarasquete et al. 2005; Puig et al. 2014; Hillengass et al. 2011; Ladetto et al. 2010; Rawstron et al. 2013; Martinez-Sanchez et al. 2008; Barlogie et al. 2008; Korthals et al. 2012; Putkonen et al. 2010; Martinelli et al. 2000). One recent pooled data analysis confirmed the value of MRD (Lahuerta et al. 2017; Flores-Montero et al. 2017). Moreover it showed that achievement of complete remission (CR) in the absence of MRD negativity was not associated with prolonged progression-free survival, clearly surpassing the prognostic value of CR achievement. Moreover it showed that the predictive value of MRD was particularly evident in patients with high-risk cytogenetics, indicating that tumor burden is critical even in neoplasms where the rapid kinetic and genetic instability of the tumor clone could theoretically impair its value.

Of particular importance were kinetic studies addressing the behavior of residual tumor burden over time. These studies were performed both in the allogeneic and autologous SCT setting. These studies indicate that achievement of molecular remission is often not stable, although cases that appear devoid of molecular disease for prolonged periods are recorded especially in the allogeneic transplantation setting (Ladetto et al. 2015; Ferrero et al. 2015). Another important point which has been observed is that clinical relapse is in the majority of cases heralded by the reappearance of molecularly detectable disease with an anticipation of several months, indicating that molecular relapse is a potential window of interest where the application of experimental preemptive treatment could be applied. This strategy has been successfully tested in other B-cell disorders.

6.4.2 Elderly

The prognostic value of MRD assessment was not investigated outside of the SCT setting until recently, when the incorporation of novel agents into the treatment of patients who were not fit for HDT/ASCT showed increased CR rates and prolonged survival (Mateos et al. 2014). Puig et al. have demonstrated that among patients treated according to the PETHEMA/GEM2005MAS65 protocol, those in molecular-CR after induction had a PFS not yet reached, whereas MRD-positive patients had a significantly shorter PFS (median 31 months; $P = 0.03$) (Puig et al. 2014). Similarly, a sub-analysis performed by Martinez-Lopez on elderly patients confirmed the prognostic significance of achieving MRD negativity by NGS (Martinez-Lopez et al. 2014). Regarding MFC, in the MRC myeloma IX protocol only a few patients achieved flow-CR after induction regimens without proteasome inhibitors, and these showed nonsignificantly superior PFS (Rawstron et al. 2013). In contrast, in the PETHEMA/GEM2005MAS65 study patients were monitored after 6 induction cycles with bortezomib, melphalan, prednisone (VMP), or bortezomib, thalidomide, prednisone (VTP), and, within a subset of 102 cases in CR/VGPR, 30% attained MRD-negativity with PFS and OS rates at 3 years of 90% and 94%, respectively (de Larrea et al. 2009). A recent update of this study (Mateos et al. 2014) after a median follow-up >5 years shows median PFS and OS rates not yet reached for patients in flow-CR after VMP (but not VTP) induction. These results suggest that MRD monitoring is also clinically relevant in elderly patients. Since MRD-negative cases after two different regimens should experience similar outcomes (Böttcher et al. 2012), this study also unraveled that the four-color MFC assay originally performed was underpowered for ultrasensitive detection of MRD (Mateos et al. 2014). This has been recently confirmed by comparing deep-sequencing vs. four-color MFC-based MRD monitoring in younger and elderly MM patients, indicating that MRD prognostication is improved when more sensitive (i.e., lower) limits of detection (i.e.: ≤ 1 tumor cell in 100,000 vs. 10,000 normal cells; 10^{-5} vs. 10^{-4}) are reached (Martinez-Lopez et al. 2014).

Accordingly, in 2016 we reported that second-generation flow-MRD monitoring was clinically meaningful in a series of 162 transplant-ineligible patients enrolled in the phase II GEM2010MAS65 study. Noteworthy, we showed that by applying the limit of detection reached with first-generation flow (ie, 10^{-4}), up to 30% of patients with persistent MRD detectable by second-generation flow would had been wrongly classified as MRD negative. We also showed that the ability to monitor MRD up to 10^{-5} was clinically relevant, because this level identifies a subset of patients (those between 10^{-4} and 10^{-5}) with inferior survival than MRD-negative cases, and like that of MRD-positive patients at the $\geq 10^{-4}$ level.

6.5 Future Perspectives

So far no clinical trial has randomized MM patients according to their MRD status, in order to investigate the role of MRD to individualize therapy. Overall, the experience of several cooperative groups using different MRD techniques indicates that persistence of MRD is always an adverse prognostic feature, even among CR patients. Consequently, it would be safer to take clinical decisions based on MRD positivity rather than on MRD negativity, since the patchy pattern of BM infiltration typically observed in MM leads to a degree of uncertainty regarding MRD-negative results: Does this guarantee absence of tumor cells or is it the result of a non-representative BM sample due to patchy tumor infiltration? Many studies have shown the value of MRD to evaluate the efficacy of specific treatment phases and, therefore, to support potential treatment decisions. For example, both the Spanish PETHEMA and the UK MRC study groups have shown that MRD kinetics before and after HDT/ASCT allow identification of chemosensitive vs. chemoresistant patients (Rawstron et al. 2013; Paiva et al. 2008). For the latter, it could be hypothesized that consolidation with alternative therapies would be needed to improve outcomes. Following consolidation physicians face another treatment decision: maintenance vs no maintenance and duration? Ladetto et al. reported PFS rates of 100% vs. 57% for patients in molecular-CR vs. MRD-positive cases after consolidation, respectively (Ladetto et al. 2010). Since no maintenance therapy was given in the GIMEMA VEL-03-096 study, one might hypothesize that for those cases failing to reach MRD negativity despite being in CR/nCR after consolidation, maintenance may represent an effective approach to eradicate MRD levels and improve outcome. Accordingly, Rawstron et al. have shown that one out of four MRD-positive patients randomized to the maintenance arm of the MRC-myeloma IX (intensive) study turned into MRD negative, and experienced significantly prolonged PFS vs. the abstention arm (Rawstron et al. 2013). However, because even MRD-negative patients receiving maintenance continue to show late relapses (Rawstron et al. 2013), it may be envisioned that we need to increase the sensitivity of MRD techniques to better monitoring "theoretically MRD-negative" patients during maintenance therapy; moreover, if treatment decisions are taken according to patients' MRD status, follow-up MRD studies would also become useful to detect MRD reappearance preceding clinical relapse (Ferrero et al. 2015). This approach is likely to imply serial MRD assessment which, at the moment, would require the need of invasive and inconvenient multiple BM aspirates. Most recently, NGS has been evaluated in PB (i.e., plasma) from MM patients after induction, and this would represent an attractive minimally invasive approach. However, preliminary data indicates that clonotypic sequences identified at baseline become undetectable with just a few cycles of chemotherapy, even among electrophoresis-positive patients. Thus, further research is warranted to establish the feasibility of PB (e.g., cell- or free DNA-based) MRD monitoring. Furthermore, our knowledge on clonal tiding (i.e., disappearance of pre-existing or occurrence of new clones), during maintenance or progression-free periods without therapy, is very limited if existing at all, and the concept of clonal tiding should also be taken into consideration while designing such treatment strategies.

The choice of MRD technology for monitoring will depend on how individual centers' priorities adjust to the specific advantages that each tool has to offer. In turn, extensive research is still warranted to determine how to best integrate medullary and extramedullary MRD monitoring. In other hematological malignancies, baseline risk factors and MRD monitoring have an established and complementary role to individualize treatment. Over the last two decades, several groups have consistently confirmed the added value of MRD in MM, and the time has come to establish the role of baseline risk factors plus MRD monitoring for tailored therapy. This requires the introduction of standardized, highly sensitive, cost-effective, and broadly available MRD techniques in clinical trials.

References

Abola MV, Prasad V, Jena AB (2014) Association between treatment toxicity and outcomes in oncology clinical trials. Ann Oncol 25(11):2284–2289. https://doi.org/10.1093/annonc/mdu444

Almeida J, Orfao A, Ocqueteau M, Mateo G, Corral M, Caballero MD et al (1999) High-sensitive immunophenotyping and DNA ploidy studies for the investigation of minimal residual disease in multiple myeloma. Br J Haematol 107(1):121–131. http://www.ncbi.nlm.nih.gov/pubmed/10520032

Barlogie B, Anaissie E, Haessler J et al (2008) Complete remission sustained 3 years from treatment initiation is a powerful surrogate for extended survival in multiple myeloma. Cancer 113:355–359

Bartel TB, Haessler J, Brown TLY, Shaughnessy JD, van Rhee F, Anaissie E et al (2009) F18-fluorodeoxyglucose positron emission tomography in the context of other imaging techniques and prognostic factors in multiple myeloma. Blood 114(10):2068–2076. http://www.bloodjournal.org/cgi/doi/10.1182/blood-2009-03-213280

Bladé J, de Larrea CF, Rosiñol L (2012) Extramedullary involvement in multiple myeloma. Haematologica 97(11):1618–1619. http://www.haematologica.org/cgi/doi/10.3324/haematol.2012.078519

Böttcher S, Ritgen M, Fischer K, Stilgenbauer S, Busch RM, Fingerle-Rowson G et al (2012) Minimal residual disease quantification is an independent predictor of progression-free and overall survival in chronic lymphocytic leukemia: a multivariate analysis from the randomized GCLLSG CLL8 trial. J Clin Oncol 30(9):980–988. http://ascopubs.org/doi/10.1200/JCO.2011.36.9348

Brüggemann M, Schrauder A, Raff T, Pfeifer H, Dworzak M, Ottmann OG, Asnafi V, Baruchel A, Bassan R, Benoit Y, Biondi A, Cavé H, Dombret H, Fielding AK, Foà R, Gökbuget N, Goldstone AH, Goulden N, Henze G, Hoelzer D, Janka-Schaub GE, Macintyre EA, Pieters R, Rambaldi A, Ribera JM, Schmiegelow K, Spinelli O, Stary J, von Stackelberg A, Kneba M, Schrappe M, van Dongen JJ, European Working Group for Adult Acute Lymphoblastic Leukemia (EWALL).; International Berlin-Frankfurt-Münster Study Group (I-BFM-SG) (2010) Standardized MRD quantification in European ALL trials: proceedings of the second international symposium on MRD assessment in Kiel, Germany, 18–20 September 2008. Leukemia 24(3):521–535. https://doi.org/10.1038/leu.2009.268

Caers J, Withofs N, Hillengass J, Simoni P, Zamagni E, Hustinx R et al (2014) The role of positron emission tomography-computed tomography and magnetic resonance imaging in diagnosis and follow up of multiple myeloma. Haematologica 99(4):629–637. http://www.haematologica.org/cgi/doi/10.3324/haematol.2013.091918

Corradini P, Ladetto M, Astolfi M, Voena C, Tarella C, Bacigalupo A, Pileri A (1996) Clinical and molecular remission after allogeneic blood cell transplantation in a patient with mantle-cell lymphoma. Br J Haematol 94(2):376–378

Dahl IMS, Rasmussen T, Kauric G, Husebekk A (2002) Differential expression of CD56 and CD44 in the evolution of extramedullary myeloma. Br J Haematol 116(2):273–277. http://www.ncbi.nlm.nih.gov/pubmed/11841427

Davies FE, Forsyth PD, Rawstron AC, Owen RG, Pratt G, Evans PA et al (2001) The impact of attaining a minimal disease state after high-dose melphalan and autologous transplantation for multiple myeloma. Br J Haematol 112(3):814–819. http://www.ncbi.nlm.nih.gov/pubmed/11260088

de Larrea CF, Cibeira MT, Elena M, Arostegui JI, Rosiñol L, Rovira M et al (2009) Abnormal serum free light chain ratio in patients with multiple myeloma in complete remission has strong association with the presence of oligoclonal bands: implications for stringent complete remission definition. Blood 114(24):4954–4956. http://www.bloodjournal.org/cgi/doi/10.1182/blood-2009-06-224832

Derlin T, Weber C, Habermann CR, Herrmann J, Wisotzki C, Ayuk F et al (2012) 18F-FDG PET/CT for detection and localization of residual or recurrent disease in patients with multiple myeloma after stem cell transplantation. Eur J Nucl Med Mol Imaging 39(3):493–500. http://link.springer.com/10.1007/s00259-011-1993-8

Derlin T, Peldschus K, Münster S, Bannas P, Herrmann J, Stübig T et al (2013) Comparative diagnostic performance of 18F-FDG PET/CT versus whole-body MRI for determination of remission status in multiple myeloma after stem cell transplantation. Eur Radiol 23(2):570–578. http://link.springer.com/10.1007/s00330-012-2600-5

Dhakal B, Vesole DH, Hari PN (2016) Allogeneic stem cell transplantation for multiple myeloma: is there a future? Bone Marrow Transplant 51(4):492–500. https://doi.org/10.1038/bmt.2015.325. Epub 2016 Jan 4

Dimopoulos M, Terpos E, Comenzo RL, Tosi P, Beksac M, Sezer O et al (2009) International myeloma working group consensus statement and guidelines regarding the current role of imaging techniques in the diagnosis and monitoring of multiple myeloma. Leukemia 23(9):1545–1556. http://www.nature.com/doifinder/10.1038/leu.2009.89

Dongen JJM, Seriu T, Panzer-Grümayer ER, Biondi A, Pongers-Willemse MJ, Corral L, Stolz F, Schrappe M, Masera G, Kamps WA, Gadner H, Van Wering ER, Ludwig W-D, Basso G, MAC DB, Cazzaniga G, Hettinger K, Van der Does-van den Berg A, WCJ H, Riehm H, Bartram CR (1998) Prognostic value of minimal residual disease in acute lymphoblastic leukaemia in childhood. Lancet 352:1731–1738

Dores GM, Landgren O, KA MG, Curtis RE, Linet MS, Devesa SS (2009) Plasmacytoma of bone, extramedullary plasmacytoma, and multiple myeloma: incidence and survival in the United States, 1992–2004. Br J Haematol 144(1):86–94. http://doi.wiley.com/10.1111/j.1365-2141.2008.07421.x

Drandi D, Kubiczkova-Besse L, Ferrero S, Dani N, Passera R, Mantoan B, Gambella M, Monitillo L, Saraci E, Ghione P, Genuardi E, Barbero D, Omedè P, Barberio D, Hajek R, Vitolo U, Palumbo A, Cortelazzo S, Boccadoro M, Inghirami G, Ladetto M (2015) Minimal residual disease detection by droplet digital PCR in multiple myeloma, mantle cell lymphoma, and follicular lymphoma: a comparison with real-time PCR. J Mol Diagn 17(6):652–660. https://doi.org/10.1016/j.jmoldx.2015.05.007. Epub 2015 Aug 28

Durie BGM, Harousseau J-L, Miguel JS, Bladé J, Barlogie B, Anderson K et al (2006) International uniform response criteria for multiple myeloma. Leukemia 20(9):1467–1473. http://www.ncbi.nlm.nih.gov/pubmed/16855634

Elliott BM, Peti S, Osman K, Scigliano E, Lee D, Isola L et al (2011) Combining FDG-PET/CT with laboratory data yields superior results for prediction of relapse in multiple myeloma. Eur J Haematol 86(4):289–298. http://doi.wiley.com/10.1111/j.1600-0609.2010.01575.x

Ferrero S et al (2011) Minimal residual disease detection in lymphoma and multiple myeloma: impact on therapeutic paradigms. Hematol Oncol 29(4):167–176

Ferrero S, Ladetto M, Drandi D, Cavallo F, Genuardi E, Urbano M et al (2015) Long-term results of the GIMEMA VEL-03-096 trial in MM patients receiving VTD consolidation after ASCT: MRD kinetics' impact on survival. Leukemia 29(3):689–695. http://www.nature.com/doifinder/10.1038/leu.2014.219

Figueiredo A, Atkins H, Kekre N, Kew A, McCurdy A (2016) Allogeneic stem cell transplantation for multiple myeloma: a single center experience. Blood 128:5874

Flanders A, Stetler-Stevenson M, Landgren O (2013) Minimal residual disease testing in multiple myeloma by flow cytometry: major heterogeneity. Blood 122(6):1088–1089. http://www.bloodjournal.org/cgi/doi/10.1182/blood-2013-05-506170

Flores-Montero J, Sanoja-Flores L, Paiva B, Puig N, García-Sánchez O, Böttcher S, van der Velden VH, Pérez-Morán JJ, Vidriales MB, García-Sanz R, Jimenez C, González M, Martínez-López J, Corral-Mateos A, Grigore GE, Fluxá R, Pontes R, Caetano J, Sedek L, Del Cañizo MC, Bladé J, Lahuerta JJ, Aguilar C, Bárez A, García-Mateo A, Labrador J, Leoz P, Aguilera-Sanz C, San-Miguel J, Mateos MV, Durie B, van Dongen JJ, Orfao A (2017) Next generation flow for highly sensitive and standardized detection of minimal residual disease in multiple myeloma. Leukemia 31(10):2094–2103. https://doi.org/10.1038/leu.2017.29

Fraioli F, Punwani S (2014) Clinical and research applications of simultaneous positron emission tomography and MRI. Br J Radiol 87(1033):20130464. http://www.birpublications.org/doi/10.1259/bjr.20130464

García-Sanz R, Orfão A, González M, Tabernero MD, Bladé J, Moro MJ et al (1999) Primary plasma cell leukemia: clinical, immunophenotypic, DNA ploidy, and cytogenetic characteristics. Blood 93(3):1032–1037. http://www.ncbi.nlm.nih.gov/pubmed/9920853

Giarin MM, Giaccone L, Sorasio R, Sfiligoi C, Amoroso B, Cavallo F et al (2009) Serum free light chain ratio, total kappa/lambda ratio, and immunofixation results are not prognostic factors after stem cell transplantation for newly diagnosed multiple myeloma. Clin Chem 55(8):1510–1516. http://www.clinchem.org/cgi/doi/10.1373/clinchem.2009.124370

Gribben JG, Freedman AS, Neuberg D, Roy DC, Blake KW, Woo SD, Grossbard ML, Rabinowe SN, Coral F, Freeman GJ et al (1991) Immunologic purging of marrow assessed by PCR before autologous bone marrow transplantation for B-cell lymphoma. N Engl J Med 325(22):1525–1533

Harousseau J-L, Attal M, Avet-Loiseau H (2009) The role of complete response in multiple myeloma. Blood 114:3139–3146. https://doi.org/10.1182/blood-2009-03-201053

Hillengass J, Landgren O (2013) Challenges and opportunities of novel imaging techniques in monoclonal plasma cell disorders: imaging "early myeloma". Leuk Lymphoma 54(7):1355–1363. http://www.tandfonline.com/doi/full/10.3109/10428194.2012.740559

Hillengass J, Bäuerle T, Bartl R, Andrulis M, McClanahan F, Laun FB et al (2011) Diffusion-weighted imaging for non-invasive and quantitative monitoring of bone marrow infiltration in patients with monoclonal plasma cell disease: a comparative study with histology. Br J Haematol 153(6):721–728. http://doi.wiley.com/10.1111/j.1365-2141.2011.08658.x

Kapoor P, Kumar SK, Dispenzieri A, Lacy MQ, Buadi F, Dingli D et al (2013) Importance of achieving stringent complete response after autologous stem-cell transplantation in multiple myeloma. J Clin Oncol 31(36):4529–4535. http://ascopubs.org/doi/10.1200/JCO.2013.49.0086

Knulst AC, Adriaansen HJ, Hählen K, Stigter JC, van den Beemd MW, Hagemeijer A, van Dongen JJ, Hooijkaas H (1993) Early diagnosis of smoldering acute lymphoblastic leukemia using immunological marker analysis. Leukemia 7(4):532–536

Korthals M, Sehnke N, Kronenwett R et al (2012) The level of minimal residual disease in the bone marrow of patients with multiple myeloma before high-dose therapy and autologous blood stem cell transplantation is an independent predictive parameter. Biol Blood Marrow Transplant 18:423–431

Kotrova M et al (2017) Is next-generation sequencing the way to go for residual disease monitoring in acute lymphoblastic leukemia? Mol Diagn Ther 21:481–492. https://doi.org/10.1007/s40291-017-0277-9

Kumar SK, Dispenzieri A, Lacy MQ, Gertz MA, Buadi FK, Pandey S et al (2014) Continued improvement in survival in multiple myeloma: changes in early mortality and outcomes in older patients. Leukemia 28(5):1122–1128. http://www.nature.com/doifinder/10.1038/leu.2013.313

Kumar S, Paiva B, Anderson KC, Durie B, Landgren O, Moreau P et al (2016) International myeloma working group consensus criteria for response and minimal residual disease assessment in multiple myeloma. Lancet Oncol 17(8):e328–e346. http://www.ncbi.nlm.nih.gov/pubmed/27511158

Ladetto M, Donovan JW, Harig S, Trojan A, Poor C, Schlossnan R, Anderson KC, Gribben JG (2000) Real-time polymerase chain reaction of immunoglobulin rearrangements for quantitative evaluation of minimal residual disease in multiple myeloma. Biol Blood Marrow Transplant 6(3):241–253

Ladetto M, Pagliano G, Ferrero S, Cavallo F, Drandi D, Santo L et al (2010) Major tumor shrinking and persistent molecular remissions after consolidation with bortezomib, thalidomide, and dexamethasone in patients with autografted myeloma. J Clin Oncol 28(12):2077–2084. http://ascopubs.org/doi/10.1200/JCO.2009.23.7172

Ladetto M, Brüggemann M, Monitillo L, Ferrero S, Pepin F, Drandi D, Barbero D, Palumbo A, Passera R, Boccadoro M, Ritgen M, Gökbuget N, Zheng J, Carlton V, Trautmann H, Faham M, Pott C (2014) Next-generation sequencing and real-time quantitative PCR for minimal residual disease detection in B-cell disorders. Leukemia 28(6):1299–1307. https://doi.org/10.1038/leu.2013.375. Epub 2013 Dec 17

Ladetto M, Ferrero S, Drandi D, Festuccia M, Patriarca F, Mordini N, Cena S, Benedetto R, Guarona G, Ferrando F, Brunello L, Ghione P, Boccasavia V, Fanin R, Omedè P, Giaccone L, Palumbo A, Passera R, Boccadoro M, Bruno B (2015) Prospective molecular monitoring of minimal residual disease after non-myeloablative allografting in newly diagnosed multiple myeloma. Leukemia 30(5):1211–1214. https://doi.org/10.1038/leu.2015.269

Lahuerta JJ, Paiva B, Vidriales MB, Cordón L, Cedena MT, Puig N, Martinez-Lopez J, Rosiñol L, Gutierrez NC, Martín-Ramos ML, Oriol A, Teruel AI, Echeveste MA, de Paz R, de Arriba F, Hernandez MT, Palomera L, Martinez R, Martin A, Alegre A, De la Rubia J, Orfao A, Mateos MV, Blade J, San-Miguel JF, GEM (Grupo Español de Mieloma)/PETHEMA (Programa para el Estudio de la Terapéutica en Hemopatías Malignas) Cooperative Study Group (2017) Depth of response in multiple myeloma: a pooled analysis of three PETHEMA/GEM clinical trials. J Clin Oncol 35(25):2900–2910. https://doi.org/10.1200/JCO.2016.69.2517

Lin P, Owens R, Tricot G, Wilson CS (2004) Flow cytometric immunophenotypic analysis of 306 cases of multiple myeloma. Am J Clin Pathol 121(4):482–488. http://www.ncbi.nlm.nih.gov/pubmed/15080299

Martinelli G, Terragna C, Zamagni E et al (2000) Molecular remission after allogeneic or autologous transplantation of hematopoietic stem cells for multiple myeloma. J Clin Oncol 18:2273–2281

Martinez-Lopez J, Lahuerta JJ, Pepin F, González M, Barrio S, Ayala R et al (2014) Prognostic value of deep sequencing method for minimal residual disease detection in multiple myeloma. Blood 123(20):3073–3079. http://www.bloodjournal.org/cgi/doi/10.1182/blood-2014-01-550020

Martinez-Lopez J, Sanchez-Vega B, Barrio S, Cuenca I, Ruiz-Heredia Y, Alonso R, Rapado I, Marin C, Cedena M-T, Paiva B, Puig N, Mateos M-V, Ayala R, Hernández M-T, Jimenez C, Rosiñol L, Martínez R, Teruel A-I, Gutiérrez N, Martin-Ramos M-L, Oriol A, Bargay J, Bladé J, San-Miguel J, Garcia-Sanz R,

Lahuerta J-J (2017) Analytical and clinical validation of a novel in-house deep-sequencing method for minimal residual disease monitoring in a phase II trial for multiple myeloma. Leukemia 31(6):1446–1449. https://doi.org/10.1038/leu.2017.58

Martinez-Sanchez P, Montejano L, Sarasquete ME et al (2008) Evaluation of minimal residual disease in multiple myeloma patients by fl uorescent-polymerase chain reaction: the prognostic impact of achieving molecular response. Br J Haematol 142:766–774

Mateo Manzanera G, San Miguel Izquierdo JF, Orfao de Matos A (2005) Immunophenotyping of plasma cells in multiple myeloma. Methods Mol Med 113:5–24. http://www.ncbi.nlm.nih.gov/pubmed/15968091

Mateo M-V, San Miguel JF (2013) How should we treat newly diagnosed multiple myeloma patients? Hematol Am Soc Hematol Educ Progr 2013(1):488–495. http://www.asheducationbook.org/cgi/doi/10.1182/asheducation-2013.1.488

Mateos M-V, Oriol A, Martínez-López J, Teruel A-I, López de la Guía A, López J et al (2014) GEM2005 trial update comparing VMP/VTP as induction in elderly multiple myeloma patients: do we still need alkylators? Blood 124(12):1887–1893. http://www.ncbi.nlm.nih.gov/pubmed/25102853

McCarthy PL, Hahn T (2013) Strategies for induction, autologous hematopoietic stem cell transplantation, consolidation, and maintenance for transplantation-eligible multiple myeloma patients. Hematol Am Soc Hematol Educ Progr 2013(1):496–503. http://www.asheducationbook.org/cgi/doi/10.1182/asheducation-2013.1.496

Moreau P, Robillard N, Jégo G, Pellat C, Le Gouill S, Thoumi S et al (2006) Lack of CD27 in myeloma delineates different presentation and outcome. Br J Haematol 132(2):168–170. http://www.ncbi.nlm.nih.gov/pubmed/16398651

Nowakowski GS, Witzig TE, Dingli D, Tracz MJ, Gertz MA, Lacy MQ et al (2005) Circulating plasma cells detected by flow cytometry as a predictor of survival in 302 patients with newly diagnosed multiple myeloma. Blood 106(7):2276–2279. http://www.ncbi.nlm.nih.gov/pubmed/15961515

Ocio EM, Richardson PG, Rajkumar SV, Palumbo A, Mateos MV, Orlowski R et al (2014) New drugs and novel mechanisms of action in multiple myeloma in 2013: a report from the international myeloma working group (IMWG). Leukemia 28(3):525–542. http://www.nature.com/doifinder/10.1038/leu.2013.350

Paiva B, Vidriales M-B, Cerveró J, Mateo G, Pérez JJ, Montalbán MA et al (2008) Multiparameter flow cytometric remission is the most relevant prognostic factor for multiple myeloma patients who undergo autologous stem cell transplantation. Blood 112(10):4017–4023. http://www.bloodjournal.org/cgi/doi/10.1182/blood-2008-05-159624

Paiva B, Almeida J, Pérez-Andrés M, Mateo G, López A, Rasillo A et al (2010) Utility of flow cytometry immunophenotyping in multiple myeloma and other clonal plasma cell-related disorders. Cytometry B Clin Cytom 78(4):239–252. http://doi.wiley.com/10.1002/cyto.b.20512

Paiva B, Martinez-Lopez J, Vidriales M-B, Mateos M-V, Montalban M-A, Fernandez-Redondo E et al (2011) Comparison of immunofixation, serum free light chain, and immunophenotyping for response evaluation and prognostication in multiple myeloma. J Clin Oncol 29(12):1627–1633. http://ascopubs.org/doi/10.1200/JCO.2010.33.1967

Paiva B, Gutierrez NC, Rosinol L, for the GEM (Grupo Español de MM)/PETHEMA (Programa para el Estudio de la Terapéutica en Hemopatías Malignas) Cooperative Study Groups et al (2012) High-risk cytogenetics and persistent minimal residual disease by multiparameter flow cytometry predict unsustained complete response after autologous stem cell transplantation in multiple myeloma. Blood 119:687–691

Paiva B, Puig N, García-Sanz R, San Miguel JF, Grupo Español de Mieloma (GEM)/Programa para el Estudio de la Terapéutica en Hemopatías Malignas (PETHEMA) cooperative study groups (2015) Is this the time to introduce minimal residual disease in multiple myeloma clinical practice? Clin Cancer Res 21(9):2001–2008. http://clincancerres.aacrjournals.org/cgi/doi/10.1158/1078-0432.CCR-14-2841

Pawlyn C, Fowkes L, Otero S, Jones JR, Boyd KD, Davies FE et al (2016) Whole-body diffusion-weighted MRI: a new gold standard for assessing disease burden in patients with multiple myeloma? Leukemia 30(6):1446–1448. http://www.nature.com/doifinder/10.1038/leu.2015.338

Pedreira CE, Costa ES, Lecrevisse Q, van Dongen JJM, Orfao A, EuroFlow Consortium (2013) Overview of clinical flow cytometry data analysis: recent advances and future challenges. Trends Biotechnol 31(7):415–425. http://linkinghub.elsevier.com/retrieve/pii/S0167779913000942

Pérez-Andrés M, Almeida J, Martín-Ayuso M, Moro MJ, Martín-Nuñez G, Galende J et al (2005) Clonal plasma cells from monoclonal gammopathy of undetermined significance, multiple myeloma and plasma cell leukemia show different expression profiles of molecules involved in the interaction with the immunological bone marrow microenvironment. Leukemia 19(3):449–455. http://www.ncbi.nlm.nih.gov/pubmed/15674420

Puig N, Sarasquete ME, Balanzategui A, Martínez J, Paiva B, García H et al (2014) Critical evaluation of ASO RQ-PCR for minimal residual disease evaluation in multiple myeloma. A comparative analysis with flow cytometry. Leukemia 28(2):391–397. http://www.nature.com/doifinder/10.1038/leu.2013.217

Putkonen M, Kairisto V, Juvonen V et al (2010) Depth of response assessed by quantitative ASO-PCR predicts the outcome after stem cell transplantation in multiple myeloma. Eur J Haematol 85:416–423

Rajkumar SV, Harousseau J-L, Durie B, Anderson KC, Dimopoulos M, Kyle R et al (2011) Consensus recommendations for the uniform reporting of clinical trials: report of the international myeloma workshop consensus panel 1. Blood 117(18):4691–4695. http://www.bloodjournal.org/cgi/doi/10.1182/blood-2010-10-299487

Rawstron AC, Barrans SL, Blythe D, English A, Richards SJ, Fenton JA et al (2001) In multiple myeloma, only a single stage of neoplastic plasma cell differentiation can be identified by VLA-5 and CD45 expression. Br J Haematol 113(3):794–802. http://www.ncbi.nlm.nih.gov/pubmed/11380472

Rawstron AC, Davies FE, DasGupta R, Ashcroft AJ, Patmore R, Drayson MT et al (2002) Flow cytometric disease monitoring in multiple myeloma: the relationship between normal and neoplastic plasma cells predicts outcome after transplantation. Blood 100(9):3095–3100. http://www.ncbi.nlm.nih.gov/pubmed/12384404

Rawstron AC, Child JA, de Tute RM, Davies FE, Gregory WM, Bell SE et al (2013) Minimal residual disease assessed by multiparameter flow cytometry in multiple myeloma: impact on outcome in the Medical Research Council myeloma IX study. J Clin Oncol 31(20):2540–2547. http://ascopubs.org/doi/10.1200/JCO.2012.46.2119

Robillard N, Pellat-Deceunynck C, Bataille R (2005) Phenotypic characterization of the human myeloma cell growth fraction. Blood 105(12):4845–4848. http://www.ncbi.nlm.nih.gov/pubmed/15741217

San Miguel JF, Almeida J, Mateo G, Bladé J, López-Berges C, Caballero D et al (2002) Immunophenotypic evaluation of the plasma cell compartment in multiple myeloma: a tool for comparing the efficacy of different treatment strategies and predicting outcome. Blood 99(5):1853–1856. http://www.ncbi.nlm.nih.gov/pubmed/11861305

San Miguel JF, Gutiérrez NC, Mateo G, Orfao A (2006) Conventional diagnostics in multiple myeloma. Eur J Cancer 42(11):1510–1519. http://www.ncbi.nlm.nih.gov/pubmed/16762540

Sarasquete ME, Garcia-Sanz R, Gonzalez D, Martinez J, Mateo G, Martinez P, Ribera JM, Hernandez JM, Lahuerta JJ, Orfao A, Gonzalez M, San Miguel JF (2005) Minimal residual disease monitoring in multiple myeloma: a comparison between allelic-specific oligonucleotide real-time quantitative polymerase chain reaction and flow cytometry. Haematologica 90:1365–1372

Sheth N, Yeung J, Chang H (2009) p53 nuclear accumulation is associated with extramedullary progression of multiple myeloma. Leuk Res 33(10):1357–1360. http://linkinghub.elsevier.com/retrieve/pii/S0145212609000174

Short KD, Rajkumar SV, Larson D, Buadi F, Hayman S, Dispenzieri A et al (2011) Incidence of extramedullary disease in patients with multiple myeloma in the era of novel therapy, and the activity of pomalidomide on extramedullary myeloma. Leukemia 25(6):906–908. http://www.nature.com/doifinder/10.1038/leu.2011.29

Shortt CP, Gleeson TG, Breen KA, McHugh J, O'Connell MJ, O'Gorman PJ et al (2009) Whole-body MRI versus PET in assessment of multiple myeloma disease activity. AJR Am J Roentgenol 192(4):980–986. http://www.ajronline.org/doi/10.2214/AJR.08.1633

Tarella C, Corradini P, Astolfi M, Bondesan P, Caracciolo D, Cherasco C, Ladetto M, Giaretta F, Ricca I, Vitolo U, Pileri A, Ferrero D (1999) Negative immunomagnetic ex vivo purging combined with high-dose chemotherapy with peripheral blood progenitor cell autograft in follicular lymphoma patients: evidence for long-term clinical and molecular remissions. Leukemia 13(9):1456

Thiago LS, Perez-Andres M, Balanzategui A, Sarasquete ME, Paiva B, Jara-Acevedo M et al (2014) Circulating clonotypic B cells in multiple myeloma and monoclonal gammopathy of undetermined significance. Haematologica 99(1):155–162. http://www.haematologica.org/cgi/doi/10.3324/haematol.2013.092817

Usmani SZ, Heuck C, Mitchell A, Szymonifka J, Nair B, Hoering A et al (2012) Extramedullary disease portends poor prognosis in multiple myeloma and is over-represented in high-risk disease even in the era of novel agents. Haematologica 97(11):1761–1767. http://www.haematologica.org/cgi/doi/10.3324/haematol.2012.065698

Usmani SZ, Mitchell A, Waheed S, Crowley J, Hoering A, Petty N et al (2013) Prognostic implications of serial 18-fluoro-deoxyglucose emission tomography in multiple myeloma treated with total therapy 3. Blood 121(10):1819–1823. http://www.bloodjournal.org/cgi/doi/10.1182/blood-2012-08-451690

van der Velden VH, Hochhaus A, Cazzaniga G, Szczepanski T, Gabert J, van Dongen JJ (2003) Detection of minimal residual disease in hematologic malignancies by real-time quantitative PCR: principles, approaches, and laboratory aspects. Leukemia 17(6):1013–1034

van der Velden VH, Cazzaniga G, Schrauder A, Hancock J, Bader P, Panzer-Grumayer ER, Flohr T, Sutton R, Cave H, Madsen HO, Cayuela JM, Trka J, Eckert C, Foroni L, Zur Stadt U, Beldjord K, Raff T, van der Schoot CE, van Dongen JJ, European Study Group on MRD detection in ALL (ESG-MRD-ALL) (2007) Analysis of minimal residual disease by Ig/TCR gene rearrangements: guidelines for interpretation of real-time quantitative PCR data. Leukemia 21(4):604–611. Epub 2007 Feb 8

van Lammeren-Venema D, Regelink JC, Riphagen II, Zweegman S, Hoekstra OS, Zijlstra JM (2012) 18F-fluoro-deoxyglucose positron emission tomography in assessment of myeloma-related bone disease: a systematic review. Cancer 118(8):1971–1981. http://doi.wiley.com/10.1002/cncr.26467

Varettoni M, Corso A, Pica G, Mangiacavalli S, Pascutto C, Lazzarino M (2010) Incidence, presenting features and outcome of extramedullary disease in multiple myeloma: a longitudinal study on 1003 consecutive patients. Ann Oncol Off J Eur Soc Med Oncol 21(2):325–330. https://academic.oup.com/annonc/article-lookup/doi/10.1093/annonc/mdp329

Voena C, Ladetto M, Astolfi M, Provan D, Gribben JG, Boccadoro M, Pileri A, Corradini P (1997) A novel nested-PCR strategy for the detection of rearranged immunoglobulin heavy-chain genes in B cell tumors. Leukemia 11(10):1793–1798

Walker RC, Brown TL, Jones-Jackson LB, De Blanche L, Bartel T (2012) Imaging of multiple myeloma and related plasma cell dyscrasias. J Nucl Med 53(7):1091–1101. http://jnm.snmjournals.org/cgi/doi/10.2967/jnumed.111.098830

Wren D, Walker B, Bruggemann M, Catherwood M, Pott C, Stamatopoulos K, Langerak A, Gonzalez D (2014) Translocations and clonality detection in lymphoproliferative disorders by capture-based next-generation sequencing. A pilot study by the euroclonality-ngs consortium. Blood 124:5169

Zamagni E, Patriarca F, Nanni C, Zannetti B, Englaro E, Pezzi A et al (2011) Prognostic relevance of 18-F FDG PET/CT in newly diagnosed multiple myeloma patients treated with up-front autologous transplantation. Blood 118(23):5989–5995. http://www.bloodjournal.org/cgi/doi/10.1182/blood-2011-06-361386

Bone Disease

7

Evangelos Terpos, Nikolaos Kanellias,
and Noopur Raje

7.1 Introduction

Multiple myeloma (MM) is a common hematological malignancy characterized by the accumulation of abnormal plasma cells in the bone marrow. Despite the improvement in survival after the introduction of novel agents (Kumar et al. 2008; Kastritis et al. 2009), MM remains an incurable plasma-cell malignancy (Jemal et al. 2010; Parker et al. 1998). MM is characterized by osteolytic bone disease due to an elevated function of osteoclasts which is not balanced by a comparable elevation of osteoblast function (Kyle et al. 2003; Terpos and Dimopoulos 2005; Raje and Roodman 2011). Osteolytic lesions are detected in 70–80% of patients at diagnosis and increase the risk for skeletal-related events (SREs: pathologic fractures, spinal cord compression (SCC), requirement for surgery or palliative radiotherapy to bone). SREs have a serious impact on the quality of life (QoL) and survival of MM patients and affect both clinical and economic aspects of their life (Coleman 2007; Roodman 2008; Croucher

and Apperley 1998; Cocks et al. 2007; Bruce et al. 1999; McCloskey et al. 1998). The novel International Myeloma Working Group (IMWG) criteria for the diagnosis of symptomatic MM have revealed the value of modern imaging for the management of MM patients, as they include (1) the presence of at least one lytic lesion detected not only by conventional radiography but also by computed tomography (CT), whole-body low-dose CT (WBLDCT), or positron emission tomography/CT (PET/CT) and (2) the presence of >1 focal bone marrow lesions on magnetic resonance imaging (MRI) studies (Rajkumar et al. 2014). Furthermore, novel imaging techniques, such as MRI and PET/CT, provide prognostic information and have been recently proven of value, for the better definition of response to anti-myeloma therapy. Bisphosphonates (BPs) are the cornerstone of therapeutic management of myeloma bone disease, offering considerable benefit in preventing or delaying skeletal-related events and relieving pain (Silbermann and Roodman 2016). This chapter reviews the latest available details of imaging and treatment of myeloma-related bone disease.

E. Terpos (✉) • N. Kanellias
Department of Clinical Therapeutics, National and Kapodistrian University of Athens, School of Medicine, Athens, Greece
e-mail: eterpos@med.uoa.gr

N. Raje
Center for Multiple Myeloma, Massachusetts General Hospital Cancer Center, Boston, MA, USA

7.2 Pathophysiology of Multiple Myeloma Bone Disease

In the adult skeleton, skeletal integrity is coordinated by the synchronized activity of three cell types. Osteoblasts create new bone matrix,

© Springer International Publishing Switzerland 2018
M. A. Dimopoulos et al. (eds.), *Multiple Myeloma and Other Plasma Cell Neoplasms*,
Hematologic Malignancies, https://doi.org/10.1007/978-3-319-25586-6_7

osteoclasts are responsible for bone resorption, and osteocytes regulate bone turnover. In MM patients, bone disease is the result of an uncoupling in bone remodeling. It consists of an increase in the osteoclast-mediated bone resorption, which is combined with suppression in the osteoblast, mediated bone mineralization, and defects on osteocyte functions (Bataille et al. 1991). Until today, several direct and indirect interactions between myeloma cells and cells of the bone marrow microenvironment have been recognized. The fact that osteolytic lesions occur close to MM cells suggests that factors secreted by tumor cells lead to direct stimulation of osteoclast-mediated bone resorption and inhibition of osteoblast-mediated bone formation (Terpos and Dimopoulos 2005). In addition to that, the increased bone resorptive progress leads to the release of growth factors that increase the growth of MM cells, leading to a vicious cycle of tumor expansion and bone destruction. Apart from that, interactions via adhesion between MM cells and bone marrow cells result in the production of factors that promote angiogenesis and make the myeloma cells resistant to chemotherapy (Abe et al. 2004; Tanaka et al. 2007). The biologic pathway of the receptor activator of nuclear factor-kappa B (RANK), its ligand (RANKL), and osteoprotegerin (OPG) which is the decoy receptor of RANKL is of major importance for the increased osteoclast activity observed in MM. Myeloma cells disrupt the balance between RANKL and OPG by increasing the expression of RANKL and decreasing the expression of OPG. The resulting increase in RANKL favors the formation and activation of osteoclasts, leading to increased bone resorption (Pearse et al. 2001; Terpos et al. 2003). More recently, activin A has been implicated in MM bone disease, through stimulating RANK expression and inducing osteoclastogenesis (Sugatani et al. 2003; Terpos et al. 2012a). On the other hand, in addition to their stimulatory effect on osteoclasts, myeloma cells have been shown to suppress bone formation (Christoulas et al. 2009). The Wingless-type (Wnt) signaling pathway is one pathway that has been shown to play a key role in osteoblast differentiation and has been implicated in osteoblast suppression in myeloma. The Wnt signaling inhibitors dickkopf-1 (Dkk-1) and sclerostin are secreted by myeloma cells and have been found to be increased in the serum of myeloma patients, leading to the block of osteoblast differentiation and activity (Tian et al. 2003; Colucci et al. 2011; Politou et al. 2006; Terpos et al. 2012b). Soluble frizzled-related protein-2 (sFRP-2), another inhibitor of Wnt signaling, has also been implicated in the suppression of bone formation in myeloma (Oshima et al. 2005). Although the circulating levels of the above molecules and mainly of sclerostin have not been found to be elevated in myeloma patients in all published studies, the importance of Wnt inhibition in the biology of myeloma-related bone disease is undoubted.

7.3 Imaging for the Diagnosis of Multiple Myeloma Bone Disease

The imaging techniques used for the diagnosis of multiple myeloma bone disease are:

1. Whole-Body X-rays (WBXR).
2. Whole-Body CT (WB-CT).
3. Magnetic resonance imaging (MRI).
4. PET/CT.

7.3.1 Whole-Body X-Rays (WBXR)

Conventional radiography has been widely used for the identification of osteolytic lesions both at diagnosis and during the course of the disease. The "skeletal survey" (whole-body X-rays, WBXR) at diagnosis should include plain radiographs of the whole skeleton (anteroposterior and lateral views of the skull; posteroanterior view of the chest; anteroposterior and lateral views of the thoracic lumbar and cervical spine (including an open mouth view), humeri and femora and anteroposterior view of the pelvis) (Dimopoulos et al. 2009a). In addition, symptomatic areas should also be specifically visualized. Osteolyses have the typical appearance of "punched-out" lesions with the absence of reactive sclerosis and are more common in the vertebrae, ribs, skull, and pelvis (Terpos et al. 2011). Although the WBXR was the standard of care for many years, it has several limitations:

1. For a lytic lesion to become apparent, >30% loss of trabecular bone must occur.
2. Difficulty of assessment of certain areas, such as the pelvis and the spine.
3. Limitations in the detection of lytic lesion response to anti-myeloma therapy because of delayed evidence of healing.
4. Reduced specificity for the differential diagnosis of myeloma-related versus benign fracture (very important, particularly in cases of new vertebral compression fractures in the absence of other criteria of relapse).
5. Observer dependency (there is very low reproducibility among centers; a higher number of osteolytic lesions detected in academic versus nonacademic centers).
6. Prolonged study length, often not tolerable from patients in severe pain (Dimopoulos et al. 2009a; Terpos et al. 2011).

Thus, the development of novel imaging methods has led to the replacement of WBXR by more advanced techniques, such as the WBLDCT in many European centers or by PET/CT in the USA.

7.3.2 Whole-Body Low-Dose CT (WBLDCT)

WBLDCT was introduced to allow the detection of osteolytic lesions in the whole skeleton with high accuracy, no need for contrast agents and low-radiation dose compared to standard CT (two- to threefold lower-radiation dose versus conventional CT) (Pianko et al. 2014; Ippolito et al. 2013). In several studies, WBLDCT was found to be superior to WBXR for the detection of osteolytic lesions (Pianko et al. 2014; Horger et al. 2005; Kropil et al. 2008; Gleeson et al. 2009; Princewill et al. 2013; Wolf et al. 2014). In one of the largest studies staging myeloma patients, 61% of patients with normal WBXR had more than one osteolytic lesions on WBLDCT (Princewill et al. 2013). According to the latest criteria for symptomatic myeloma, these patients should receive therapy. In the same study, the total number of lesions detected by WBLDCT was 968 versus 248 for WBXR ($p < 0.001$). The only limitation of this study was its retrospective origin (Princewill et al. 2013). In a more recent prospective study, which included 52 myeloma patients at diagnosis, WBLDCT revealed osteolyses in 12 patients (23%) with negative WBXR and proved to be more sensitive than WBXR mainly in the axial skeleton ($p < 0.001$). WBLDCT was superior in the detection of lesions in patients with osteopenia and osteoporosis (Wolf et al. 2014).

In total, WBLDCT advantages over WBXR include (1) superior diagnostic sensitivity for depiction of osteolytic lesions, especially in areas where the WBXR detection rate is low, i.e., pelvis and spine; (2) superiority in estimating fracture risk and bone instability; (3) duration of the examination, which is ≤5 min, an important issue for patients in extreme pain; (4) production of higher-quality 3D high-resolution images for planning biopsies and therapeutic interventions; and finally (5) demonstration of unsuspected manifestations of myeloma or other diseases, especially in the lungs and kidneys (33% in the study by Wolf et al.; 37, 31–37). Major disadvantages of WBLDCT include increased length of time required for radiologists to report their findings, lack of availability in several centers (Rajkumar et al. 2014; Pianko et al. 2014), and lack of specificity for the differential diagnosis between malignant and osteoporotic fractures, despite improvements during the last years (Cretti and Perugini 2016). Furthermore, although exposure to radiation is much lower compared to standard CT, it continues to be higher than WBXR: mean dose of WBLDCT is approximately 3.6 and 2.8 mSv for females and males, respectively, versus 1.2 mSv for WBXR (Borggrefe et al. 2015). Nevertheless, the higher diagnostic accuracy of the WBLDCT and patient comfort particularly important for the elderly, often suffering group, renders the dose/quality ratio favorable for WBLDCT. For these reasons, the European Myeloma Network has suggested that WBLDCT should replace conventional radiography as the standard imaging technique for evaluation of bone disease in MM, where available (Terpos et al. 2015a).

7.3.3 Magnetic Resonance Imaging

Techniques Several MRI techniques have been developed for the assessment of the bone marrow involvement in MM. Conventional MRI protocols include T1-weighted, T2-weighted with fat suppression, short time inversion recovery (STIR) and gadolinium T1-weighted with fat suppression (Moulopoulos and Dimopoulos 1997). Myeloma lesions show typically a low signal intensity on T1-weighted images, a high signal intensity on T2-weighted and STIR images, and often enhancement on gadolinium-enhanced images (Libshitz et al. 1992; Weininger et al. 2008).

Limitations of MRI are the prolonged acquisition time, availability issues, the high cost, the exclusion of patients with metal devices in their body, the difficulties in cases of claustrophobic patients, and the limited field of view. To override these restrictions, a WB-MRI methodology, which does not usually require contrast infusion, was developed. The time of WB-MRI is approximately 45 min. Although of interest, this newer technique is not yet widely employed.

All above MRI methods use MRI exquisite contrast and spatial resolution for the depiction of the WB anatomy and specific tissue composition in details.

Novel MRI techniques include diffusion-weighted imaging, dynamic contrast-enhanced MRI, and PET-MRI.

A novel and promising MRI sequence is the diffusion-weighted imaging (DWI-MRI) which derives its contrast mainly from differences in the diffusivity of water molecules in the tissue environment. This functional technique demonstrates alterations in intra- and extracellular water content from disruption of the transmembrane water flux that are visible before identified changes on

the morphologic routine sequences (Attariwala and Picker 2013; Muller and Edelman 1995; Wang 2000). DWI-MRI uses the calculation of apparent diffusion coefficient (ADC) values to better evaluate myeloma burden and MRI infiltration patterns (Nonomura et al. 2001; Terpos et al. 2015b). DWI can be used to detect regions with bone marrow infiltration for both diagnosis and monitoring treatment response (Xu et al. 2008), because ADC values are higher in MM patients at diagnosis compared with patients in remission 20 weeks after initiation of treatment (Messiou et al. 2012). In MM patients, the ADC was reproducible (Messiou et al. 2011) and correlated with bone marrow cellularity and microvessel density (MVD) (Hillengass et al. 2011). One disadvantage of DWI is that the ADC is not exclusively influenced by diffusion but also by perfusion. However, improved sequences are under development to differentiate both influences (Lemke et al. 2011). DWI-MRI was found superior to WBXR for the detection of bone involvement in 20 patients with relapsed/refractory MM in all areas of the skeleton except of the skull, where both examinations had equal sensitivity (Giles et al. 2015). In another small study with 24 myeloma patients (both treated and untreated), DWI-MRI was found more sensitive than F18-fluorodeoxyglucose (FDG)-PET in the detection of myeloma lesions (Sachpekidis et al. 2015a). In a recent study, 17 patients were evaluated with DWI-MRI and FDG-PET/CT, and the findings were compared with bone marrow biopsy data. In all studied regions, WB-DWI scores were higher compared to FDG-PET/CT. DWI-MRI was particularly accurate in diagnosing diffuse disease (diffuse disease was observed in 37% of regions imaged on WB-DWI scans versus only 7% on FDG-PET/CT); both techniques were equally sensitive in the detection of focal lesions (Pawlyn et al. 2015). Preliminary reports suggest that DWI-MRI may be used for the better definition of response to therapy, but this has to be confirmed in larger studies and in comparison with PET/CT results (Terpos et al. 2015b; Horger et al. 2011).

The dynamic contrast-enhanced MRI (DCE-MRI) is another MRI technique which evaluates the distribution of a contrast agent inside and outside the blood vessels. Information is assessed by computer-based analysis of repeated images over time. The analysis provides data for blood volume and vessel permeability for the assessment of microcirculation of a specific area (Hillengass et al. 2007; Hillengass and Landgren 2013). More importantly in MM patients, DCE-MRI derived parameters correlated with marrow angiogenesis, microvessel density (MVD) (Huang et al. 2012), as well as in angiogenic response to therapy (Zechmann et al. 2012). Regarding DCE-MRI sampling rate and model, there are two pharmacokinetic models (proposed by Brix and Tofts) that have been applied in the literature. However, a comparison of these models demonstrated that the Brix model is a little bit more robust (Zwick et al. 2010). Since DCE-MRI has not been established in clinical routine, no definite sequence can be recommended.

Positron emission tomography in combination with MRI (PET-MRI) represents a novel imaging modality in which the PET part detects active focal lesions, while the MRI part shows the location of the lesions and gives information on myeloma cell infiltration of the bone marrow. Especially in patients who reach a complete remission (CR), this technique might be able to localize residual sites of disease activity and therefore may help to guide treatment in the future (Fraioli and Punwani 2014). In MM, there is only one prospective study, which compared PET-MRI with PET/CT in 30 myeloma patients with both techniques performed sequentially. There was a high correlation between the two techniques, regarding number of active lesions and average SUV (Sachpekidis et al. 2015b). Further studies with PET-MRI will reveal if there is any value of this technique for MM patients.

MRI Patterns of Marrow Involvement Five MRI patterns of bone marrow infiltration in myeloma have been reported: (1) normal appearance of the bone marrow, (2) focal involvement (positive focal lesion is considered the lesion of a diameter of at least 5 mm), (3) homogeneous diffuse infiltration, (4) combined diffuse and focal infiltration, and (5) variegated or "salt-and-

pepper" pattern with inhomogeneous bone marrow with interposition of fat islands (Baur-Melnyk et al. 2005; Moulopoulos et al. 1992). Low tumor burden is usually associated with a normal MRI pattern, but a high tumor burden is usually suspected when there is diffuse hypointense change on T1-weighted images, diffuse hyperintensity on T2-weighted images, and enhancement with gadolinium injection (Moulopoulos et al. 2005). In several studies, the percentage of symptomatic patients with each of the abnormal MRI bone marrow patterns ranges from 18 to 50% for focal pattern, 25 to 43% for diffuse pattern, and 1 to 5% for variegated pattern (Hillengass and Landgren 2013). The Durie-Salmon PLUS system uses the number of focal lesions (from focal or combined focal/diffuse patterns) for the staging of a myeloma patient and not the diffuse or "salt-and-pepper" patterns (Durie 2006).

MRI Versus Conventional Radiography and Other Imaging Techniques for the Detection of Bone Involvement in Symptomatic Myeloma MRI is more sensitive compared to WBXR for the detection of bone involvement in MM. In the largest series of patients published to date, MRI was compared to WBXR in 611 patients who received tandem autologous transplantation (ASCT). MRI and WBXR detected focal and osteolytic lesions in 74% and 56% of the imaged anatomic sites, respectively. Furthermore, 52% of 267 patients with normal WBXR had focal lesions on MRI. More precisely, MRI detected more focal lesions compared to lytic lesions in WBXR in the spine (78% vs. 16%, $p < 0.001$), the pelvis (64% vs. 28%, $p < 0.001$), and the sternum (24%vs. 3%, $p < 0.001$). WBXR had better performance than MRI in the ribs (10% vs. 43%, $p < 0.001$) and the long bones (37% vs. 48%, $p = 0.006$) and equal results in the skull and the shoulders (Walker et al. 2007). Similar results had been previously reported in smaller studies, where MRI was superior to WBXR for the detection of focal vs. osteolytic lesions in the pelvis (75% vs. 46% of patients) and the spine (76% vs. 42%), especially in the lumbar spine (Ludwig et al. 1987; Ghanem et al. 2006; Lecouvet et al. 1999; Tertti et al.

1995; Narquin et al. 2013). A recent meta-analysis confirmed the superiority of MRI over WBXR regarding the detection of focal lesions and showed that MRI especially outscores WBXR in the axial skeleton but not in the ribs (Regelink et al. 2013).

Although it is clear that MRI can detect bone marrow focal lesions long before the development of osteolytic lesions in the WBXR, other imaging techniques such as PET combined with computed tomography (PET/CT), CT, or WB-CT detect more osteolytic lesions compared to WBXR (Regelink et al. 2013). Is there any evidence that MRI is superior to the other techniques in depicting bone involvement in myeloma? In a study with 41 newly diagnosed MM patients, WB-MRI was found superior to WB-CT in detecting lesions in the skeleton (Baur-Melnyk et al. 2008). In a prospective study, Zamagni et al. compared MRI of the spine and pelvis with WBXR and PET/CT in 46 MM patients at diagnosis. Although PET/CT was superior to WBXR in detecting lytic lesions in 46% of patients (19% had negative WBXR), it failed to reveal abnormal findings in 30% of patients who had abnormal MRI in the same areas, mainly of diffuse pattern. In that study, the combination of spine and pelvic MRI with PET/CT detected both medullary and extramedullary active myeloma sites in almost all patients (92%) (Zamagni et al. 2007). Nevertheless, the Arkansas group was not able to confirm any superiority of MRI over PET/CT in the detection of more focal lesions in a large number of patients ($n = 303$) within the total of three therapy protocols (Waheed et al. 2013). Still, in 188 patients who had at least 1 focal lesion in MRI, MRI was superior to PET/CT regarding the detection of a higher number of focal lesions ($p = 0.032$). Furthermore, in this study, the presence of diffuse marrow pattern was not taken into consideration as an abnormal MRI finding (Waheed et al. 2013). Compared to sestamibi technetium-99 m (MIBI) scan, WB-MRI detected more lesions in the vertebrae and the long bones produced similar results in the skull and was inferior in the ribs (Khalafallah et al. 2013). One important question in this point is the value of WB-MRI, which is not available

everywhere, over the MRI of the spine and pelvis. In 100 patients with MM and MGUS who underwent WB-MRI, 10% presented with focal lesions merely in the extra-axial skeleton. These lesions would have been ignored if only MRI of the spine and pelvis had been performed (Bauerle et al. 2009).

Other advantages of MRI over WBXR and CT include the discrimination of myeloma from a normal marrow (Moulopoulos and Dimopoulos 1997; Baur et al. 1998); this finding can help in the differential diagnosis between myeloma and benign cause of a vertebral fracture. This is of extreme importance in cases of patients with a vertebral fracture and no other CRAB criteria and no lytic lesions. The MRI can also accurately illustrate the spinal cord and/or nerve root compression for surgical intervention or radiation therapy (Dimopoulos et al. 2009a; Moulopoulos and Dimopoulos 1997). Furthermore, the presence of soft tissue extension of MM and the presence of extramedullary plasmacytomas that are developed in approximately 10–20% of patients during the course of their disease can be precisely visualized by WB-MRI (Moulopoulos et al. 1993; Dimopoulos et al. 2000; Varettoni et al. 2010; Lafforgue et al. 1993). MRI can also help in the better evaluation of avascular necrosis of the femoral head (Lafforgue et al. 1993) and the presence of soft tissue amyloid deposits (Syed et al. 2010). Moreover, the tumor load can be assessed and monitored by MRI even in patients with nonsecretory and oligosecretory MM (Carlson et al. 1995).

In conclusion, according to the latest IMWG guidelines, MRI is the gold standard imaging technique for the detection of bone marrow involvement in MM (grade A). MRI detects bone marrow involvement and not bone destruction. MRI of the spine and pelvis can detect approximately 90% of focal lesions in MM, and thus it can be used in cases where WB-MRI is not available (grade B). MRI is the procedure of choice to evaluate a painful lesion in myeloma patients, mainly in the axial skeleton, and to detect spinal cord compression (grade A). MRI is particularly useful in the evaluation of collapsed vertebrae, especially when myeloma is not active, where the possibility of osteoporotic fracture is high (grade B) (Dimopoulos et al. 2015).

Prognostic Value of MRI The prognostic significance of MRI findings in symptomatic myeloma has been evaluated. The largest study in the literature included 611 patients who received tandem ASCT-based protocols. Focal lesions are detected by spinal MRI and not seen on WBXR independently correlated with overall survival (OS). Resolution of the focal lesions on MRI posttreatment occurred in 60% of the patients who had superior survival. At disease progression after complete response (CR), MRI revealed new focal lesions in 26% of patients, enlargement of previous focal lesions in 28%, and both features in 15% of patients (Walker et al. 2007). In a more recent analysis of the same group on 429 patients, patients who had >7 focal lesions in MRI ($n = 147$) had a 73% probability of 3-year OS vs. 86% for those who had 0–7 focal lesions ($n = 235$) and 81% for those who had diffuse pattern of marrow infiltration ($n = 47$; $p = 0.04$). PET/CT and WBXR also produced similar results in the univariate analysis. In the multivariate analysis, from the imaging variables, only the presence of >2 osteolytic lesions in WBXR at diagnosis and the presence of >3 focal lesions in the PET/CT, 7 days post-ASCT had independent prognostic value for inferior OS ($p = 0.01$ and 0.03, respectively). However, we have to mention the high percentage of patients (232/429, 54%) who had no detectable osteolytic lesions by WBXR and the absence of evaluation of diffuse MRI pattern in this study (Usmani et al. 2013).

The MRI pattern of marrow infiltration has also reported to have a prognostic significance in newly diagnosed patients with symptomatic disease (Moulopoulos et al. 2005; Lecouvet et al. 1998; Moulopoulos et al. 2012). In the conventional chemotherapy (CC) era, Moulopoulos et al. published that the median OS of newly diagnosed MM patients was 24 months if they had diffuse MRI pattern versus 51, 52, and 56 months for those with focal, variegated, and normal patterns, respectively ($p = 0.001$) (Moulopoulos et al. 2005). This is possibly because diffuse MRI marrow pattern correlates

with increased angiogenesis and advanced disease features (Moulopoulos et al. 2010; Song et al. 2014). The same group also reported the prognostic value of MRI patterns in 228 symptomatic MM patients who received upfront regimens based on novel agents. Patients with diffuse pattern had inferior survival compared to patients with other MRI patterns; moreover, the combination of diffuse MRI pattern, ISS-3 stage, and high-risk cytogenetics could identify a group of patients with very poor survival: median of 21 months and a probability of 3-year OS of only 35% (Moulopoulos et al. 2012). Another study in 126 patients with newly diagnosed symptomatic myeloma who underwent an ASCT showed that the diffuse and the variegated MRI patterns had an independent predictive value for disease progression (HR: 1.922, $p = 0.008$) (Song et al. 2014). Finally, in patients with progressive or relapsed MM, an increased signal of DCE-MRI offered shorter PFS, possibly due to its association with higher MVD (Hillengass et al. 2007).

MRI and Response to Anti-myeloma Therapy An interesting finding is that a change in MRI pattern correlates with response to therapy. Moulopoulos et al. firstly reported in the era of CC that CR is characterized by complete resolution of the preceding marrow abnormality, while partial response (PR) is characterized by changeover of diffuse pattern to variegated or focal patterns (Moulopoulos et al. 1994). In a retrospective study that was conducted in the era of novel agents, response to treatment was compared with changes in infiltration patterns of WB-MRI before and after ASCT ($n = 100$). There was a strong correlation between response to anti-myeloma therapies and changes in both diffuse ($p = 0.004$) and focal ($p = 0.01$) MRI patterns. Furthermore, the number of focal lesions at second MRI was of prognostic significance for OS ($p = 0.001$) (Hillengass et al. 2012). Another study in 33 patients who underwent an ASCT showed that WB-MRI data demonstrated progressive disease in ten patients (30%) and response to high-dose therapy in 23 (70%). Eight (80%) of the ten patients with progressive disease revealed intramedullary lesions, and two patients

(20%) had intra- and extramedullary lesions. WB-MRI had a sensitivity of 64%, specificity of 86%, positive predictive value of 70%, negative predictive value of 83%, and accuracy of 79% for detection of remission (Bannas et al. 2012). This study supports that one of the disadvantages of MRI is that it often provides false-positive results because of persistent nonviable lesions. Thus, PET/CT might be more suitable than MRI for determination of remission status (Derlin et al. 2013). Indeed in a large study of 191 patients, PET/CT revealed faster change of imaging findings than MRI in patients who responded to therapy (Spinnato et al. 2012). It seems that the PET/CT normalization after treatment can offer more information compared to MRI for the better definition of CR (Bartel et al. 2009).

To improve the results of MRI for the most accurate detection of remission, the DW-MRI has been recently used. In the first preliminary report, ADC values in active myeloma were significantly higher than marrow in remission (Messiou et al. 2012). Furthermore, the mean ADC increased in 95% of responding patients and decreased in all ($n = 5$) non-responders ($p = 0.002$). An increase of ADC by 3.3% was associated with a positive response, having a sensitivity of 90% and specificity of 100%. Furthermore, there was a negative correlation between changes of ADC and changes of biochemical markers of response ($r = -0.614$, $p = 0.001$) (Giles et al. 2014). Large prospective clinical studies are definitely justified by these results.

The Value of MRI in the Definition of Smoldering/Asymptomatic Myeloma The presence of lytic lesions by WBXR is included in the definition of symptomatic myeloma, based on studies showing that patients with at least one lytic lesion in WBXR have a median time to progression (TTP) of 10 months (Dimopoulos et al. 1993). However, in patients with no osteolytic lesions in WBXR, the MRI reveals abnormal marrow appearance in 20–50% of them (Moulopoulos et al. 1992; Moulopoulos et al. 2005; Moulopoulos et al. 1995; Hillengass et al. 2010; Kastritis et al. 2013); these patients are at a higher risk for progression. Moulopoulos et al.

reported that patients with SMM and abnormal MRI studies required therapy after a median of 16 vs. 43 months for those with normal MRI ($p < 0.01$) (Moulopoulos et al. 1995). Hillengass and colleagues evaluated WB-MRI in 149 SMM patients. Focal lesions were detected in 42 (28%) patients, while >1 focal lesion was present in 23 patients (15%) who had high risk of progression (HR = 4.05, $p < 0.001$). The median TTP was 13 months, and the progression rate at 2 years was 70%. On multivariate analysis, the presence of >1 focal lesion remained a significant predictor of progression after adjusting for other risk factors including bone marrow plasmacytosis, serum and urine M protein levels, and suppression of uninvolved immunoglobulins. In the same study, the diffuse marrow infiltration on MRI was also associated with increased risk for progression (HR = 3.5, $p < 0.001$) (Hillengass et al. 2010). Kastritis and colleagues also showed in 98 SMM patients that abnormal marrow pattern in the MRI of the spine, which was present in 21% of patients, was associated with high risk of progression with a median TTP to symptomatic myeloma of 15 months ($p = 0.001$) (Kastritis et al. 2013).

An important issue is whether patients who have two or more small focal lesions (<5 mm) should be considered as patients with symptomatic myeloma and how to manage them. The Heidelberg group analyzed very recently data of 63 SMM patients who had at least two WB-MRIs performed for follow-up before progression into symptomatic disease. The definition of radiological progression according to MRI findings included one of the following: (1) development of a new focal lesion, (2) increase of the diameter of an existing focal lesion, and (3) detection of novel or progressive diffuse MRI pattern. The second MRI was performed 3–6 months after the performance of the first MRI. Evaluation of response according to IMWG criteria was also performed. Progressive disease according to MRI was observed in approximately 50% of patients, while 40% of patients developed symptomatic MM based on the CRAB criteria. In the multivariate analysis, MRI-PD was an independent prognostic factor for progression. Patients with stable MRI findings had no higher risk of progression, even when focal lesions were present at the initial MRI (Merz et al. 2014). Prospective clinical trials should be conducted to confirm the above findings.

MRI Findings in Monoclonal Gammopathy of Undetermined Significance (MGUS) MGUS by definition is characterized by the absence of osteolytic lesions. However, MGUS patients have higher incidence of osteoporosis and vertebral fractures compared to normal population (Pepe et al. 2006; Van de Donk et al. 2014). In a small study which included 37 patients with MGUS or SMM, MRI abnormalities were detected in 20% of them. These patients had a higher time to progression (TTP) to symptomatic myeloma compared to patients with a normal MRI who did not progress after a median follow-up of 30 months (Vande Berg et al. 1997). A prospective study in 331 patients with MGUS or SMM revealed that the detection of multiple (>1) focal lesions by MRI conferred an increased risk of progression (Dhodapkar et al. 2014). In another large study, which included only MGUS patients ($n = 137$) who underwent a WB-MRI at diagnosis, a focal infiltration pattern was detected in 23% of them. Independent prognostic factors for progression to symptomatic myeloma included the presence and number of focal lesions and the value of M protein (Hillengass et al. 2014).

MRI and Solitary Plasmacytoma of the Bone (SPB) The diagnosis of SBP includes the presence of a solitary bone lesion, with a confirmed infiltration by plasma cells in the biopsy of the lesion, absence of clonal plasma cells in the trephine bone marrow biopsy, and no CRAB criteria. Although definitive radiotherapy usually eradicates the local disease, the majority of patients will develop MM because of the growth of previously occult lesions which have not been detected by WBXR (Dimopoulos et al. 2000). Moulopoulos et al. published that spinal MRI revealed additional focal lesions in 4/12 SBP patients. After treatment with radiotherapy to the painful lesion, three patients developed systemic

disease within 18 months from diagnosis (Moulopoulos et al. 1993). Furthermore, Liebross et al. observed that among SBP patients with spinal disease, 7/8 staged by WBXR alone developed MM compared to only 1/7 patients who also had spinal MRI (Liebross et al. 1998).

7.3.4 PET-CT

PET/CT Detection of Bone Involvement in Myeloma FDG-PET/CT is a functional imaging method, which combines demonstration of hypermetabolic activity in intramedullary and extramedullary sites (PET) with evidence of osteolysis (CT). Several studies have shown that PET/CT is more sensitive compared to WBXR for the detection of osteolytic lesions in MM (Zamagni et al. 2007; Bredella et al. 2005; Lütje et al. 2009; Breyer et al. 2006). This has been confirmed by the largest meta-analysis in the field (Regelink et al. 2013). The higher detection rate of PET/CT over WBXR for the presence of osteolytic lesions is especially important for patients with SMM. In one study with 120 patients with SMM based on the previous IMWG criteria (Zamagni et al. 2007), 16% of patients with normal WBXR had positive PET/CT results. The median time to progression (TTP) for PET/CT-positive patients was 1.1 years versus 4.5 for patients with negative PET/CT, while the probability of progression at 2 years for PET/CT-positive patients was 58% (Zamagni et al. 2015a). The largest study in the field involved 188 with suspected SMM examined with PET/CT. PET/CT was positive in 39% of patients. The probability of progression to symptomatic MM within 2 years was 75% for patients with a positive PET/CT under observation versus only 30% for patients with a negative PET/CT. This probability was higher if hypermetabolic activity was combined with underlying osteolysis (2-year progression rate: 87%). The median TTP was 21 versus 60 months for PET/CT-positive and negative patients, respectively (Siontis et al. 2015). The results of these two studies support the integration of changes in imaging requirements in the new IMWG diagnostic criteria for MM;

detection of osteolytic lesions by PET/CT is a criterion for symptomatic MM (Rajkumar et al. 2014).

Compared to MRI, as mentioned previously, PET/CT performs equally well in detecting focal lesions, but MRI is better in detecting diffuse disease (Baur-Melnyk et al. 2008; Zamagni et al. 2007; Breyer et al. 2006).

Value of PET/CT for Better Definition of Complete Response to Anti-myeloma Therapy Data obtained from PET/CT in 40 MM patients, including average SUV and FDG kinetic parameters K1, influx, and fractal dimension, correlated significantly with the percentage of bone marrow infiltration on trephine biopsies (PC %) (Sachpekidis et al. 2015c). Furthermore, PET/CT efficiently detected extramedullary disease in patients both at diagnosis and at relapse (Tirumani et al. 2016). Consequently, PET/CT was tested for better definition of CR in 282 MM patients. It was performed at diagnosis and every 12–18 months afterward. At diagnosis, 42% of MM patients had >3 focal lesions; in 50% of these patients, SUV max was >4.2. After treatment, PET/CT was negative in 70% of patients, while 53% of patients achieved CR according to IMWG criteria. Approximately 30% of patients at CR had positive PET/CT. More importantly, PET/CT negativity was an independent predictor for prolonged PFS and OS in CR patients; median PFS was 50 months for PET/CT-positive and 90 months for PET/CT-negative CR patients (Zamagni et al. 2015b). PET/CT, therefore, provides more accurate definition of CR, and it has been suggested that it should be incorporated to the CR criteria (Paiva et al. 2015).

Prognostic Significance of PET/CT Several studies have confirmed the value of PET/CT as an independent factor for survival in MM patients both at diagnosis and posttreatment (Bartel et al. 2009; Zamagni et al. 2011; Patriarca et al. 2015; Fonti et al. 2015; Lapa et al. 2014; Cascini et al. 2013). In 192 newly diagnosed patients who underwent ASCT, the presence of extramedullary disease and SUV max >4.2 on PET/CT performed at diagnosis and the persistence of FDG uptake post-ASCT were independent variables,

adversely affecting PFS (Zamagni et al. 2011). In the largest study in the field, 429 patients who were treated with total therapy protocols in Arkansas were evaluated with both MRI and PET/CT at diagnosis and 7 days post-ASCT. From the imaging variables, in the multivariate analysis, only the detection of >2 osteolytic lesions by WBXR at diagnosis and the detection of >3 focal lesions by PET/CT, 7 days post-ASCT, were independent prognostic factors for inferior OS. Limitation of this study was the exclusion of diffuse MRI pattern from the analysis (Usmani et al. 2013). Despite this limitation, studies reported to date support the role of PET/CT after therapy, deeming it the best imaging technique for the follow-up of myeloma patients. Indeed, in a recent study which has been reported only in an abstract form, 134 patients who were eligible for treatment with ASCT were randomized to receive eight cycles of bortezomib-lenalidomide-dexamethasone (VRD) followed by 1-year maintenance with lenalidomide or three cycles of VRD followed by ASCT plus two cycles of VRD consolidation and 1-year lenalidomide maintenance. PET/CT and WB-MRI were performed after induction and before maintenance. Both techniques were positive at diagnosis in more than 90% of patients. After induction therapy and before maintenance, more patients continued to have positive MRI than PET/CT (93% versus 55% and 83% versus 21%, respectively), possibly due to earlier reduction of activity of PET/CT lesions. Both after induction and before maintenance, normalization of PET/CT and not of MRI could predict for PFS, while only normalization of PET/CT before maintenance could predict for OS (30-month OS rate: 70% in PET/CT-positive patients versus 94.6% in patients with negative PET/CT, $p = 0.01$) (Moreau et al. 2015).

At this point, it is crucial to mention that one of the major limitations of PET/CT is the lack of standardization and the controversies regarding SUV level of positivity. Recently, an Italian panel of experts introduced novel criteria for the interpretation of PET/CT images (Nanni et al. 2016). Large, multicenter, studies with prospective evaluation of these new criteria will reveal their clinical impact.

Other PET/CT Indications and Limitations PET/CT may be used for the workup of patients with SBP at diagnosis (Fouquet et al. 2014). However, it is not clear whether PET/CT or MRI is more suitable in this setting, since restaging PET/CT after radiotherapy has a number of false-positive findings (Alongi et al. 2015). PET/CT also has a role in patients with nonsecretory or oligosecretory myeloma for the detection of active lesions in the body (Lonial and Kaufman 2013). Major limitations of PET/CT include high cost, lack of availability in many centers and countries, and false-positive results due to inflammation of other underlying pathology.

7.4 Management of Multiple Myeloma Bone Disease

Bisphosphonates (BPs) are the mainstay in the management of MM bone disease. They are artificial analogues of pyrophosphates. In comparison with natural pyrophosphates, bisphosphonates are resistant to phosphatase-induced hydrolysis (Rogers et al. 2000). Bisphosphonates cause osteoclast suppression. They bind to calcium-containing molecules such as hydroxyapatite (Terpos et al. 2009). Osteoclast-induced bone resorption causes exposure of hydroxyapatite. Bisphosphonates bind to the exposed molecules of hydroxyapatite. This fact leads to increased concentration of bisphosphonates within the lytic lesions (Terpos et al. 2009; Boonekamp et al. 1986; Rowe et al. 1999). There are two main groups of bisphosphonates, each with a differently proposed mechanism of action (Terpos et al. 2009). Nonnitrogen-containing bisphosphonates induce osteoclast apoptosis via their cytotoxic ATP analogues. On the other hand, nitrogen-containing bisphosphonates downregulate osteoclast activity by inhibiting the HMG-CoA reductase pathway. Etidronate and clodronate (CLO) are nonnitrogen-containing bisphosphonates. Zoledronic acid (ZOL), ibandronate, pamidronate (PAM), and risedronate are nitrogen-containing bisphosphonates. All bisphosphonates have similar physicochemical properties; however, their anti-resorbing activity is different. Their activity is drastically increased when an amino group is entered into the aliphatic carbon chain. Thus, pamidronate is 100- and 700-fold more potent than etidronate, both in vitro and in vivo, while zoledronic acid and ibandronate show 10,000- to 100,000-fold greater potency than etidronate (Terpos et al. 2014). Bisphosphonates also appear to affect the microenvironment in which tumor cells grow and may have direct anti-tumor activity (Mundy and Yoneda 1998; Yin et al. 1999; Diel et al. 1998; Aparicio et al. 1998; Shipman et al. 1997; Dhodapkar et al. 1998). Possible mechanisms include the reduction of IL-6 secretion by bone marrow stromal cells or the expansion of gamma/delta T cells with possible anti-MM activity. The aim of bisphosphonates use is the reduction of SREs in patients with myeloma bone disease (Christoulas et al. 2009).

According to the latest IMWG Guidelines, bisphosphonates should be initiated in MM patients, with (grade A) or without (grade B) detectable osteolytic bone lesions in conventional radiography, who are receiving anti-myeloma therapy, as well as patients with osteoporosis (grade A) or osteopenia (grade C) due to myeloma. The beneficial effect of zoledronic acid in patients without detectable bone disease by MRI or PET/CT is not known. Oral clodronate, intravenous pamidronate, and intravenous zoledronic acid have been licensed for the management of myeloma bone disease. Etidronate and ibandronate were found to be ineffective for the treatment of bone disease in myeloma patients (Daragon et al. 1993; Menssen et al. 2002). Several studies have evaluated the effects of bisphosphonates (BPs) on SREs and bone pain in patients with MM (Terpos et al. 2013a).

7.4.1 Etidronate

Etidronate was found to be ineffective in two placebo-controlled studies in myeloma patients (Daragon et al. 1993; Belch et al. 1991).

7.4.2 Ibandronate

Ibandronate is ineffective in reducing SREs or improving bone pain in patients with MM (Menssen et al. 2002).

7.4.3 Clodronate

The oral BP, clodronate, reduced the proportion of patients with MM who experienced progression of osteolytic lesions by 50% compared with placebo (24% vs. 12%, $p = 0.026$) and reduced the time to first SRE and the rate of nonvertebral fracture (6.8% vs. 13.2% for placebo, $p = 0.04$) in patients with newly diagnosed MM (McCloskey et al. 1998). Two major, placebo-controlled, randomized trials have been performed in MM. Lahtinen et al. reported reduction of the development of new osteolytic lesions by 50% in myeloma patients who received oral CLO for 2 years that was independent of the presence of lytic lesions at baseline (Lahtinen et al. 1992). In the other study, although there was no difference in overall survival (OS) between CLO and placebo patients, patients who received CLO and did not have vertebral fractures at baseline appeared to have a survival advantage (59 vs. 37 months). Both vertebral and nonvertebral fractures as well as the time to first nonvertebral fracture and severe hypercalcemia were reduced in the CLO group after 1 year of follow-up, and at 2 years, the patients who received CLO had better performance status and less myeloma-related pain than patients treated with placebo (McCloskey et al. 2001).

7.4.4 Pamidronate

PAM is an amino-bisphosphonate, which has been administered either orally or intravenously. In one trial, patients with advanced disease and at least one lytic lesion were randomized to placebo or intravenous PAM (Berenson et al. 1998). Administration of PAM resulted in a significant reduction in skeletal-related events (SREs, 24%) versus placebo (41%, $p < 0.001$). Patients receiving PAM also experienced reduced bone pain and no deterioration in the quality of life (QoL) during the 2-year study. By contrast, administration of oral PAM failed to reduce SREs relative to placebo (Brincker et al. 1998). However, patients treated with oral PAM experienced fewer episodes of severe pain. The overall negative result of this study was attributed to the low absorption of orally administered BPs (Brincker et al. 1998). A recent study for patients with newly diagnosed MM demonstrated that PAM 30 mg monthly had comparable time with SREs and SRE-free survival time as compared with PAM 90 mg monthly. After a minimum of 3 years, patients receiving PAM 30 mg showed a trend toward lower risks of osteonecrosis of the jaw (ONJ) and nephrotoxicity compared with the higher dose. However, the study was not powered to show SRE differences between the two PAM dosages but only to show QoL differences (Gimsing et al. 2010).

7.4.5 Zoledronic Acid (ZOL)

In a non-inferiority randomized phase II trial published by Berenson et al. escalating doses of ZOL were tested in comparison with 90 mg of PAM; in 280 patients, 108 of them affected by MM (the other had metastatic breast cancer to the bone). Both ZOL (at doses of 2 and 4 mg) and PAM significantly reduced SREs in contrast to 0.4 mg ZOL (Berenson et al. 2001). This phase II trial failed to show any superiority of ZOL compared with PAM in terms of SREs, but it was not powered to show differences between the groups.

Bisphosphonates Head to Head There are only two large randomized studies comparing two different BPs. A Phase III, randomized, double-blind, study was performed to compare the effects of zoledronic acid with pamidronate for patients with myeloma and lytic bone disease or with metastatic breast cancer to the bone (Rosen et al. 2001; Rosen et al. 2003). In the myeloma cohort, there was no difference between the two treatment arms regarding incidence and time to first SRE. However, N-terminal cross-linking telopeptide of collagen type I (NTX) levels, a sensitive marker of bone resorption, normalized more often in the zoledronic acid arm compared with pamidronate-treated patients. More recently, the Medical Research Council (MRC) of the UK compared zoledronic acid (4 mg intravenous every 3–4 weeks or at doses according to creatinine clearance [CrCl] rates) and oral clodronate (1600 mg orally daily) for patients with newly diagnosed, symptomatic MM, who were treated with anti-myeloma therapy (n = 1960 evaluable for efficacy). Zoledronic acid reduced the incidence of SREs both in myeloma patients with or without bone lesions as assessed using conventional radiography, compared with clodronate (Morgan et al. 2010; Morgan et al. 2012). After a median follow-up of 3.7 years, 35% of patients receiving clodronate had experienced SREs versus 27% of patients receiving zoledronic acid (p = 0.004). More importantly, zoledronic acid reduced mortality and extended median survival. Further, subset analysis showed this that treatment extended survival by 10 months over clodronate for patients with osteolytic disease at diagnosis, whereas myeloma patients without bone disease at diagnosis as assessed using conventional radiography had no survival advantage with zoledronic acid (Morgan et al. 2012). These results confirm preclinical studies suggesting indirect and direct anti-myeloma effects of zoledronic acid (Croucher et al. 2003). Possible mechanisms for the anti-myeloma effects of zoledronic acid include direct cytotoxic effect on the tumor cells, the reduction of IL-6 secretion by bone marrow stromal cells, the expansion of gamma/delta T cells with possible anti-MM activity, anti-angiogenic effects, and inhibitory effects in the adhesion molecules. In specific subsets of patients, other BPs have also been associated with improved survival: patients receiving second-line anti-myeloma chemotherapy and treated with pamidronate experienced a borderline improvement in OS over placebo (Berenson et al. 1998), whereas clodronate had an OS advantage in patients without vertebral fractures at presentation relative to placebo (McCloskey et al. 2001). Nevertheless, a Cochrane Database meta-analysis showed that zoledronic acid was the only BP associated with superior OS compared with placebo (hazard ratio, 0.61; 95% CI, 0.28–0.98), but not compared with other BPs (Mhaskar et al. 2012).

Patients with Asymptomatic Myeloma (AMM) Intravenous PAM (60–90 mg monthly for 12 months) in patients with AMM reduced bone involvement at progression but did not decrease the risk and increase the time to progression (D'Arena et al. 2011). Similarly, intravenous ZOL (4 mg monthly for 12 months) reduced the SRE risk at progression but did not influence the risk of progression of AMM patients (Musto et al. 2008).

Several studies have reported the value of MRI (presence of >1 focal lesion and presence of diffuse pattern of marrow infiltration) in detecting patients with AMM at high risk for progression (Moulopoulos et al. 1995; Hillengass et al. 2010). Since there is no data supporting PFS advantage with bisphosphonates in AMM, bisphosphonates should not be recommended except for a clinical trial of high-risk patients.

Patients with MGUS MGUS patients are at high risk for developing osteoporosis and pathological fractures (Bida et al. 2009; Kristinsson et al. 2010). Three doses of ZOL (4 mg intravenously every 6 months) increased bone mineral density (BMD) by 15% in the lumbar spine and by 6% in the femoral neck in MGUS patients with osteopenia or osteoporosis (Berenson et al. 2008). Oral alendronate (70 mg/weekly) also increased BMD of the lumbar spine and total femur by 6.1% and 1.5%, respectively, in 50 MGUS patients with vertebral fractures and/or osteoporosis (Pepe et al. 2008).

Patients with Solitary Plasmacytoma (SPB) Patients with solitary plasmacytoma and no evidence of MM do not require therapy with bisphosphonates. However, these patients should have a whole-body MRI since in a study of 17 patients diagnosed with a solitary plasmacytoma, all showed additional focal lesions or a diffuse infiltration on MRI, leading to a classification as stage I MM (76%), stage II MM (12%), or stage

III MM (12%) using the Durie-Salmon PLUS system (Fechtner et al. 2010).

Route of Administration Strict adherence to dosing recommendations is required for bisphosphonate therapy to effectively reduce and delay SREs in patients with MM. Each patient prescribed bisphosphonate therapy should be instructed about the crucial importance of adherence to the dosing regimen. Although a few randomized, placebo-controlled clinical studies suggest that long-term compliance with oral bisphosphonates such as CLO is satisfactory in MM patients (McCloskey et al. 1998; Lahtinen et al. 1992), compliance with oral bisphosphonate therapy is generally suboptimal (Cramer et al. 2007). Further, the MRC-IX data strongly support the use of intravenous ZOL over CLO in all outcomes measured, including reduction of SREs and improvement in OS (Morgan et al. 2010; Morgan et al. 2012; Morgan et al. 2011). According to the latest IMWG guidelines, intravenous administration of BPs is the preferred choice (grade A). However, oral administration remains an option for patients who cannot receive regular hospital care or in-home nursing visits (grade D) (Terpos et al. 2013a).

Treatment Duration Intravenous bisphosphonates should be administered at 3- to 4-week intervals to all patients with active MM (grade A). ZOL improves OS and reduces SREs over CLO in patients who received treatment for more than 2 years; thus, it should be given until disease progression in patients not in complete remission (CR) or a very good partial remission (VGPR) and further continued at relapse (grade B). There is no similar evidence for PAM. PAM may be continued in patients with active disease at the physician's discretion (grade D), and PAM therapy should be resumed after disease relapse (grade D). For patients in CR/VGPR, the optimal treatment duration of BPs is not clear; according to the IMWG BPs should be given for at least 12 months and up to 24 months and then at the physician's discretion (grade D, panel consensus).

According to the latest IMWG guidelines and due to higher reported rates of ONJ with extended duration of therapy, ZOL or PAM should be discontinued after 1–2 years in patients who have achieved CR or VGPR (grade D, panel consensus) (Terpos et al. 2013a).

7.4.6 Adverse Events

Even though bisphosphonate therapy is well tolerated in patients with MM, clinicians should be alert for symptoms and signs suggesting adverse events (AEs), and patients and healthcare professionals should be instructed on how to prevent and recognize AEs. Potential AEs associated with bisphosphonate administration include hypocalcemia and hypophosphatemia, gastrointestinal events after oral administration, inflammatory reactions at the injection site, and acute-phase reactions after IV administration of amino-bisphosphonates. Renal impairment and ONJ represent infrequent but potentially serious AEs with bisphosphonate use.

Hypocalcemia Hypocalcemia is usually relatively mild and asymptomatic with bisphosphonate use in most MM patients. The incidence of symptomatic hypocalcemia is much lower in MM patients compared to patients with solid tumors. Although severe hypocalcemia has been observed in some patients (Roux et al. 2003), these events are usually preventable via the administration of oral calcium and vitamin D3. Patients should routinely receive calcium (600 mg/day) and vitamin D3 (400 IU/day) supplementation since 60% of MM patients have vitamin D deficiency or insufficiency (Badros et al. 2008a; Laroche et al. 2010). In vitamin D-deficient patients, there is an increase in bone remodeling. This fact shows that MM patients should be calcium and vitamin D sufficient (Ross et al. 2011). Calcium supplementation should be used with caution in patients with renal insufficiency.

Renal Impairment Bisphosphonate infusions are associated with both dose- and infusion rate-dependent effects on renal function. The potential for renal damage is dependent on the concentration of bisphosphonate in the bloodstream, and the highest risk is observed after administration of high dosages or rapid infusion. Both ZOL and PAM have been associated with acute renal damage or increases in serum creatinine (Rosen et al. 2001; Berenson et al. 1996). Patients should be closely monitored for compromised renal function by measuring CrCl before administration of each IV bisphosphonate infusion. Current guideline recommendations (Terpos et al. 2013a) states that the dosages of zoledronic acid and clodronate, when administered intravenously, should be reduced for patients who have preexisting renal impairment (CrCl 30–60 mL/min), but there are no clinical studies demonstrating the efficacy of this approach. For patients with CrCl between 30 and 60 mL/min, zoledronic acid dose should be adjusted. Zoledronic acid has not been studied for patients presented with severe renal impairment (CrCl <30 mL/min), and it is not recommended for patients with severe renal impairment (CrCl <30 mL/min). We suggest that pamidronate may be given at a dose of 90 mg infused over 4–6 h for myeloma patients with osteolytic disease and renal insufficiency. Furthermore, serum creatinine and CrCl should be measured before each infusion of pamidronate or zoledronic acid, while BPs should not be administered in short infusion times (<2 h for pamidronate and less than 15 min for zoledronic acid). Bisphosphonate therapy can be resumed, after withholding zoledronic acid or pamidronate for patients who develop renal deterioration during therapy, when serum creatinine returns to within 10% of the baseline (Terpos et al. 2013a).

Osteonecrosis of the Jaw It is an uncommon complication of intravenous bisphosphonates. It is potentially serious and its main characteristic is the presence of exposed bone in the mouth. Incidence may vary from 2% to 10% (Bamias et al. 2005; Dimopoulos et al. 2006). Longer exposure increases the cumulative incidence of ONJ. One of the main risk factors for the development of ONJ is the invasive dental procedures (Bamias et al. 2005). Other risk factors include poor oral hygiene, age, and duration of myeloma. Zoledronic acid was associated with a higher incidence of ONJ in retrospective evaluations (Zervas et al. 2006). In approximately one half of patients, ONJ lesions will heal (Badros et al. 2008b), but approximately one half of patients who restart bisphosphonate therapy after having stopped it will develop recurrence of ONJ. According to recent IMWG guidelines (Coleman et al. 2005), preventive strategies should be adopted to avoid ONJ. A dental examination is necessary before beginning of bisphosphonate's course. Patients should also be alerted regarding dental hygiene (grade C, panel consensus). All existing dental condition should be treated before initiation of bisphosphonate therapy (grade C, panel consensus). After bisphosphonate treatment initiation, unnecessary invasive dental procedures should be avoided, and dental health status should be monitored on annual basis (grade C). Patients' dental health status should be monitored by a physician and a dentist (grade D, panel consensus). Dental problems should be managed conservatively if possible (grade C). If invasive dental procedures are necessary, there should be temporary suspension of bisphosphonate treatment (grade D). The panel consensus suggests the interruption of bisphosphonates before and after dental procedures for a total of 180 days (90 days before and 90 days after procedures such as tooth extraction, dental implants, and surgery to the jaw). Bisphosphonates do not need to be discontinued for routine dental procedures including root canal. Initial treatment of ONJ should include discontinuation of bisphosphonates until healing occurs (grade C). The physician should consider the advantages and disadvantages of continued treatment with bisphosphonates, especially in the relapsed/refractory MM setting (grade D). Preventive measures during bisphosphonate treatment have the potential to reduce the incidence of ONJ about 75% (Dimopoulos et al. 2009b). Prophylactic antibiotic treatment may prevent ONJ occurrence after dental procedures (Montefusco et al. 2008). Management of patients depends on ONJ stage. Stage I (asymptomatic exposed bone, no soft tissue infection) can be managed conservatively with oral antimicrobial rinses. Stage II (exposed bone and associated pain/swelling and/or soft tissue infection) requires culture-directed long-term and maintenance antimicrobial therapy, analgesic management, and, occasionally, minor bony debridement. Stage III disease (pathological fracture and exposed bone or soft tissue infection not manageable with antibiotics) requires surgical resection in order to reduce the volume of necrotic bone in addition to the measures described in stage II (Migliorati et al. 2005). When ONJ occurs, initial therapy should include discontinuation of bisphosphonates until healing occurs (Terpos et al. 2009). The administration of medical ozone (O3) as an oil suspension directly to the ONJ lesions that are below ≤2.5 cm may be another possible therapeutic strategy for those patients who fail to respond to conservative treatment. In such patients, there are reports suggesting that ONJ lesions resolved with complete reconstitution of oral and jaw tissue, with three to ten applications (Ripamonti et al. 2011; Agrillo et al. 2012). In addition, treatment with hyperbaric oxygen has been reported to be helpful.

7.4.7 Future Treatment Options

7.4.7.1 RANKL/RANK Pathway Regulators: Targeting the Osteoclast

RANKL Antagonists Preclinical models of MM demonstrated that RANKL inhibition can prevent bone destruction from MM. RANKL inhibition with recombinant RANK-Fc protein not only reduced MM-induced osteolysis but also caused a marked decline in tumor burden (Yaccoby et al. 2002; Croucher et al. 2001). Similar results were obtained using recombinant OPG for the treatment of MM-bearing animals (Vanderkerken et al. 2003). These data gave the rationale for using RANKL inhibition in the clinical setting.

Denosumab A fully human monoclonal antibody has showed high affinity and specificity in binding RANKL and inhibits RANKL-RANK interaction, mimicking the endogenous effects of OPG. In knock-in mice with chimeric (murine/ human) RANKL expression, denosumab showed inhibition of bone resorption (Kostenuik et al. 2009).

In a phase I trial, 54 patients with breast cancer ($n = 29$) or MM ($n = 25$) with radiologically confirmed bone lesions received a single dose of either denosumab or pamidronate. Denosumab decreased bone resorption within 24 h of administration, as reflected by levels of urinary and serum NTX. That was similar in magnitude but more sustained than with intravenous pamidronate (Body et al. 2006). These results were confirmed in another phase I trial, in which denosumab was given at multiple doses (Yonemori et al. 2008).

In a phase II trial, the ability of denosumab (120 mg given monthly as a subcutaneous injection) to affect bone resorption markers and monoclonal protein levels in MM patients who relapsed after response to prior therapy and in patients with response to most recent therapy and who had stable disease for at least 3 months was evaluated. No patients experienced complete or partial response (≥ 50% reduction in M protein), but seven patients had maximum reduction of ≥25% in serum M protein. Bone resorption markers were reduced by more than 50% with denosumab (Vij et al. 2007).

In another phase II trial, Fizazi et al. evaluated the effect of denosumab in patients with bone metastases and elevated urinary NTX levels despite ongoing intravenous bisphosphonate therapy. Patients were stratified by tumor type (total 111 patients: 9 patients with multiple myeloma, 50 patients with prostate cancer, 46 patients with breast cancer, and 6 patients with another solid tumor) and screening NTX levels and randomly assigned to receive subcutaneous denosumab 180 mg every 4 or every 12 weeks or continue intravenous bisphosphonates every 4 weeks. Denosumab normalized urinary NTX levels more frequently than the continuation of intravenous bisphosphonate (64% vs. 37% respectively, $p = 0.01$), while fewer patients receiving denosumab experienced on-study SREs than those receiving intravenous bisphosphonate (8% vs. 17%) (Fizazi et al. 2009). This study showed that denosumab inhibits bone resorption and prevents SREs even in patients who are refractory to bisphosphonate therapy.

A meta-analysis of major phase III studies comparing denosumab versus zoledronic acid including mainly patients with solid tumors showed that denosumab was superior in terms of delaying the time to first on-study SRE by 8 months and reducing the risk of the first SRE by 17%. No difference between the two drugs was reported regarding disease progression and overall survival. Hypocalcaemia was more common in denosumab arm, while ONJ was similar with the two drugs (Lipton et al. 2012).

Denosumab appears to have little toxicity, mainly asthenia, and multiple phase III trials of denosumab in patients with bone metastasis are ongoing. However, it is crucial to mention that RANKL is involved in dendritic cell survival and that the anti-RANKL strategy may have an effect on the immune system and a possible increase in infection rate, especially in cancer patients who have already had severe immunodeficiency. For MM patients, while denosumab was comparable to zoledronic acid with respect to the occurrence of SREs, inferior survival occurred in denosumab compared to zoledronic acid-treated patients, but this was a subset analysis from a large phase III trial that involved mostly solid tumor patients with metastatic bone disease (Henry et al. 2011). Interpretation is limited based on the small numbers of MM patients who were enrolled on the trial and imbalance in baseline disease characteristics.

7.4.7.2 Activin-A Inhibitors

Sotatercept (ACE-011) is a fusion protein of the extracellular domain of the high-affinity activin receptor IIA (ActRIIA) and human immunoglobulin G (IgG) Fc domain with potent inhibitory effect on activin, enhancing the deposition of new bone tissue and preventing bone loss. In the preclinical setting, RAP-011, a murine counterpart of sotatercept, prevented the formation of osteolytic lesions in a murine MM model by stimulating bone formation through osteoblasts,

while having no effect on osteoclast activity (Chantry et al. 2010).

In a phase I study, in healthy postmenopausal volunteers, single-dose sotatercept was associated with increased serum levels of the bone formation marker bone-specific alkaline phosphatase (bALP) and decreased bone resorption markers CTX and tartrate-resistant acid phosphatase isoform 5b (TRACP-5b), reflecting a decrease in bone resorption and an increase in bone formation (Ruckle et al. 2009). No safety concerns were noted in this study.

In a multicenter phase II trial, patients with osteolytic bone lesions due to MM were randomized to receive either four 28-day cycles of sotatercept or placebo as subcutaneous injection with concomitant anticancer therapy consisting of oral melphalan, prednisolone, and thalidomide (MPT). Sotatercept treatment demonstrated clinically significant increases in biomarkers of bone formation, decreases in bone pain, and anti-tumor activity as well as increase in hemoglobin levels (Chantry et al. 2010), but further research is needed to support these findings. Moreover, increased activin-A secretion was induced by lenalidomide and was canceled by the addition of an activin-A-neutralizing antibody. This effectively restored osteoblast function and subsequently inhibited myeloma-related osteolysis without abrogating the cytotoxic effects of lenalidomide on malignant cells (Scullen et al. 2013) and thus supporting the combination of lenalidomide with an anti-activin-A molecule.

7.4.7.3 Future Agents Targeting the Osteoclast

The pathophysiology of myeloma bone disease is complex. Interactions between myeloma cells, stromal cells, osteoclasts, and osteoblasts create vicious cycles that lead to the development of osteolytic disease and support the myeloma cell growth and survival. The better understanding of this biology has revealed several other pathways that enhance osteoclastogenesis, including the PI3K/AKT/mTOR pathway, the extracellular signal-regulated kinase 1/2 pathway, the nuclear export protein

CRM1/XPO1 signaling, the MAPK pathways, the parathyroid hormone-related protein, chemokines and their receptors such as the C-C chemokine receptor types I and II (CCR1 and -2), the C-C motif ligand 3 (CCL-3, previously known as macrophage inflammatory protein 1a) pathways, and others (Christoulas et al. 2009; Oranger et al. 2013; Cao et al. 2013; Breitkreutz et al. 2007; Tai et al. 2013; Cafforio et al. 2013; Moreaux et al. 2011; Choi et al. 2001; Roussou et al. 2009). This knowledge has led to the development of novel drugs that may be used in the near future for the management of lytic bone disease in myeloma patients. AKT pathway is upregulated in marrow monocytes from MM patients, leading to a sustained high expression of RANK in osteoclast precursors. AKT inhibition blocks this upregulation of RANK expression and the subsequent osteoclast formation. In the clinical setting, the novel AKT inhibitor LY294002 blocked the formation of myeloma masses in the bone marrow cavity and dramatically reduced osteoclast formation and osteolytic lesions in SCID mice, suggesting a potential role in the management of MM patients with bone disease in the future (Cao et al. 2013). AZD6244 is a mitogen-activated or extracellular signal-regulated protein kinase (MEK) inhibitor. It has been reported in preclinical models that AZD6244 blocked osteoclast formation in a dose-dependent manner and inhibited bone resorption targeting a later stage of osteoclast differentiation (Breitkreutz et al. 2007). Novel, oral, irreversible, selective nuclear export inhibitors (SINEs) that target CRM1 have shown strong anti-myeloma activity, and they inhibit the MM-induced osteolysis. SINEs have direct anti-osteoclastic function through the blockade of RANKL-induced NF-kB and NFATc1, with almost no impact on osteoblasts, supporting their clinical development for myeloma-related bone disease (Tai et al. 2013). MLN3897 is a novel antagonist of the chemokine receptor CCR1 that demonstrated reduction of osteoclast formation and function by inhibiting the AKT signaling and the CCL-3 pathway in preclinical models (Vallet et al. 2007).

7.4.7.4 Wnt Pathway Regulators: Helping the Osteoblast

DKK-1 Antagonists DKK-1 plays an important role in the dysfunction of osteoblasts observed in MM. The production of this soluble Wnt inhibitor by MM cells inhibits osteoblast activity, and its serum level reflects the extension of focal bone lesions in MM (Durie 2006; Brincker et al. 1998). Serum DKK-1 is increased not only in symptomatic MM patients at diagnosis but also in relapsed MM, correlating with advanced disease features and the presence of lytic lesions, while serum DKK-1 levels of asymptomatic patients at diagnosis and plateau do not differ from control values (Politou et al. 2006; Terpos et al. 2010a).

BHQ880, an IgG antibody, the first in class, fully human anti-Dkk-1 neutralizing antibody, seems to promote bone formation, and thus it has been shown to inhibit tumor-induced osteolytic disease in preclinical studies (Lipton et al. 2012). Inhibiting Dkk-1 with BHQ880 in the 5T2MM murine model of myeloma reduced the development of osteolytic bone lesions and in vivo growth of MM cells (Steinman et al. 2005). A phase I/II study of BHQ880 in combination with zoledronic acid in relapsed or refractory myeloma patients is ongoing as well as phase II studies in patients with high-risk smoldering MM or untreated MM and renal insufficiency. Results are highly anticipated.

Sclerostin Antagonists Sclerostin is another Wnt inhibitor, specifically expressed by osteocytes, which inhibits osteoblast-driven bone formation and induces mature osteoblast apoptosis (Moester et al. 2010). Sclerostin deficiency leads to the development of rare bone sclerosing disorders, including sclerosteosis and van Buchem disease. On the other hand, elevated sclerostin is implicated in the mechanisms of bone loss in metabolic bone diseases, such as postmenopausal osteoporosis and thalassemia-associated osteoporosis (Polyzos et al. 2012; Voskaridou et al. 2012). Elevated circulating sclerostin levels correlate with advanced disease features and abnormal bone remodeling in symptomatic myeloma (Terpos et al. 2012b). In particular, MM patients who presented with fractures at diagnosis had very high levels of circulating sclerostin compared with all others ($p < 0.01$), while sclerostin serum levels correlated negatively with bALP ($r = -0.541, p < 0.0001$) and positively with CTX ($r = 0.524, p < 0.0001$) (Terpos et al. 2012b). Romosozumab (AMG 785, CDP7851), an investigational humanized monoclonal antibody that inhibits the activity of sclerostin, has been used in phase II clinical studies in postmenopausal women with low bone mineral density (BMD), demonstrating significant increases in lumbar spine BMD after 12 months (Lewiecki 2011). Studies in MM are planned to start soon.

7.5 Anti-Myeloma Agents

7.5.1 Bortezomib

Bortezomib is the first proteasome inhibitor with established activity against myeloma, with subsequent effects on osteoclasts that leads to reduced bone resorption (von Metzler et al. 2007; Boissy et al. 2008). For patients with relapsed/refractory MM, bortezomib reduces circulating RANKL, osteoclast function, and bone resorption, as assessed by TRACP-5b and CTX serum levels, respectively (Terpos et al. 2006). Furthermore, bortezomib increases osteoblast activity and bone formation both in vitro and for patients with relapsed/refractory MM (Giuliani et al. 2007; Zangari et al. 2005). More specifically, bortezomib increased bone formation markers such as bALP; this increase was observed both among responders and non-responders to bortezomib suggesting a direct effect of bortezomib on osteoblastic activity (Heider et al. 2006). Another proteasome inhibitor, carfilzomib, has been reported to increase bALP in patients with relapsed/refractory MM that responded to therapy (Zangari et al. 2011). Bortezomib in combination with zoledronic acid increased BMD in a subset of MM patients at first relapse even in the presence of dexamethasone (Terpos et al. 2010b). However, when bortezomib was given in combination with other anti-myeloma drugs, such as melphalan and thalidomide (VMDT regimen), no increase in bALP and osteocalcin was observed suggesting that in such combinations, bortezomib seems to lose its beneficial effect on osteoblasts (Terpos et al. 2008). Even in post-autologous stem cell transplantation patients with low myeloma burden, bortezomib in combination with thalidomide and dexamethasone as consolidation therapy failed to produce a significant bone anabolic effect (Terpos et al. 2013b). Nevertheless, in this specific cohort of patients who did not receive BPs during consolidation, bone resorption was reduced, and there were no SREs in responding patients. In a subanalysis of a phase III study in newly diagnosed patients (VISTA trial), bortezomib in combination with melphalan and prednisone (VMP) reduced substantially DKK-1 in responding patients, while the MP regimen increased DKK-1 even in responders (Delforge et al. 2011). In the same study, there was evident bone formation effect in conventional radiography in a subset of VMP patients but not in MP patients (Delforge et al. 2011).

These findings suggest that proteasome inhibition and especially bortezomib, in addition to its antineoplastic effects on tumor cells, may directly stimulate osteoblast differentiation and function and lead to increased bone formation and increased BMD, at least in responders. However, it is unclear if bortezomib alone is sufficient to reverse bone disease in MM patients and heal lytic lesions as evidence of the effect of bortezomib on clinical end points specific to the bone, such as SREs is limited, possibly as a result of relatively short follow-up periods. Prospective trials that specifically investigate end points related to bone formation are needed.

7.5.2 Immunomodulatory Agents

Immunomodulatory agents (IMiDs), such as thalidomide, lenalidomide, and pomalidomide, are highly active agents in the treatment of both newly diagnosed and relapsed/refractory MM. These agents also alter interactions between bone marrow microenvironment and malignant plasma cells and modify abnormal bone metabolism in MM (Christoulas et al. 2009).

Thalidomide Thalidomide almost completely blocks RANKL-induced osteoclast formation in vitro. In relapsed/refractory MM patients, intermediate dose of thalidomide (200 mg/d) in combination with dexamethasone produced a significant reduction of serum markers of bone resorption [C-telopeptide of collagen type I (CTX) and tartrate-resistant acid phosphatase isoform-5b (TRACP-5b)] and also of sRANKL/OPG ratio (Terpos et al. 2005).

Lenalidomide Lenalidomide also inhibited osteoclast formation, by targeting PU.1, a critical transcription factor for the development of osteoclasts, and downregulating cathepsin K. The downregulation of PU.1 in hematopoietic progenitor cells resulted in a complete shift of lineage development toward granulocytes. Lenalidomide also reduced the serum levels of sRANKL/OPG ratio in MM patients (Breitkreutz et al. 2008).

Pomalidomide Pomalidomide, like thalidomide, blocks RANKL-induced osteoclastogenesis in vitro, even at concentrations of 1 μM, which is similar or even lower than that achieved in vivo after the therapeutic administration of this agent. Pomalidomide downregulates transcription factor PU.1, affecting the lineage commitment of osteoclast precursors toward granulocytes instead of mature osteoclasts (Anderson et al. 2006).

7.5.3 Other Novel Agents

Panobinostat is a histone deacetylase inhibitor, which has shown significant preclinical anti-myeloma activity and is currently in phase III trials for relapsed MM. Recently, a potent synergistic antiproliferative effect of panobinostat with zoledronic acid was described in three myeloma cell lines and may result in clinical trials in myeloma patients (Bruzzese et al. 2013).

Bruton's tyrosine kinase (BTK) has been reported to play an important role in myeloma cell homing to the bone and the subsequent myeloma-induced bone disease (Bam et al. 2013). Several BTK inhibitors have been developed including ibrutinib, which was recently approved for the treatment of mantle cell lymphoma. This new category of drugs has entered into clinical trials in myeloma patients and may be used in the future in patients with bone disease.

Other novel anti-myeloma agents have also shown effects on bone disease in preclinical models. Antibodies against B-cell-activating factor (anti-BAFF) have produced direct anti-myeloma effects and reductions in tartrate-resistant acid phosphatase-positive osteoclasts and in lytic lesions in anti-BAFF-treated animals (Neri et al. 2007). Similarly, SCIO-469, a selective p38a MAPK inhibitor, inhibited MM growth and prevented bone disease in the 5T2MM and 5T33MM animal models (Vanderkerken et al. 2007).

7.6 Kyphoplasty and Vertebroplasty

Several studies have demonstrated that balloon kyphoplasty (BKP) and vertebroplasty are well-tolerated and effective procedures that provide pain relief and improve functional outcomes in patients with painful neoplastic spinal fractures. A single randomized study of 134 patients with bone metastases due to solid tumors and MM demonstrated that treatment of VCFs with BKP was associated with clinically meaningful improvements in physical functioning, back pain, QoL, and ability to perform daily activities relative to nonsurgical management. These benefits persisted throughout the 12-month study (Berenson et al. 2011). A meta-analysis of seven nonrandomized studies of patients with MM or osteolytic metastasis revealed that BKP was associated with reduced pain and improved functional outcomes, benefits that were maintained up to 2 years post-procedure ($N = 306$). BKP also improved early vertebral height loss and spinal deformity, but these effects were not long term (Bouza et al. 2009). Similarly, a retrospective review of 67 patients with MM-related vertebral compression fractures (VCFs) demonstrated that vertebroplasty provided clinically meaningful improvements in physical functioning, pain, and mobility throughout 12 months of follow-up (McDonald et al. 2008). Several small nonrandomized studies of BKP or BKP and vertebroplasty generated comparable results (Huber et al. 2009; Zou et al. 2010; Dalbayrak et al. 2010). However, the role of vertebroplasty for myeloma patients remains debatable in the absence of prospective data (Zou et al. 2010), as two randomized trials failed to show any benefit of vertebroplasty in patients with osteoporotic fractures versus conservative therapy (Buchbinder et al. 2009; Kallmes et al. 2009). Furthermore, a meta-analysis of 59 studies (56 case series) showed that BKP appears to be more effective than vertebroplasty in relieving pain secondary to cancer-related VCFs and is associated with lower rates of cement leakage (Bhargava et al. 2009).

7.7 Radiation Therapy

Several studies, the majority of which were retrospective and included relatively small patient cohorts, demonstrated that radiotherapy provided pain relief, decreased analgesic use, promoted recalcification, reduced neurologic symptoms, and improved motor function and QoL in patients with MM (Rades et al. 2006; Hirsch et al. 2011; Balducci et al. 2011). In addition, the total administered dose should be limited and the field of therapy restricted, especially when the aim of treatment is pain relief rather than treatment or prevention of pathologic fractures. A single 8–10 Gy fraction is generally recommended. Indeed, single fractions are increasingly preferred to fractionated treatment. No difference in rapidity of onset or duration of pain relief was observed between a single 8 Gy fraction and a fractionated 2-week course of 30 Gy in a randomized study of 288 patients with widespread bony metastases, including 23 patients with MM (Price et al. 1986).

MM accounts for 11% of the most prevalent cancer diagnoses causing spinal cord compression (SCC) (Mak et al. 2011). In the largest retrospective series to date, radiotherapy alone improved motor function in 75% of patients with MM and SCC. One-year local control was 100%, and 1-year survival was 94% (Rades et al. 2007).

7.8 Surgery

Surgery is usually directed toward preventing or repairing axial fractures, unstable spinal fractures, and SCC in myeloma patients. Decompression laminectomy is rarely required in MM patients, but radioresistant MM or retropulsed bone fragments may require surgical intervention (Wedin 2001). In a relatively large study, 75 MM patients were treated surgically (83 interventions) for skeletal complications of the disease. Most of the lesions were in the axial skeleton or the proximal extremities apart from one distal lesion of the fibula, and most surgery was performed in the spine (35 patients). Surgical treatment in these patients was mostly limited to a palliative approach and was well tolerated (Utzschneider et al. 2011).

References

Abe M, Hiura K, Wilde J et al (2004) Osteoclasts enhance myeloma cell growth and survival via cell-cell contact: a vicious cycle between bone destruction and myeloma expansion. Blood 104(8):2484–2491

Agrillo A, Filiaci F, Ramieri V et al (2012) Bisphosphonate-related osteonecrosis of the jaw (BRONJ): 5 year experience in the treatment of 131 cases with ozone therapy. Eur Rev Med Pharmacol Sci 16(12):1741–1747

Alongi P, Zanoni L, Incerti E et al (2015) 18F-FDG PET/CT for early post-radiotherapy assessment in solitary bone plasmacytomas. Clin Nucl Med 40:e399–e404

Anderson G, Gries M, Kurihara N et al (2006) Thalidomide derivative CC-4047 inhibits osteoclast formation by down-regulation of PU.1. Blood 107(8):3098–3105

Aparicio A, Gardner A, Tu Y et al (1998) In vitro cytoreductive effects on multiple myeloma cells induced by bisphosphonates. Leukemia 12:220

Attariwala R, Picker W (2013) Whole body MRI: improved lesion detection and characterization with diffusion weighted techniques. J Magn Reson Imaging 38:253–268

Badros A, Goloubeva O, Terpos E et al (2008a) Prevalence and significance of vitamin D deficiency in multiple myeloma patients. Br J Haematol 142:492–494

Badros A, Terpos E, Katodritou E et al (2008b) Natural history of osteonecrosis of the jaw in patients with multiple myeloma. J Clin Oncol 26(36):5904–5909

Balducci M, Chiesa S, Manfrida S et al (2011) Impact of radiotherapy on pain relief and recalcification in plasma cell neoplasms: long-term experience. Strahlenther Onkol 187:114–119

Bam R, Ling W, Khan S et al (2013) Role of Bruton's tyrosine kinase in myeloma cell migration and induction of bone disease. Am J Hematol 88(6):463–471

Bamias A, Kastritis E, Bamia C et al (2005) Osteonecrosis of the jaw in cancer after treatment with bisphosphonates: incidence and risk factors. J Clin Oncol 23(34):8580–8587

Bannas P, Hentschel HB, Bley TA et al (2012) Diagnostic performance of whole-body MRI for the detection of persistent or relapsing disease in multiple myeloma after stem cell transplantation. Eur Radiol 22:2007–2012

Bartel TB, Haessler J, Brown TL et al (2009) F18-fluorodeoxyglucose positron emission tomography in the context of other imaging techniques and prognostic factors in multiple myeloma. Blood 114:2068–2076

Bataille R, Chappard D, Marcelli C et al (1991) Recruitment of new osteoblasts and osteoclasts is the earliest critical event in the pathogenesis of human multiple myeloma. J Clin Invest 88(1):62–66

Bauerle T, Hillengass J, Fechtner K et al (2009) Multiple myeloma and monoclonal gammopathy of undetermined significance: importance of whole-body versus spinal MR imaging. Radiology 252:477–485

Baur A, Stabler A, Bruning R et al (1998) Diffusion-weighted MR imaging of bone marrow: differentiation of benign versus pathologic compression fractures. Radiology 207:349–356

Baur-Melnyk A, Buhmann S, Durr HR et al (2005) Role of MRI for the diagnosis and prognosis of multiple myeloma. Eur J Radiol 55:56–63

Baur-Melnyk A, Buhmann S, Becker C et al (2008) Whole-body MRI versus whole-body MDCT for staging of multiple myeloma. AJR Am J Roentgenol 190:1097–1104

Belch AR, Bergsagel DE, Wilson K et al (1991) Effect of daily etidronate on the osteolysis of multiple myeloma. J Clin Oncol 9(8):1397–1402

Berenson J, Pflugmacher R, Jarzem P et al (2011) Balloon kyphoplasty versus non-surgical fracture management for treatment of painful vertebral body compression fractures in patients with cancer: a multicentre, randomised controlled trial. Lancet Oncol 12:225–3596

Berenson JR, Lichtenstein A, Porter L et al (1996) Efficacy of pamidronate in reducing skeletal events in patients with advanced multiple myeloma. Myeloma Aredia Study Group. N Engl J Med 334(8):488–493

Berenson JR, Lichtenstein A, Porter L et al (1998) Long-term pamidronate treatment of advanced multiple myeloma patients reduces skeletal events. Myeloma Aredia Study Group. J Clin Oncol 16(2):593–602

Berenson JR, Rosen LS, Howell A et al (2001) Zoledronic acid reduces skeletal-related events in patients with osteolytic metastases. Cancer 91(7):1191–1200

Berenson JR, Yellin O, Boccia RV et al (2008) Zoledronic acid markedly improves bone mineral density for patients with monoclonal gammopathy of undetermined significance and bone loss. Clin Cancer Res 14:6289–6295

Bhargava A, Trivedi D, Kalva L et al (2009) Management of cancer-related vertebral compression fracture: comparison of treatment options: a literature meta-analysis. J Clin Oncol (Meeting Abstracts) 27:e20529

Bida JP, Kyle RA, Therneau TM et al (2009) Disease associations with monoclonal gammopathy of undetermined significance: a population-based study of 17,398 patients. Mayo Clin Proc 84:685–693

Body JJ, Facon T, Coleman RE et al (2006) A study of the biological receptor activator of nuclear factor-kappaB ligand inhibitor, denosumab, in patients with multiple myeloma or bone metastases from breast cancer. Clin Cancer Res 12(4):1221–1228

Boissy P, Andersen TL, Lund T et al (2008) Pulse treatment with the proteasome inhibitor bortezomib inhibits osteoclast resorptive activity in clinically relevant conditions. Leuk Res 32(11):1661–1668

Boonekamp PM, van der Wee-Pals LJ, van Wijk-van Lennep MM et al (1986) Two modes of action of bisphosphonates on osteoclastic resorption of mineralized matrix. Bone Miner 1:27

Borggrefe J, Giravent S, Campbell G et al (2015) Association of osteolytic lesions, bone mineral loss and trabecular sclerosis with prevalent vertebral fractures in patients with multiple myeloma. Eur J Radiol 84:2269–2274

Bouza C, Lopez-Cuadrado T, Cediel P et al (2009) Balloon kyphoplasty in malignant spinal fractures: a systematic review and meta-analysis. BMC Palliat Care 8:12

Bredella MA, Steinbach L, Caputo G et al (2005) Value of FDG PET in the assessment of patients with multiple myeloma. AJR Am J Roentgenol 184:1199–1204

Breitkreutz I, Raab MS, Vallet S et al (2007) Targeting MEK1/2 blocks osteoclast differentiation, function and cytokine secretion in multiple myeloma. Br J Haematol 139(1):55–63

Breitkreutz I, Raab MS, Vallet S et al (2008) Lenalidomide inhibits osteoclastogenesis, survival factors and bone-remodeling markers in multiple myeloma. Leukemia 22(10):1925–1932

Breyer RJ 3rd, Mulligan ME, Smith SE et al (2006) Comparison of imaging with FDG PET/CT with other imaging modalities in myeloma. Skelet Radiol 35:632–640

Brincker H, Westin J, Abildgaard N et al (1998) Failure of oral pamidronate to reduce skeletal morbidity in multiple myeloma: a double-blind placebo-controlled trial. Danish-Swedish co-operative study group. Br J Haematol 101(2):280–286

Bruce NJ, McCloskey EV, Kanis JA et al (1999) Economic impact of using clodronate in the management of patients with multiple myeloma. Br J Haematol 104:358–364

Bruzzese F, Pucci B, Milone MR et al (2013) Panobinostat synergizes with zoledronic acid in prostate cancer and multiple myeloma models by increasing ROS and modulating mevalonate and p38-MAPK pathways. Cell Death Dis 4:e878

Buchbinder R, Osborne RH, Ebeling PR et al (2009) A randomized trial of vertebroplasty for painful osteoporotic vertebral fractures. N Engl J Med 361:557–568

Cafforio P, Savonarola A, Stucci S et al (2013) PTHrP produced by myeloma plasma cells regulates their survival and pro-osteoclast activity for bone disease progression. J Bone Miner Res 29(1):55–66

Cao H, Zhu K, Qiu L et al (2013) Critical role of AKT protein in myeloma-induced osteoclast formation and osteolysis. J Biol Chem 288(42):30399–30410

Carlson K, Aström G, Nyman R et al (1995) MR imaging of multiple myeloma in tumour mass measurement at diagnosis and during treatment. Acta Radiol 36:9–14

Cascini GL, Falcone C, Console D et al (2013) Whole-body MRI and PET/CT in multiple myeloma patients during staging and after treatment: personal experience in a longitudinal study. Radiol Med 118(6):930–948

Chantry AD, Heath D, Mulivor AW et al (2010) Inhibiting activin-a signaling stimulates bone formation and prevents cancer-induced bone destruction in vivo. J Bone Miner Res 25(12):2633–2646

Choi SJ, Oba Y, Gazitt Y et al (2001) Antisense inhibition of macrophage inflammatory protein 1-alpha blocks bone destruction in a model of myeloma bone disease. J Clin Invest 108(12):1833–1841

Christoulas D, Terpos E, Dimopoulos MA (2009) Pathogenesis and management of myeloma bone disease. Expert Rev Hematol 2:385–398

Cocks K, Cohen D, Wisloff F et al (2007) An international field study of the reliability and validity of a disease-specific questionnaire module (the QLQ-MY20) in assessing the quality of life of patients with multiple myeloma. Eur J Cancer 43:1670–1678

Coleman RE (2007) Skeletal complications of malignancy. Cancer 80:1588–1594

Coleman RE, Major P, Lipton A et al (2005) Predictive value of bone resorption and formation markers in cancer patients with bone metastases receiving the bisphosphonate zoledronic acid. J Clin Oncol 23(22):4925–4935

Colucci S, Brunetti G, Oranger A et al (2011) Myeloma cells suppress osteoblasts through sclerostin secretion. Blood Cancer J 1:e27

Cramer JA, Gold DT, Silverman SL et al (2007) A systematic review of persistence and compliance with bisphosphonates for osteoporosis. Osteoporos Int 18:1023–1031

Cretti F, Perugini G (2016) Patient dose evaluation for the whole-body low-dose multidetector CT (WBLDMDCT) skeleton study in multiple myeloma (MM). Radiol Med 121(2):93–105

Croucher PI, Apperley JF (1998) Bone disease in multiple myeloma. Br J Haematol 103:902–910

Croucher PI, Shipman CM, Lippitt J et al (2001) Osteoprotegerin inhibits the development of osteolytic bone disease in multiple myeloma. Blood 98(13):3534–3540

Croucher PI, De Hendrik R, Perry MJ et al (2003) Zoledronic acid treatment of 5T2MM-bearing mice inhibits the development of myeloma bone disease: evidence for decreased osteolysis, tumor burden and angiogenesis, and increased survival. J Bone Miner Res 18(3):482–492

D'Arena G, Gobbi PG, Broglia C et al (2011) Pamidronate versus observation in asymptomatic myeloma: final results with long-term follow-up of a randomized study. Leuk Lymphoma 52:771–775

Dalbayrak S, Onen M, Yilmaz M et al (2010) Clinical and radiographic results of balloon kyphoplasty for treatment of vertebral body metastases and multiple myelomas. J Clin Neurosci 17:219–224

Daragon A, Humez C, Michot C et al (1993) Treatment of multiple myeloma with etidronate: results of a multicentre double-blind study. Eur J Med 2(8):449–452

Delforge M, Terpos E, Richardson PG et al (2011) Fewer bone disease events, improvement in bone remodeling, and evidence of bone healing with Bortezomib plus melphalan-prednisone vs. melphalan-prednisone in the phase III VISTA trial in multiple myeloma. Eur J Haematol 86:372–384

Derlin T, Peldschus K, Münster S et al (2013) Comparative diagnostic performance of ^{18}F-FDG PET/CT versus whole-body MRI for determination of remission status in multiple myeloma after stem cell transplantation. Eur Radiol 23:570–578

Dhodapkar MV, Singh J, Mehta J et al (1998) Anti-myeloma activity of pamidronate in vivo. Br J Haematol 103:530

Dhodapkar MV, Sexton R, Waheed S et al (2014) Clinical, genomic, and imaging predictors of myeloma progression from asymptomatic monoclonal gammopathies (SWOG S0120). Blood 123:78–85

Diel IJ, Solomayer EF, Costa SD et al (1998) Reduction in new metastases in breast cancer with adjuvant clodronate treatment. N Engl J Med 339:357

Dimopoulos M, Terpos E, Comenzo RL et al (2009a) International myeloma working group consensus statement and guidelines regarding the current role of imaging techniques in the diagnosis and monitoring of multiple Myeloma. Leukemia 23:1545–1556

Dimopoulos MA, Kastritis E, Bamia C et al (2009b) Reduction of osteonecrosis of the jaw (ONJ) after implementation of preventive measures in patients with multiple myeloma treated with zoledronic acid. Ann Oncol 20(1):117–120

Dimopoulos MA, Moulopoulos A, Smith T et al (1993) Risk of disease progression in asymptomatic multiple myeloma. Am J Med 94:57–61

Dimopoulos MA, Moulopoulos LA, Maniatis A et al (2000) Solitary plasmacytoma of bone and asymptomatic multiple myeloma. Blood 96:2037–2044

Dimopoulos MA, Kastritis E, Anagnostopoulos A et al (2006) Osteonecrosis of the jaw in patients with multiple myeloma treated with bisphosphonates: evidence of increased risk after treatment with zoledronic acid. Haematologica 91(7):968–971

Dimopoulos MA, Hillengass J, Usmani S et al (2015) Role of magnetic resonance imaging in the management of patients with multiple myeloma: a consensus statement. J Clin Oncol 33(6):657–664. https://doi.org/10.1200/JCO.2014.57.9961

Durie BGM (2006) The role of anatomic and functional staging in myeloma: description of Durie/Salmon plus staging system. Eur J Cancer 42:1539–1543

Fechtner K, Hillengass J, Delorme S et al (2010) Staging monoclonal plasma cell disease: comparison of the Durie-Salmon and the Durie-Salmon PLUS staging systems. Radiology 257:195–204

Fizazi K, Lipton A, Mariette X et al (2009) Randomized phase II trial of denosumab in patients with bone metastases from prostate cancer, breast cancer, or other neoplasms after intravenous bisphosphonates. J Clin Oncol 27(10):1564–1571

Fonti R, Pace L, Cerchione C et al (2015) 18F-FDG PET/CT, 99mTc-MIBI, and MRI in the prediction of outcome of patients with multiple myeloma: a comparative study. Clin Nucl Med 40:303–308

Fouquet G, Guidez S, Herbaux C et al (2014) Impact of initial FDG-PET/CT and serum-free light chain on transformation of conventionally defined solitary plasmacytoma to multiple myeloma. Clin Cancer Res 20:3254–3260

Fraioli F, Punwani S (2014) Clinical and research applications of simultaneous positron emission tomography and MRI. Br J Radiol 87:20130464

Ghanem N, Lohrmann C, Engelhardt M et al (2006) Whole-body MRI in the detection of bone marrow infiltration in patients with plasma cell neoplasms in comparison to the radiological skeletal survey. Eur Radiol 16:1005–1014

Giles SL, Messiou C, Collins DJ et al (2014) Whole-body diffusion-weighted MR imaging for assessment of treatment response in myeloma. Radiology 271(3):785–794

Giles SL, deSouza NM, Collins DJ et al (2015) Assessing myeloma bone disease with whole-body diffusion-weighted imaging: comparison with x-ray skeletal survey by region and relationship with laboratory estimates of disease burden. Clin Radiol 70:614–621

Gimsing P, Carlson K, Turesson I et al (2010) Effect of pamidronate 30 mg versus 90 mg on physical function in patients with newly diagnosed multiple myeloma (Nordic Myeloma Study Group): a double-blind, randomised controlled trial. Lancet Oncol 11(10):973–982

Giuliani N, Morandi F, Tagliaferri S et al (2007) The proteasome inhibitor bortezomib affects osteoblast differentiation in vitro and in vivo in multiple myeloma patients. Blood 110(1):334–338

Gleeson TG, Moriarty J, Shortt CP et al (2009) Accuracy of whole-body low-dose multidetector CT (WBLDCT) versus skeletal survey in the detection of myclomatous lesions, and correlation of disease distribution with whole-body MRI (WBMRI). Skelet Radiol 38:225–236

Heider U, Kaiser M, Muller C et al (2006) Bortezomib increases osteoblast activity in myeloma patients irrespective of response to treatment. Eur J Haematol 77(3):233–238

Henry DH, Costa L, Goldwasser F et al (2011) Randomized, double-blind study of denosumab versus zoledronic acid in the treatment of bone metastases in patients with advanced cancer (excluding breast and prostate cancer) or multiple myeloma. J Clin Oncol 29(9):1125–1132

Hillengass J, Landgren O (2013) Challenges and opportunities of novel imaging techniques in monoclonal plasma cell disorders: imaging "early myeloma". Leuk Lymphoma 54:1355–1363

Hillengass J, Wasser K, Delorme S et al (2007) Lumbar bone marrow microcirculation measurements from dynamic contrast-enhanced magnetic resonance imaging is a predictor of event-free survival in progressive multiple myeloma. Clin Cancer Res 13:475–481

Hillengass J, Fechtner K, Weber MA et al (2010) Prognostic significance of focal lesions in whole-body magnetic resonance imaging in patients with asymptomatic multiple myeloma. J Clin Oncol 28:1606–1610

Hillengass J, Bäuerle T, Bartl R et al (2011) Diffusion-weighted imaging for non-invasive and quantitative monitoring of bone marrow infiltration in patients with monoclonal plasma cell disease: a comparative study with histology. Br J Haematol 153:721–728

Hillengass J, Ayyaz S, Kilk K et al (2012) Changes in magnetic resonance imaging before and after autologous stem cell transplantation correlate with response and survival in multiple myeloma. Haematologica 97:1757–1760

Hillengass J, Weber MA, Kilk K et al (2014) Prognostic significance of whole-body MRI in patients with monoclonal gammopathy of undetermined significance. Leukemia 28:174–178

Hirsch AE, Jha RM, Yoo AJ et al (2011) The use of vertebral augmentation and external beam radiation therapy in the multimodal management of malignant vertebral compression fractures. Pain Physician 14:447–458

Horger M, Claussen CD, Bross-Bach U et al (2005) Whole-body low-dose multidetector row-CT in the diagnosis of multiple myeloma: an alternative to conventional radiography. Eur J Radiol 54:289–297

Horger M, Weisel K, Horger W et al (2011) Whole-body diffusion-weighted MRI with apparent diffusion coefficient mapping for early response monitoring in multiple myeloma: preliminary results. AJR Am J Roentgenol 196:W790–W795

Huang SY, Chen BB, HY L et al (2012) Correlation among DCE-MRI measurements of bone marrow angiogenesis, microvessel density, and extramedullary disease in patients with multiple myeloma. Am J Hematol 87:837–839

Huber F, McArthur N, Tanner M et al (2009) Kyphoplasty for patients with multiple myeloma is a safe surgical procedure: results from a large patient cohort. Clin Lymphoma Myeloma 9:375–380

Ippolito D, Besostri V, Bonaffini PA et al (2013) Diagnostic value of whole-body low-dose computed tomography (WBLDCT) in bone lesions detection in patients with multiple myeloma. Eur J Radiol 82:2322–2327

Jemal A, Siegel R, Xu J et al (2010) Cancer statistics. CA Cancer J Clin 60:277–300

Kallmes DF, Comstock BA, Heagerty PJ et al (2009) A randomized trial of vertebroplasty for osteoporotic spinal fractures. N Engl J Med 361:569–579

Kastritis E, Zervas K, Symeonidis A et al (2009) Improved survival of patients with multiple myeloma after the introduction of novel agents and the applicability of the International Staging System (ISS): an analysis of the Greek Myeloma Study Group (GMSG). Leukemia 23:1152–1157

Kastritis E, Terpos E, Moulopoulos L et al (2013) Extensive bone marrow infiltration and abnormal free light chain ratio identifies patients with asymptomatic myeloma at high risk for progression to symptomatic disease. Leukemia 27:947–953

Khalafallah AA, Snarski A, Heng R et al (2013) Assessment of whole body MRI and sestamibi technetium-99m bone marrow scan in prediction of multiple myeloma disease progression and outcome: a prospective comparative study. BMJ Open 3:pii: e002025

Kostenuik P, Nguyen H, McCabe J et al (2009) Denosumab, a fully human monoclonal antibody to RANKL, inhibits bone resorption and increases bone density in knock-in mice that express chimeric (murine/human) RANKL. J Bone Miner Res 24(2):182–195

Kristinsson SY, Tang M, Pfeiffer RM et al (2010) Monoclonal gammopathy of undetermined significance and risk of skeletal fractures: a population-based study. Blood 116:2651–2655

Kropil P, Fenk R, Fritz LB et al (2008) Comparison of whole- body 64-slice multidetector computed tomography and conventional radiography in staging of multiple myeloma. Eur Radiol 18:51–58

Kumar SK, Rajkumar SV, Dispenzieri A et al (2008) Improved survival in multiple myeloma and the impact of novel therapies. Blood 111:2516–2520

Kyle RA, Gertz MA, Witzig TE et al (2003) Review of 1027 patients with newly diagnosed multiple myeloma. Mayo Clin Proc 78:21–33

Lafforgue P, Dahan E, Chagnaud C et al (1993) Early-stage avascular necrosis of the femoral head: MR imaging for prognosis in 31 cases with at least 2 years of follow-up. Radiology 187:199–204

Lahtinen R, Laakso M, Palva I et al (1992) Randomised, placebo-controlled multicentre trial of clodronate in multiple myeloma. Lancet 340(8832):1049–1052

Lapa C, Lückerath K, Malzahn U et al (2014) 18 FDG-PET/CT for prognostic stratification of patients with multiple myeloma relapse after stem cell transplantation. Oncotarget 5(17):7381–7391

Laroche M, Lemaire O, Attal M (2010) Vitamin D deficiency does not alter biochemical markers of bone metabolism before or after autograft in patients with multiple myeloma. Eur J Haematol 85:65–67

Lecouvet FE, Vande Berg BC, Michaux L et al (1998) Stage III multiple myeloma: clinical and prognostic value of spinal bone marrow MR imaging. Radiology 209:653–660

Lecouvet FE, Malghem J, Michaux L et al (1999) Skeletal survey in advanced multiple myeloma: radiographic versus MR imaging survey. Br J Haematol 106:35–39

Lemke A, Stieltjes B, Schad LR et al (2011) Toward an optimal distribution of b values for intravoxel incoherent motion imaging. Magn Reson Imaging 29:766–776

Lewiecki EM (2011) Sclerostin: a novel target for intervention in the treatment of osteoporosis. Discov Med 12(65):263–273

Libshitz HI, Malthouse SR, Cunningham D et al (1992) Multiple myeloma: appearance at MR imaging. Radiology 182:833–837

Liebross RH, Ha CS, Cox JD et al (1998) Solitary bone plasmacytoma: outcome and prognostic factors following radiotherapy. Int J Radiat Oncol Biol Phys 41:1063–1067

Lipton A, Fizazi K, Stopeck AT et al (2012) Superiority of denosumab to zoledronic acid for prevention of skeletal-related events: a combined analysis of 3 pivotal, randomised, phase 3 trials. Eur J Cancer 48(16):3082–3092

Lonial S, Kaufman JL (2013) Non-secretory myeloma: a clinician's guide. Oncology (Williston Park) 27:924–928

Ludwig H, Frühwald F, Tscholakoff D et al (1987) Magnetic resonance imaging of the spine in multiple myeloma. Lancet 2:364–366

Lütje S, de Rooy JW, Croockewit S et al (2009) Role of radiography, MRI and FDG-PET/CT in diagnosing, staging and therapeutical evaluation of patients with multiple myeloma. Ann Hematol 88:1161–1168

Mak KS, Lee LK, Mak RH et al (2011) Incidence and treatment patterns in hospitalizations for malignant spinal cord compression in the United States, 1998–2006. Int J Radiat Oncol Biol Phys 80:824–831

McCloskey EV, MacLennan IC, Drayson MT et al (1998) A randomized trial of the effect of clodronate on skeletal morbidity in multiple myeloma. MRC Working Party on Leukaemia in Adults. Br J Haematol 100:317–325

McCloskey EV, Dunn JA, Kanis JA et al (2001) Long-term follow-up of a prospective, double-blind, placebo-controlled randomized trial of clodronate in multiple myeloma. Br J Haematol 113(4):1035–1043

McDonald RJ, Trout AT, Gray LA et al (2008) Vertebroplasty in multiple myeloma: outcomes in a large patient series. AJNR Am J Neuroradiol 29:642–648

Menssen HD, Sakalova A, Fontana A et al (2002) Effects of long-term intravenous ibandronate therapy on skeletal-related events, survival, and bone resorption markers in patients with advanced multiple myeloma. J Clin Oncol 20(9):2353–2359

Merz M, Hielscher T, Wagner B et al (2014) Predictive value of longitudinal whole-body magnetic resonance imaging in patients with smoldering multiple myeloma. Leukemia 28(9):1902–1908

Messiou C, Collins DJ, Morgan VA et al (2011) Optimising diffusion weighted MRI for imaging metastatic and myeloma bone disease and assessing reproducibility. Eur Radiol 21:1713–1718

Messiou C, Giles S, Collins DJ et al (2012) Assessing response of myeloma bone disease with diffusion-weighted MRI. Br J Radiol 85:e1198–e1203

Mhaskar R, Redzepovic J, Wheatley K et al (2012) Bisphosphonates in multiple myeloma: a network meta-analysis. Cochrane Database Syst Rev 5:CD003188

Migliorati CA, Casiglia J, Epstein J et al (2005) Managing the care of patients with bisphosphonate-associated osteonecrosis an American Academy of Oral Medicine position paper. J Am Dent Assoc 136(12):1658–1668

Moester MJ, Papapoulos SE, Löwik CW et al (2010) Sclerostin: current knowledge and future perspectives. Calcif Tissue Int 87(2):99–107

Montefusco V, Gay F, Spina F et al (2008) Antibiotic prophylaxis before dental procedures may reduce the incidence of osteonecrosis of the jaw in patients with multiple myeloma treated with bisphosphonates. Leuk Lymphoma 49(11):2156–2162

Moreau P, Attal M, Karlin L et al (2015) Prospective evaluation of MRI and PET-CT at diagnosis and before maintenance therapy in symptomatic patients with Multiple Myeloma included in the IFM/DFCI 2009 trial. Blood 126:395. (ASH abstract)

Moreaux J, Hose D, Kassambara A et al (2011) Osteoclast-gene expression profiling reveals osteoclast-derived CCR2 chemokines promoting myeloma cell migration. Blood 117(4):1280–1290

Morgan GJ, Davies FE, Gregory WM et al (2010) First-line treatment with zoledronic acid as compared with clodronic acid in multiple myeloma (MRC Myeloma IX): a randomised controlled trial. Lancet 376(9757):1989–1999

Morgan GJ, Child JA, Gregory WM et al (2011) Effects of zoledronic acid versus clodronic acid on skeletal morbidity in patients with newly diagnosed multiple myeloma (MRC Myeloma IX): secondary outcomes from a randomised controlled trial. Lancet Oncol 12:743–752

Morgan GJ, Davies FE, Gregory WM et al (2012) Effects of induction and maintenance plus long-term bisphosphonates on bone disease in patients with multiple myeloma: MRC Myeloma IX trial. Blood 119(23):5374–5383

Moulopoulos LA, Dimopoulos MA (1997) Magnetic resonance imaging of the bone marrow in hematologic malignancies. Blood 90:2127–2147

Moulopoulos LA, Varma DG, Dimopoulos MA et al (1992) Multiple myeloma: spinal MR imaging in patients with untreated newly diagnosed disease. Radiology 185:833–840

Moulopoulos LA, Dimopoulos MA, Weber D et al (1993) Magnetic resonance imaging in the staging of solitary plasmacytoma of bone. J Clin Oncol 11:1311–1315

Moulopoulos LA, Dimopoulos MA, Alexanian R et al (1994) Multiple myeloma: MR patterns of response to treatment. Radiology 193:441–446

Moulopoulos LA, Dimopoulos MA, Smith TL et al (1995) Prognostic significance of magnetic resonance imaging in patients with asymptomatic multiple myeloma. J Clin Oncol 13:251–256

Moulopoulos LA, Gika D, Anagnostopoulos A et al (2005) Prognostic significance of magnetic resonance imaging of bone marrow in previously untreated patients with multiple myeloma. Ann Oncol 16:1824–1828

Moulopoulos LA, Dimopoulos MA, Christoulas D et al (2010) Diffuse MRI marrow pattern correlates with increased angiogenesis, advanced disease features and poor prognosis in newly diagnosed myeloma treated with novel agents. Leukemia 24:1206–1212

Moulopoulos LA, Dimopoulos MA, Kastritis E et al (2012) Diffuse pattern of bone marrow involvement on magnetic resonance imaging is associated with high risk cytogenetics and poor outcome in newly diagnosed, symptomatic patients with multiple myeloma: a single center experience on 228 patients. Am J Hematol 87:861–864

Muller MF, Edelman RR (1995) Echo planar imaging of the abdomen. Top Magn Reson Imaging 7:112–119

Mundy GR, Yoneda T (1998) Bisphosphonates as anti-cancer drugs. N Engl J Med 339:398

Musto P, Petrucci MT, Bringhen S et al (2008) A multicenter, randomized clinical trial comparing zoledronic acid versus observation in patients with asymptomatic myeloma. Cancer 113:1588–1595

Nanni C, Zamagni E, Versari A et al (2016) Image interpretation criteria for FDG PET/CT in multiple myeloma: a new proposal from an Italian expert panel. IMPeTUs (Italian Myeloma criteria for PET USe). Eur J Nucl Med Mol Imaging 43:414–421

Narquin S, Ingrand P, Azais I et al (2013) Comparison of whole-body diffusion MRI and conventional radiological assessment in the staging of myeloma. Diagn Interv Imaging 94:629–636

Neri P, Kumar S, Fulciniti MT et al (2007) Neutralizing B-cell activating factor antibody improves survival and inhibits osteoclastogenesis in a severe combined immunodeficient human multiple myeloma model. Clin Cancer Res 13(19):5903–5909

Nonomura Y, Yasumoto M, Yoshimura R et al (2001) Relationship between bone marrow cellularity and apparent diffusion coefficient. J Mag Reson Imaging 13:757–760

Oranger A, Carbone C, Izzo M et al (2013) Cellular mechanisms of multiple myeloma bone disease. Clin Dev Immunol 2013:289458

Oshima T, Abe M, Asano J et al (2005) Myeloma cells suppress bone formation by secreting a soluble Wnt inhibitor, sFRP-2. Blood 106:3160–3165

Paiva B, van Dongen JJ, Orfao A et al (2015) New criteria for response assessment: role of minimal residual disease in multiple myeloma. Blood 125:3059–3068

Parker SL, Davis KJ, Wingo PA et al (1998) Cancer statistics by race and ethnicity. CA Cancer J Clin 48:31–48

Patriarca F, Carobolante F, Zamagni E et al (2015) The role of positron emission tomography with 18F-fluorodeoxyglucose integrated with computed tomography in the evaluation of patients with multiple myeloma undergoing allogeneic stem cell transplantation. Biol Blood Marrow Transplant 21:1068–1073

Pawlyn C, Fowkes L, Otero S et al (2015) Whole-body diffusion-weighted MRI: a new gold standard for assessing disease burden in patients with multiple myeloma? Leukemia 30(6):1446–1448. https://doi.org/10.1038/leu.2015.338

Pearse RN, Sordillo EM, Yaccoby S et al (2001) Multiple myeloma disrupts the TRANCE/osteoprotegerin cytokine axis to trigger bone destruction and promote tumor progression. Proc Natl Acad Sci U S A 98:11581–11586

Pepe J, Petrucci MT, Nofroni I et al (2006) Lumbar bone mineral density as the major factor determining increased prevalence of vertebral fractures in monoclonal gammopathy of undetermined significance. Br J Haematol 134:485–490

Pepe J, Petrucci MT, Mascia ML et al (2008) The effects of alendronate treatment in osteoporotic patients affected by monoclonal gammopathy of undetermined significance. Calcif Tissue Int 82:418–426

Pianko MJ, Terpos E, Roodman GD et al (2014) Whole-body low-dose computed tomography and advanced imaging techniques for multiple myeloma bone disease. Clin Cancer Res 20:5888–5897

Politou MC, Heath DJ, Rahemtulla A et al (2006) Serum concentrations of Dickkopf-1 protein are increased in patients with multiple myeloma and reduced after autologous stem cell transplantation. Int J Cancer 119:1728–1731

Polyzos SA, Anastasilakis AD, Bratengeier C et al (2012) Serum sclerostin levels positively correlate with lumbar spinal bone mineral density in postmenopausal women—the six-month effect of risedronate and teriparatide. Osteoporos Int 23(3):1171–1176

Price P, Hoskin PJ, Easton D et al (1986) Prospective randomised trial of single and multifraction radiotherapy schedules in the treatment of painful bony metastases. Radiother Oncol 6:247–255

Princewill K, Kyere S, Awan O et al (2013) Multiple myeloma lesion detection with whole body CT versus radiographic skeletal survey. Cancer Investig 31:206–211

Rades D, Hoskin PJ, Stalpers LJ et al (2006) Short-course radiotherapy is not optimal for spinal cord compression due to myeloma. Int J Radiat Oncol Biol Phys 64:1452–1457

Rades D, Veninga T, Stalpers LJ et al (2007) Outcome after radiotherapy alone for metastatic spinal cord compression in patients with oligometastases. J Clin Oncol 25:50–56

Raje N, Roodman GD (2011) Advances in the biology and treatment of bone disease in multiple myeloma. Clin Cancer Res 17:1278–1286

Rajkumar SV, Dimopoulos MA, Palumbo A et al (2014) International Myeloma Working Group updated criteria for the diagnosis of multiple myeloma. Lancet Oncol 15:e538–e548

Regelink JC, Minnema MC, Terpos E et al (2013) Comparison of modern and conventional imaging techniques in establishing multiple myeloma-related bone disease: a systematic review. Br J Haematol 162:50–61

Ripamonti CI, Cislaghi E, Mariani L et al (2011) Efficacy and safety of medical ozone (O(3)) delivered in oil suspension applications for the treatment of osteonecrosis of the jaw in patients with bone metastases treated with bisphosphonates: preliminary results of a phase I-II study. Oral Oncol 47(3):185–190

Rogers MJ, Gordon S, Benford HL et al (2000) Cellular and molecular mechanisms of action of bisphosphonates. Cancer 88:2961

Roodman GD (2008) Novel targets for myeloma bone disease. Expert Opin Ther Targets 12:1377–1387

Rosen LS, Gordon D, Kaminski M et al (2001) Zoledronic acid versus pamidronate in the treatment of skeletal metastases in patients with breast cancer or osteolytic lesions of multiple myeloma: a phase III, double-blind, comparative trial. Cancer J 7(5):377–387

Rosen LS, Gordon D, Kaminski M et al (2003) Long-term efficacy and safety of zoledronic acid compared with pamidronate disodium in the treatment of skeletal complications in patients with advanced multiple myeloma or breast carcinoma: a randomized, double-blind, multicenter, comparative trial. Cancer 98(8):1735–1744

Ross AC, Manson JE, Abrams SA et al (2011) The 2011 report on dietary reference intakes for calcium and vitamin D from the Institute of Medicine: what clinicians need to know. J Clin Endocrinol Metab 96:53–58

Roussou M, Tasidou A, Dimopoulos MA et al (2009) Increased expression of macrophage inflammatory protein-1alpha on trephine biopsies correlates with extensive bone disease, increased angiogenesis and advanced stage in newly diagnosed patients with multiple myeloma. Leukemia 23(11):2177–2181

Roux S, Bergot C, Fermand JP et al (2003) Evaluation of bone mineral density and fat-lean distribution in patients with multiple myeloma in sustained remission. J Bone Miner Res 18:231–236

Rowe DJ, Etre LA, Lovdahl MJ et al (1999) Relationship between bisphosphonate concentration and osteoclast activity and viability. In Vitro Cell Dev Biol Anim 35:383

Ruckle J, Jacobs M, Kramer W et al (2009) Single-dose, randomized, double-blind, placebo-controlled study of ACE-011 (ActRIIA-IgG1) in postmenopausal women. J Bone Miner Res 24(4):744–752

Sachpekidis C, Mosebach J, Freitag MT et al (2015a) Application of (18)F-FDG PET and diffusion weighted imaging (DWI) in multiple myeloma: comparison of functional imaging modalities. Am J Nucl Med Mol Imaging 5:479–492

Sachpekidis C, Hillengass J, Goldschmidt H et al (2015b) Comparison of (18)F-FDG PET/CT and PET/MRI in patients with multiple myeloma. Am J Nucl Med Mol Imaging 5:469–478

Sachpekidis C, Mai EK, Goldschmidt H et al (2015c) (18) F-FDG dynamic PET/CT in patients with multiple myeloma: patterns of tracer uptake and correlation with bone marrow plasma cell infiltration rate. Clin Nucl Med 40:e300–e307

Scullen T, Santo L, Vallet S et al (2013) Lenalidomide in combination with an activin A-neutralizing antibody: preclinical rationale for a novel anti-myeloma strategy. Leukemia 27(8):1715–1721

Shipman CM, Rogers MJ, Apperley JF et al (1997) Bisphosphonates induce apoptosis in human myeloma cell lines: a novel anti-tumour activity. Br J Haematol 98:665

Silbermann R, Roodman GD (2016) Current controversies in the management of myeloma bone disease. J Cell Physiol 231(11):2374–2379. https://doi.org/10.1002/jcp.25351

Siontis B, Kumar S, Dispenzieri A et al (2015) Positron emission tomography-computed tomography in the diagnostic evaluation of smoldering multiple myeloma: identification of patients needing therapy. Blood Cancer J 5:e364

Song MK, Chung JS, Lee JJ et al (2014) Magnetic resonance imaging pattern of bone marrow involvement as a new predictive parameter of disease progression in newly diagnosed patients with multiple myeloma eligible for autologous stem cell transplantation. Br J Haematol 165(6):777–785

Spinnato P, Bazzocchi A, Brioli A et al (2012) Contrast enhanced MRI and ¹⁸F-FDG PET-CT in the assessment of multiple myeloma: a comparison of results in different phases of the disease. Eur J Radiol 81:4013–4018

Steinman RM, Bonifaz L, Fujii S et al (2005) The innate functions of dendritic cells in peripheral lymphoid tissues. Adv Exp Med Biol 560:83–97

Sugatani T, Alvarez UM, Hruska KA (2003) Activin A stimulates IkappaB-alpha/NFkappaB and RANK expression for osteoclast differentiation, but not AKT survival pathway in osteoclast precursors. J Cell Biochem 90:59–67

Syed IS, Glockner JF, Feng D et al (2010) Role of cardiac magnetic resonance imaging in the detection of cardiac amyloidosis. JACC Cardiovasc Imaging 3:155–164

Tai YT, Landesman Y, Acharya C et al (2013) CRM1 inhibition induces tumor cell cytotoxicity and impairs osteoclastogenesis in multiple myeloma: molecular mechanisms and therapeutic implications. Leukemia 28(1):155–165

Tanaka Y, Abe M, Hiasa M et al (2007) Myeloma cell-osteoclast interaction enhances angiogenesis together with bone resorption: a role for vascular endothelial cell growth factor and osteopontin. Clin Cancer Res 13(3):816–823

Terpos E, Dimopoulos MA (2005) Myeloma bone disease: pathophysiology and management. Ann Oncol 16:1223–1231

Terpos E, Szydlo R, Apperley JF et al (2003) Soluble receptor activator of nuclear factor kappaB ligand-osteoprotegerin ratio predicts survival in multiple myeloma: proposal for a novel prognostic index. Blood 102:1064–1069

Terpos E, Mihou D, Szydlo R et al (2005) The combination of intermediate doses of thalidomide with dexamethasone is an effective treatment for patients with refractory/relapsed multiple myeloma and normalizes abnormal bone remodeling, through the reduction of sRANKL/osteoprotegerin ratio. Leukemia 19(11):1969–1976

Terpos E, Heath DJ, Rahemtulla A et al (2006) Bortezomib reduces serum dickkopf-1 and receptor activator of nuclear factor-kappaB ligand concentrations and normalises indices of bone remodelling in patients with relapsed multiple myeloma. Br J Haematol 135(5):688–692

Terpos E, Kastritis E, Roussou M et al (2008) The combination of bortezomib, melphalan, dexamethasone and intermittent thalidomide is an effective regimen for relapsed/refractory myeloma and is associated with improvement of abnormal bone metabolism and angiogenesis. Leukemia 22(12):2247–2256

Terpos E, Sezer O, Croucher PI et al (2009) The use of bisphosphonates in multiple myeloma recommendations of an expert panel on behalf of the European Myeloma Network. Ann Oncol 20:1303

Terpos E, Christoulas D, Papatheodorou A et al (2010a) Dickkopf-1 is elevated in newly-diagnosed, symptomatic patients and in relapsed patients with multiple myeloma; correlations with advanced disease features: a single-center experience in 284 patients. Presented at: 15th Congress of the European Hematology Association, Barcelona, Spain, 10–13 June 2010

Terpos E, Christoulas D, Kokkoris P et al (2010b) Increased bone mineral density in a subset of patients with relapsed multiple myeloma who received the combination of bortezomib, dexamethasone and zoledronic acid. Ann Oncol 21(7):1561–1562

Terpos E, Moulopoulos LA, Dimopoulos MA (2011) Advances in imaging and the management of myeloma bone disease. J Clin Oncol 29:1907–1915

Terpos E, Kastritis E, Christoulas D et al (2012a) Circulating activin-A is elevated in patients with advanced multiple myeloma and correlates with extensive bone involvement and inferior survival; no alterations post-lenalidomide and dexamethasone therapy. Ann Oncol 23:2681–2686

Terpos E, Christoulas D, Katodritou E et al (2012b) Elevated circulating sclerostin correlates with advanced disease features and abnormal bone remodeling in symptomatic myeloma: reduction post-bortezomib monotherapy. Int J Cancer 131:1466–1471

Terpos E, Morgan G, Dimopoulos MA et al (2013a) International Myeloma Working Group recommendations for the treatment of multiple myeloma-related bone disease. J Clin Oncol 31(18):2347–2357

Terpos E, Christoulas D, Kastritis E et al (2013b) VTD consolidation, without bisphosphonates, reduces bone resorption and is associated with a very low incidence of skeletal-related events in myeloma patients post-ASCT. Leukemia 28(4):928–934

Terpos E, Berenson J, Raje N et al (2014) Management of bone disease in multiple myeloma. Expert Rev Hematol 7(1):113–125

Terpos E, Kleber M, Engelhardt M et al (2015a) European Myeloma Network guidelines for the management of multiple myeloma-related complications. Haematologica 100:1254–1266

Terpos E, Koutoulidis V, Fontara S et al (2015b) Diffusion-Weighted Imaging improves accuracy in the diagnosis of MRI patterns of marrow involvement in newly diagnosed myeloma: results of a prospective study in 99 patients. Blood 126:4178. (ASH abstract)

Tertti R, Alanen A, Remes K (1995) The value of magnetic resonance imaging in screening myeloma lesions of the lumbar spine. Br J Haematol 91:658–660

Tian E, Zhan F, Walker R et al (2003) The role of the Wnt-signaling antagonist DKK1 in the development of osteolytic lesions in multiple myeloma. N Engl J Med 349:2483–2494

Tirumani SH, Sakellis C, Jacene H et al (2016) Role of FDG-PET/CT in extramedullary multiple myeloma: correlation of FDG-PET/CT findings with clinical outcome. Clin Nucl Med 41:e7–e13

Usmani SZ, Mitchell A, Waheed S et al (2013) Prognostic implications of serial 18-fluoro-deoxyglucose emission tomography in multiple myeloma treated with total therapy. Blood 121:1819–1823

Utzschneider S, Schmidt H, Weber P et al (2011) Surgical therapy of skeletal complications in multiple myeloma. Int Orthop 35:1209–1213

Vallet S, Raje N, Ishitsuka K et al (2007) MLN3897, a novel CCR1 inhibitor, impairs osteoclastogenesis and inhibits the interaction of multiple myeloma cells and osteoclasts. Blood 110(10):3744–3752

Van de Donk NW, Palumbo A, Johnsen HE et al (2014) The clinical relevance and management of monoclonal gammopathy of undetermined significance and related disorders: recommendations from the European Myeloma Network. Haematologica 99(6):984–996

Vande Berg BC, Michaux L, Lecouvet FE et al (1997) Nonmyelomatous monoclonal gammopathy: correlation of bone marrow MR images with laboratory findings and spontaneous clinical outcome. Radiology 202:247–251

Vanderkerken K, De Leenheer E, Shipman C et al (2003) Recombinant osteoprotegerin decreases tumor burden and increases survival in a murine model of multiple myeloma. Cancer Res 63(2):287–289

Vanderkerken K, Medicherla S, Coulton L et al (2007) Inhibition of p38alpha mitogen-activated protein kinase prevents the development of osteolytic bone disease, reduces tumor burden, and increases survival in murine models of multiple myeloma. Cancer Res 67(10):4572–4577

Varettoni M, Corso A, Pica G et al (2010) Incidence, presenting features and outcome of extramedullary disease in multiple myeloma: a longitudinal study on 1003 consecutive patients. Ann Oncol 21:325–330

Vij R, Horvath N, Spencer A, Kitagawa K et al (2007) An open-label, Phase 2 trial of denosumab in the treatment of relapsed (R) or plateau-phase (PP) multiple myeloma (MM). Presented at: 49th ASH Annual Meeting and Exposition, 8–11 Dec 2007, Atlanta, GA, USA

von Metzler I, Krebbel H, Hecht M et al (2007) Bortezomib inhibits human osteoclastogenesis. Leukemia 21(9):2025–2034

Voskaridou E, Christoulas D, Plata E et al (2012) High circulating sclerostin is present in patients with thalassemia-associated osteoporosis and correlates with bone mineral density. Horm Metab Res 44(12):909–913

Waheed S, Mitchell A, Usmani S et al (2013) Standard and novel imaging methods for multiple myeloma: correlates with prognostic laboratory variables including gene expression profiling data. Haematologica 98:71–78

Walker R, Barlogie B, Haessler J et al (2007) Magnetic resonance imaging in multiple myeloma: diagnostic and clinical implications. J Clin Oncol 25:1121–1128

Wang Y (2000) Description of parallel imaging in MRI using multiple coils. Magn Reson Med 44:495–499

Wedin R (2001) Surgical treatment for pathologic fracture. Acta Orthop Scand Suppl 72(2p):1–29

Weininger M, Lauterbach B, Knop S et al (2008) Whole-body MRI of multiple myeloma: comparison of different MRI sequences in assessment of different growth patterns. Eur J Radiol 69:339–345

Wolf MB, Murray F, Kilk K et al (2014) Sensitivity of whole-body CT and MRI versus projection radiography in the detection of osteolyses in patients with monoclonal plasma cell disease. Eur J Radiol 83:1222–1230

Xu X, Ma L, Zhang JS et al (2008) Feasibility of whole body diffusion weighted imaging in detecting bone metastasis on 3.0T MR scanner. Chin Med Sci J 23:151–157

Yaccoby S, Pearse RN, Johnson CL et al (2002) Myeloma interacts with the bone marrow microenvironment to induce osteoclastogenesis and is dependent on osteoclast activity. Br J Haematol 116(2):278–290

Yin JJ, Selander K, Chirgwin JM et al (1999) TGF-beta signaling blockade inhibits PTHrP secretion by breast cancer cells and bone metastases development. J Clin Invest 103:197

Yonemori K, Fujiwara Y, Minami H et al (2008) Phase 1 trial of denosumab safety, pharmacokinetics, and pharmacodynamics in Japanese women with breast cancer-related bone metastases. Cancer Sci 99(6):1237–1242

Zamagni E, Nanni C, Patriarca F et al (2007) A prospective comparison of 18F-fluorodeoxyglucose positron emission tomography-computed tomography, magnetic resonance imaging and whole-body planar radiographs in the assessment of bone disease in newly diagnosed multiple myeloma. Haematologica 92:50–55

Zamagni E, Patriarca F, Nanni C et al (2011) Prognostic relevance of 18-F FDG PET/CT in newly diagnosed multiple myeloma patients treated with up-front autologous transplantation. Blood 118:5989–5995

Zamagni E, Nanni C, Gay F et al (2015a) 18F-FDG PET/CT focal, but not osteolytic, lesions predict the progression of smoldering myeloma to active disease. Leukemia 30(2):417–422

Zamagni E, Nanni C, Mancuso K et al (2015b) PET/CT improves the definition of complete response and allows to detect otherwise unidentifiable skeletal progression in multiple myeloma. Clin Cancer Res 21:4384–4390

Zangari M, Esseltine D, Lee CK et al (2005) Response to bortezomib is associated to osteoblastic activation in patients with multiple myeloma. Br J Haematol 131(1):71–73

Zangari M, Aujay M, Zhan F et al (2011) Alkaline phosphatase variation during carfilzomib treatment is associated with best response in multiple myeloma patients. Eur J Haematol 86(6):484–487

Zechmann CM, Traine L, Meissner T et al (2012) Parametric histogram analysis of dynamic contrast-enhanced MRI in multiple myeloma: a technique to evaluate angiogenic response to therapy? Acad Radiol 19:100–108

Zervas K, Verrou E, Teleioudis Z et al (2006) Incidence, risk factors and management of osteonecrosis of the jaw in patients with multiple myeloma: a single-centre experience in 303 patients. Br J Haematol 134(6):620–623

Zou J, Mei X, Gan M et al (2010) Kyphoplasty for spinal fractures from multiple myeloma. J Surg Oncol 102:43–47

Zwick S, Brix G, Tofts PS et al (2010) Simulation-based comparison of two approaches frequently used for dynamic contrast-enhanced MRI. Eur Radiol 20:432–442

Other Complications of Multiple Myeloma

8

Heinz Ludwig, Meletios-Athanasios Dimopoulos, and Evangelos Terpos

8.1 Renal Impairment

8.1.1 Epidemiology

Comparison of data on the epidemiology of renal failure is limited because criteria used for definition of renal impairment vary between individual reports. This limitation should be overcome in the future by widespread use of the AKIN (acute kidney injury network) or the RIFLE (risk, injury, failure, loss, and end-stage kidney disease) criteria for classification of renal impairment as recommended by a recent report of the IMWG (International Multiple Myeloma Working Group) (Dimopoulos et al. 2016a).

Renal impairment is one of the defining markers of symptomatic multiple myeloma according to the CRAB criteria (hypercalcemia, renal impairment, anemia, bone disease) and a frequent complication throughout the course of the disease. In a small proportion of patients, acute severe renal impairment is the key symptom mandating emergency care (Johnson et al. 1990; Torra et al. 1995) and prompt diagnostic work-up. Mild to moderate myeloma-induced renal impairment has been reported in 20–50% of patients (Eleutherakis-Papaiakovou et al. 2007; Knudsen et al. 1994) but seems to be less frequent now with earlier diagnosis and more effective therapies for multiple myeloma. Moderate myeloma-induced renal impairment often improves with successful anti-myeloma therapy but may aggravate or develop de novo during progressive disease.

8.1.2 Pathogenesis

Renal insufficiency in multiple myeloma is the consequence of the destructive effect of monoclonal free light chains (FLCs) on renal structures, mainly on the tubular apparatus, and—less frequently—on glomerular mesangium, and even less often on tubular and vascular basement membranes. Hypercalcemia, dehydration, infection, nephrotoxic drugs, and contrast agents may provoke the manifestation of clinical sequels or lead to their intensification (Dimopoulos et al. 2008; Pirani et al. 1987).

Two general types of FLC-induced renal injury can be distinguished: Firstly, deposits of FLCs precipitate as amorphous non-amyloid structures as seen in cast nephropathy, Fanconi syndrome, or

H. Ludwig (✉)
Department of Medicine I, Center for Oncology and Hematology, Wilhelminen Cancer Research Institute, Vienna, Austria
e-mail: heinz.ludwig@aon.at

M.-A. Dimopoulos • E. Terpos
Department of Clinical Therapeutics, National and Kapodistrian University of Athens, School of Medicine, Athens, Greece

© Springer International Publishing Switzerland 2018
M. A. Dimopoulos et al. (eds.), *Multiple Myeloma and Other Plasma Cell Neoplasms*, Hematologic Malignancies, https://doi.org/10.1007/978-3-319-25586-6_8

monoclonal immunoglobulin deposit disease, and secondly amyloidogenic FLC fibrils aggregate as seen in amyloidosis (Sanders et al. 1991). In cast nephropathy, the most frequent form of renal injury, the abundantly circulating monoclonal FLCs are filtered through the glomeruli and bind to Tamm-Horsfall glycoprotein (uromodulin), thereby forming aggregates and casts which congest the lumen of the distal nephrons leading to tubular obstruction, necrosis of tubular cells, interstitial inflammation, and fibrosis (Fig. 8.1) (Sanders et al. 1991; Myatt et al. 1994). The binding affinity of FLCs to uromodulin depends on a nine amino acid epitope on the CDR3 region of the free light chains (Hutchison et al. 2011). This explains the great variability of FLCs in forming tubular casts and cast nephropathy. Acquired adult Fanconi syndrome affects the proximal renal tubules and renal reabsorption resulting in various degrees of glucosuria, aminoaciduria, hypouricemia, hypophosphatemia, and loss of bicarbonate (Ma et al. 2004). Most of these changes remain asymptomatic, but bicarbonate loss may result in tubular acidosis and long-standing hypophosphatemia in rickets. FLCs found in Fanconi syndrome are structurally unorganized, often fragmented,

and usually of kappa light chain type that do not bind Tamm-Horsfall glycoprotein. This explains why cast nephropathy and Fanconi syndrome rarely coexist (Leboulleux et al. 1995). Fanconi syndrome is less frequently associated with multiple myeloma and more often found in monoclonal gammopathy of undetermined significance (MGUS). Monoclonal immunoglobulin deposition disease (MIDD), mainly due to monoclonal light chains (LCDD) and less frequently due to heavy chains (HCDD) or a combination of both light and heavy chains (LHDD), features amorphous granular deposits in multiple organs, with the kidneys being most likely affected (Leung et al. 2012). In amyloidosis, structurally organized (fibrillous β-pleated sheet) light chain amyloid (AL-amyloid) protein is deposited predominantly in the glomerular mesangium with massive fibrillary involvement (Bahlis and Lazarus 2006). The terminology of monoclonal gammopathy of renal significance (MGRS) has recently been introduced to describe B-cell monoclonal disorders that do not meet the criteria for the diagnosis of multiple myeloma or lymphoma but produce monoclonal proteins that cause permanent renal injury (Bridoux et al. 2015).

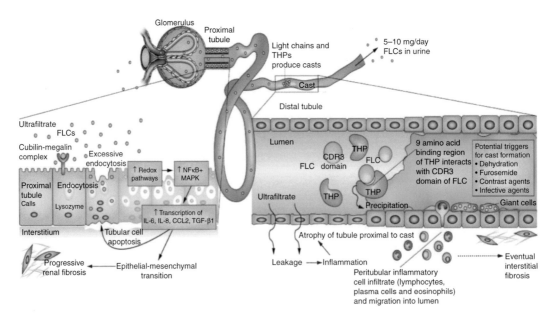

Fig. 8.1 Mechanism of free light chain-induced injury (with kind permission from Hutchison CA, et al., Nat. Rev. Nephrol. 2011 (Hutchison et al. 2011))

8.1.3   Diagnostic Work-Up

Determination of renal function, monoclonal components, and electrolytes in serum and urine at presentation is essential. Glomerular function should be estimated using the MDRD (modification of diet in renal disease) or the CKD-EPI (chronic kidney disease epidemiology collaboration) formula (Terpos et al. 2015). Immunoglobulins, albumin, β2-microglobulin, and FLCs should be measured in serum; electrophoresis should be run in serum and urine; and 24-h proteinuria needs to be determined. Immunofixation of both serum and urine should be performed in newly diagnosed patients and in those with low urinary protein excretion. The electrophoresis of the urinary proteins usually reveals a pattern, which either is characteristic for glomerular or tubular injury. In patients with tubular injury (cast nephropathy), FLCs will pass through the glomeruli and will, to most part, be excreted in the urine. These large amounts of filtered FLCs will appear as a large spike in the gamma region of the electrophoretic curve; urine immunofixation and/or the FLC tests will show kappa or lambda light chains. In cases with glomerular injury (AL-amyloidosis), albumin will predominate the electrophoretic curve and appear as a large, usually broader-based spike. Patients with amyloidosis usually have only little light chain excretion and levels are even lower in those with MIDD/LCDD. In the latter patients, urine immunofixation may be negative; therefore, FLCs should be determined in the urine of those patients as well. Monoclonal light chains of lambda type are more frequently associated with amyloidosis, while kappa type monoclonal light chains predominate in patients with LCDD. For definitive diagnosis, a biopsy should be carried out in those patients, where the nature of the renal damage cannot be established with noninvasive diagnostic procedures (Kastritis et al. 2013).

8.1.4   Treatment

Acute renal insufficiency is a medical emergency, and every effort must be taken to restore renal function rapidly. Symptomatic treatment should include hydration, urine alkalinization, therapy of hypercalcemia and, where indicated, dialysis. Prompt initiation of effective anti-myeloma therapy for rapid reduction of pathogenic light chains is the most important measure. Bortezomib-based combination regimens exert significant activity in reversing renal impairment (Table 8.1) (Burnette et al. 2011; Badros et al. 2013). A retrospective comparison found superior activity of bortezomib-based regimens over thalidomide- or lenalidomide-based combinations with significantly higher rates of reversal of renal function (Dimopoulos et al. 2014a). This favorable activity may partly be due to a significant anti-inflammatory effect of bortezomib that may ameliorate the intra- and peritubular inflammation induced by tubular damage as shown in an experimental mouse model (Hainz et al. 2012). Clearance of bortezomib and the newer proteasome inhibitors carfilzomib and ixazomib are independent of renal function, obviating the need for dose adaption to renal function. Substantial experience with bortezomib did not reveal any nephrotoxicity.

Bortezomib in combination with alkylating agents, IMiDs, anthracyclines, and bendamustine revealed high anti-myeloma activity and renal recovery in about 20–45% of patients with severe renal impairment (Dimopoulos et al. 2009a, b; Jagannath et al. 2005; San-Miguel et al. 2008; Blade et al. 2008; Ludwig et al. 2010; Morabito et al. 2010; Ponisch et al. 2013; Scheid et al. 2014). In patients tolerating more intensive therapy, a three-drug combination is preferred. In order to enhance the response rate and to expedite the reduction of light chains, dexamethasone should be administered in the traditional high-dose regimen during the first cycle, but this strategy should be restricted to fit patients only, because of the heightened risk for infections and other complications such as fluid retention, psychotropic effects, and cardiotoxicity in elderly patients.

Carfilzomib is presently considered the most potent proteasome inhibitor. Based on its activity and pharmacokinetic profile (Badros et al. 2013), it should be the ideal backbone for combination

Table 8.1 Selected studies with bortezomib- or lenalidomide-based regimens reporting renal response rates in patients with renal impairment

Main study drug	Study	No. of patients with RI	Patients on dialysis	Disease status	Regimen	Myeloma response[a]	Renal response
Bortezomib	Dimopoulos et al. (2009b)	46 (sCr >2 mg/dL; eGFR <40 mL/min)	9	Nd (n = 10) Rel/Ref (n = 36)	VD (n = 17) VMPT (n = 14) PAD (n = 6) VTD (n = 5) VRD (n = 4)	ORR: 76%	ORR: 59% 2 of 9 became dialysis independent
	Dimopoulos et al. (2009a)	227 (34 with eGFR <30 mL/min)	0	Nd, ineligible for ASCT	VMP (n = 111) MP (n = 116)	ORR: VMP 74% pts. (eGFR <30 mL/min) MP 47% pts (eGFR <30 mL/min)	ORR: VMP 44% MP 34%
	Ludwig et al. (2010)	68 (eGFR <50 mL/min; sCR ≥ 2 mg/dL)	9	Nd (n = 50) Rel/Ref (n = 18)	PAD	ORR: 72% CR/nCR: 38% VGPR: 15% PR: 13%	ORR: 62% eGFR (median) increased from 20.5 to 48.4 mL/min; 3 of 9 became dialysis independent
	Ponisch et al. (2013)	36 (eGFR <60 mL/min)	16 (eGFR <15 mL/min)	Rel/Ref	BPV	ORR: 67%	ORR: 87% CR: 31% PR: 14% MR: 42%
	Scheid et al. (2014)	81 (sCR ≥2 mg/dL)	0	Nd	PAD (n = 36) VAD (n = 45)	ORR: PAD 89% VAD 64%; CR: PAD 36% VAD 13%	ORR: PAD 81% VAD 63%
Lenalidomide	Ludwig et al. (2015)	35 (eGFR <50 mL/min; sCR ≥2 mg/dL)	13	Nd (n = 28) Rel/Ref (n = 7)	Ld	ORR: 68.6% CR: 20% VGPR: 8.6% PR: 40%	ORR: 45.7% CR: 14.2% PR: 11.4% MR: 20%

Nd newly diagnosed, *Rel/Ref* relapsed/refractory, *ORR* objective response rate, *CR* complete response, *PR* partial response, *MR* minor response, *eGFR* estimated glomerular filtration rate, *sCR* serum creatinine, *BPV* bendamustine-prednisone-bortezomib, *MP* melphalan-prednisone, *PAD* bortezomib-doxorubicin-dexamethasone, *VAD* vincristine-doxorubicin-dexamethasone, *VD* bortezomib-dexamethasone, *VMPT* bortezomib-melphalan-prednisone-thalidomide, *VRD* bortezomib-lenalidomide-dexamethasone, *VTD* bortezomib-thalidomide-dexamethasone

[a]CR: increase in eGFR >60 mL/min, PR: eGFR increase from <15 to 30–59 mL/min, MR: eGFR increase from <15 by >100% to 1–29 mL/min

regimens. Results from a randomized trial comparing carfilzomib-dexamethasone with bortezomib-dexamethasone, which enrolled patients with a GFR $\geq$15 mL/min (Dimopoulos et al. 2016b) showed slightly more frequent grade 3/4 renal toxicities with the former regimen (7% vs. 4%). Hence, further data are required to establish its safety in patients with severe renal insufficiency (Jhaveri and Wanchoo 2015).

Thalidomide and pomalidomide (Dimopoulos et al. 2014b) are not cleared by renal pathways and do not require dose modification in patients with renal insufficiency. Thalidomide in combination with high-dose steroids resulted in unusual toxicity with hypokalemia (possibly because of high-dose glucocorticosteroids) but yielded renal recovery ranging from 55% to 75% in newly diagnosed patients and approximately 60% of patients with relapsed or refractory multiple myeloma (Dimopoulos et al. 2013; Kastritis et al. 2007; Fakhouri et al. 2004; Tosi et al. 2004).

Lenalidomide is excreted by renal pathways and requires dose modifications in patients with renal impairment (Dimopoulos et al. 2011). Phase II trials including patients with renal insufficiency or acute renal failure showed improvement in renal function in 72% and 45% of patients, respectively (Dimopoulos et al. 2010; Ludwig et al. 2015). Clearance of pomalidomide is not dependent on renal function; its potential in patients with renal failure is presently evaluated in several trials. Ixazomib likewise does not require dose modification in renal failure and has been found to be safe in patients with GFR >30 mL/min (Moreau et al. 2016).

Stem cell transplantation with high-dose melphalan is an additional option, but not feasible in patients with acute renal failure if stem cells have not been collected before. When ASCT is considered in patients with slowly emerging or chronic renal failure, the melphalan dose should be reduced to 100–140 mg/m^2.

Therapeutic plasma exchange for rapid removal of pathogenic light chains did not improve the outcome in two of three randomized trials (including the largest) (Burnette et al. 2011). Prolonged hemodialysis with a high cutoff dialysis membrane to enhance mechanical

elimination of free light chains unfortunately did not fulfill its early promise and was found to be ineffective and to increase mortality in the EuLITE trial (Cook et al. 2016). Similarly, in the MYRE study, no significant increase in dialysis indpendency was noted with the intensified dialysis at 3 months after enrollment in the study (Bridoux et al. 2017). Treatment options for patients with MGRS are similar to those recommended above and recently have been discussed in detail by Fermand et al. (2013).

8.2 Anemia

Anemia due to multiple myeloma with a Hb level <10 g/dL or below the lower limit of normal by >2 g/dL is a myeloma-defining event and as such included in the CRAB criteria and an indication for anti-myeloma therapy (Rajkumar et al. 2014).

8.2.1 Epidemiology

Anemia is a frequent complication of multiple myeloma and one of the most frequent adverse events of modern myeloma therapy. Depending on various factors such as stage of the disease, patient's age, renal function, and tumor therapy, anemia can be observed in up to 85% of patients. Its incidence may even increase further in patients with refractory progressive disease and in those subjected to ASCT (Birgegard et al. 2006; Beguin et al. 1992; Kyle et al. 2003).

8.2.2 Pathogenesis

The pathogenesis of anemia in multiple myeloma is multifactorial and involves mechanisms of chronic anemia of cancer, mainly an increased release of inflammatory cytokines (TNF-α, IL-1, IL-6, interferon-γ), resulting in impaired renal erythropoietin production, reduced sensitivity of erythroid precursors to erythropoietin, impaired iron supply (Weinstein et al. 2002), and premature apoptosis. Other relevant causes are the

myelosuppressive effect of chemo- and radiotherapy (Kyle et al. 2003). In addition, in aggressive disease, myeloma cells exert a direct
apoptotic effect on erythroid precursors via Fas-L
and tumor necrosis factor-related apoptosis-
inducing ligand (TRAIL) interaction (Silvestris
et al. 2002).

8.2.3 Treatment

Treatment is recommended in patients with
symptomatic anemia and concomitant anti-
myeloma therapy. Treatment options are the
administration of erythropoiesis-stimulating
agents (ESAs) or red blood cell transfusions
(RBCTs). RBCTs are associated with significant
risks, such as thromboembolic complications,
transfusion reactions due to blood group incom-
patibility, transfusion-related purpura, immunosuppression of the recipient with an increased
risk for infections, and very rarely, graft-versus-
host disease, and transfer of infections (Taylor
et al. 2008; Schrijvers 2011). RBCTs, therefore
are considered as treatment reserved for patients
with severe symptomatic anemia, i.e., in patients
with Hb <8 g/dL and in those severely symptomatic due to anemia needing rapid improvement.

ESAs increase Hb levels by ≥ 2 g/dL in
60–75% of anemic patients with multiple
myeloma, improve their quality of life, and
reduce their transfusion requirements (Ludwig
et al. 1990; Dammacco et al. 2001; Osterborg
et al. 2002; Hedenus et al. 2003; Beguin et al.
2013). However, ESAs are associated with side
effects as well such as increased thromboembolic complications (HR: 1.5), occasional hypertension, and—when administered outside the
approved indication—increased mortality. ESAs
should be administered to prevent the need for
RBCTs and to improve quality of life. Therapy
should be initiated at Hb level of ≤ 10 g/dL. The
dose of ESAs recommended in the package
inserts varies between different types of ESAs.
Epoetin theta should be administered at a dose of
20.000 IU, Epoetin beta at 30.000 IU, Epoetin
alpha or zeta at 40.000 IU, and Darbepoetin at
150 µg once per week. Darbepoetin can also be
given at a dose 500 µg once every 3 weeks. The
Hb target level should not exceed 12 g/dL,
because previous reports showed an increased
risk of thromboembolic events and mortality in
cancer patients in whom Hb levels were
increased with ESAs widely exceeding this target level (Tonia et al. 2012). True or functional
iron deficiency, which has been reported in about
40% of patients with multiple myeloma, should
adequately be corrected with intravenous iron.
In case of inadequate response to ESA therapy
(increase to Hb levels ≥ 10 g – ≤ 12/dL or Hb
increase by >2 g/dL within 6–8 weeks) treatment
should be discontinued (Rizzo et al. 2010).

8.3 Infections

8.3.1 Epidemiology

A history of an increased incidence of infections
is one of the lead symptoms of multiple myeloma,
mandating adequate diagnostic work-up.
Infections are the second most frequent cause of
death, outnumbered only by progressing multiple
myeloma; they account for 22% of deaths within
the first year and up to 42% overall (Blimark
et al. 2015; Salonen and Nikoskelainen 1993). A
large population-based study of 9253 myeloma
patients found an infection rate of 40%, with an
overall sevenfold increased risk of bacterial and a
tenfold risk of viral infections compared to
matched controls (Blimark et al. 2015).
Interestingly a twofold increased risk of infections is already noted in patients with MGUS
(Kristinsson et al. 2012a). A characteristic pattern
of different types of infections along the different
phases of treatment of multiple myeloma has
been documented in a recent study on 199 multiple myeloma patients with 771 infectious episodes. After initiation of therapy, bacterial
infections prevail. Their incidence decreases subsequently with viral infections or reactivation of
latent viral infections becoming slightly more
common. Fungal infections usually are observed
only after high-dose dexamethasone therapy or
after allogeneic transplantation (Fig. 8.2) (Teh
et al. 2015).

8.3.2   Pathogenesis

Haemophilus influenzae, Streptococcus pneumonia, Gram-negative bacilli, and viruses (influenza and herpes zoster) are the most frequent pathogenic germs found in myeloma patients (Blimark et al. 2015). Viral infections are most frequently due to newly acquired upper respiratory viruses or reactivation of viruses belonging to the herpes family. In multiple myeloma infection with less aggressive approximately 40%, respectively viruses, such as rhinovirus or parainfluenza virus, usually results in a self-limited illness (Hammond et al. 2012), which can lead to significant morbidity and even mortality. These viruses tend to spread to the lower respiratory tract, cause additional immunosuppression, and serve as door openers for the development of secondary infections with bacteria or rarely fungi or other germs. Dormant viruses (including herpes simplex and zoster in about 90%, CMV in roughly 60%, and EBV in approximately 40%, respectively) kept under control by a healthy immune system are frequently found in the general population. Suppression of the subtle immune surveillance by anti-myeloma therapy and/or the disease itself may result in their reactivation with or without clinical symptoms (Arvin et al. 2007). Other risk factors for infections are uncontrolled myeloma, high age, comorbidity, hypoventilation, immobilization, RBCTs, and indwelling catheters such as Port-A-Cath's (Nucci and Anaissie 2009).

8.3.3   Diagnostic Work-Up

Infections, particularly those with unspecific clinical symptoms easily can be overlooked in multiple myeloma and not rarely are diagnosed with some delay only. Because of these risks, patients with active, uncontrolled disease should be monitored carefully, and fever should be considered as symptom of an underlying infection until proven otherwise. Respective diagnostic work-up is mandatory in patients with sudden onset of weakness, night sweats, diarrhea, or respiratory symptoms (Nucci and Anaissie 2009). Testing for viral infections should include herpes simplex and zoster virus, influenza, CMV, EBV, Adeno- and RSV viruses and others if indicated and should aim for direct detection of viral DNA by PCR, because antibody testing is less reliable due to frequently impaired immune response. Traditional detection of bacteria still depends on investigation of samples from various specimens of suspected infection and on investigation of blood cultures, but in future will be substituted by modern technology detecting germ-specific nucleic acid sequence.

8.3.4   Treatment and Prevention

Appropriate prophylaxis is an essential element in the management of myeloma patients and encompasses vaccination, antiviral prophylaxis in all patients on proteasome inhibitors, and antibacterial prophylaxis in selected patients (Table 8.2).

Ideally, patients should be vaccinated already during the precursor phase of myeloma when presenting with MGUS or at times of significant disease control. All patients, their family members, and caregivers should be vaccinated against influenza. In addition, vaccination against *Streptococcus pneumoniae, Haemophilus influenzae*, and hepatitis B is recommended (Anaissie 2011). Response to vaccination is frequently impaired in patients with myeloma (Robertson et al. 2000; Hargreaves et al. 1995); this is why antibody formation to vaccines should be evaluated and patients should be revaccinated in case of insufficient response. Importantly, live vaccines—such as yellow fever, varicella zoster, oral polio, intranasal influenza, bacillus Calmette–Guérin (BCG), typhoid fever, and measles-mumps-rubella (MMR)—should be avoided, unless in MGUS and smoldering myeloma or when the patient is in remission and >6 months after termination of chemotherapy (Khalafallah et al. 2010). Viral prophylaxis with acyclovir, valganciclovir, famvir, or similar drugs is mandatory in all patients on proteasome inhibitor therapy and in those subjected to high-dose therapy with autologous or allogeneic stem

Table 8.2 Prophylaxis and treatment of infections (modified according to Nucci et al. (Hargreaves et al. 1995) and Ludwig et al. (Palumbo et al. 2014))

Prophylaxis		Treatment
Viral infections		
Herpes simplex	Indication: mandatory during proteasome inhibitor treatment	Acyclovir, Valacyclovir, Famcyclovir usually 7–14 days
Herpes zoster	Agents: Acyclovir, Valacyclovir, Famcyclovir	
CMV	Indication: allotransplantation, in CMV pos. patients and in CMV neg. patients with a CMV pos. donor	Gancyclovir, Valgancyclovir, Foscarnet, 14–21 days
	Agents: Valgancyclovir	
Influenza	Indication: recommended in all patients, family members, and caregivers	Oseltamivir for 5–7 days
	Agents: vaccination	
RSV	No prophylaxis available	Ribavirin 200 mg tid for 14 days
Bacterial infections		
Pneumoccoci	Indication: recommended in all patients	Penicillin F, Cephalosporin (Ceftriaxone, Cefotaxime, Vancomycin, Rifampicin)
	Agents: vaccination	
Haemophilus influenzae	Indication: recommended in all patients	Aminopenicillin, Macrolide, Fluorchinolone
	Agents: vaccination	
Any bacterial infections	Indication: elderly patients, patients with a history of frequent episodes of infections, patients with uncontrolled myeloma, and high risk of neutropenia	Broad spectrum AB (Fluorchinolone, β-lactam AB). In case of suspected bacterial infection and active disease, start AB TX promptly
	Limit prophylaxis to episodes of poorly controlled myeloma	
	Agents: Fluorchinolone, TMP-SMX, Amoxicillin	
Clostridium	Consider Metronidazole in relapsing clostridia infections	Vancomycin, Metronidazole (Fidaxomicin)
Fungal infections		
Candidiasis[a] (oropharyngeal)	Amphotericin solution, fluconazole	Fluconazole
Pneumocystis Jirovecii[b]	Trimethoprim-sulfamethoxazole	Trimethoprim-sulfamethoxazole

CMV cytomegalovirus, *RSV* respiratory syncytial virus, *AB* antibiotic, *TX* treatment
[a]Only in selected patients on high-dose dexamethasone TX
[b]Only in patients receiving allogeneic transplantation Table 8.3 recommendations for dose reduction or treatment discontinuation and strategies for PNP symptom control and (Becker 2011; Briani et al. 2013; Ludwig et al. 2014)

cell transplantation. Prophylactic treatment should be continued during active anti-myeloma therapy.

Antibiotic prophylaxis is indicated in very elderly patients (usually above age 75) and in those with a history of frequent episodes of bacterial infections and in patients with highly marrow suppressive treatment. Generally, antibiotic prophylaxis should be limited to episodes of poorly controlled myeloma. In case of suspected bacterial infection and active disease, prompt action should be taken and antibiotic treatment initiated even before availability of results of diagnostic work-up. Intravenous (IV) immunoglobulins have been shown to reduce infection rates in myeloma patients (Kristinsson et al. 2012a; Teh et al. 2015; Hammond et al. 2012; Arvin et al. 2007; Nucci and Anaissie 2009; Anaissie 2011; Robertson et al. 2000; Hargreaves et al. 1995; Khalafallah et al. 2010; Gordon et al.

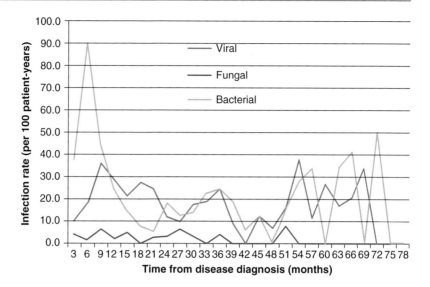

Fig. 8.2 Incidence of bacterial, viral, and fungal infections during the course of multiple myeloma (with kind permission from Teh BW et al., Br J Haematology, 2015 (Teh et al. 2015))

1984; Chapel et al. 1994; Richardson et al. 2012), and may be considered in individual patients with frequent episodes of bacterial infections (Fig. 8.2).

8.4 Peripheral Neuropathy

8.4.1 Epidemiology

Peripheral neuropathy (PNP) is a frequent complication in patients with multiple myeloma, particularly in those on thalidomide or bortezomib therapy. About 20% of patients present with PNP due to causes other than neurotoxic therapy already before start of any myeloma therapy, but the incidence increases up to 75% depending on the use of thalidomide and/or bortezomib, the dose administered, the duration of therapy, individual susceptibility, and in case of bortezomib, on the route of administration (Gorson and Ropper 1997).

8.4.2 Pathophysiology

The pathomechanisms accounting for neurologic symptoms in multiple myeloma vary, depending on the cause of the PNP (Becker 2011). Thalidomide, bortezomib, and other chemotherapy drugs induce axonal neuropathies affecting myelin sheaths and Schwann cells. In myeloma, patients with concomitant AL amyloidosis, endoneurial deposits of amyloidogenic FLCs can impair neuronal function. Polyclonal antibodies against myelin-associated glycoprotein on Schwann cells (anti-MAG antibodies) usually are associated with monoclonal gammopathy and are rarely observed in patients with multiple myeloma. A few studies showed an association between certain single nucleotide polymorphisms (SNPs) and the risk for drug-induced PNP (Magrangeas et al. 2016), while a single SNP conferring a roughly twofold increased risk for bortezomib-induced polyneuropathy has been described in a recent genome-wide association study (Moreau et al. 2011). Targeting the involved gene PKNOX1 may allow the development of protective strategies.

8.4.3 Clinical Presentation

Disease-associated symptoms are predominantly symmetric and include sensory, sensorimotor, or motor symptoms such as paranesthesia, numbness, burning sensation, weakness, or the "myeloma chin" meaning periorbital numbness. Treatment-emergent symptoms usually are symmetric and affect distal extremities first, but may progress proximally with relevant differences between thalidomide-induced and bortezomib-induced PNP. Thalidomide-induced PNP is cumulative, dose dependent, and often permanent. Symptoms are largely sensorimotor. Bortezomib-induced PNP affects small nerve fibers as well and is perceived as sensory PNP mainly, prevailing in the lower extremities (Delforge et al. 2010), and importantly improves or even is resolved completely after discontinuation of therapy (Becker 2011; Briani et al. 2013). Lenalidomide and carfilzomib are not associated with substantial rates of new-onset PNP or exacerbation of previous or existing PNP (Martin 2013; Dimopoulos et al. 2009c).

8.4.4 Diagnostic Work-Up

Careful attention of treating physicians to evolvement of PNP is essential. Physicians usually underestimate the impact of PNP on the individual patient. Therefore, it is important to obtain patient's self-assessment. Electrophysiological testing (electromyograms, EMG) may help to determine whether PNP is treatment-emergent or myeloma-associated, because the latter is primarily demyelinating, whereas treatment-emergent PNP is largely axonal. In addition, steroid-induced myopathy can be distinguished from motor neuropathy by EMG (Gorson and Ropper 1997).

8.4.5 Treatment

Informing patients about the risk of PNP and instructing them to report emerging symptoms is important. They should be encouraged to seek advice promptly in case of onset or aggravation of PNP (Magrangeas et al. 2016; Briani et al. 2013; Ludwig et al. 2014; Palumbo et al. 2014; Coppola et al. 2011). The principal treatment goal is to prevent emergence and/or progression of PNP and to reduce the severity of neuropathic symptoms. (Wolf et al. 2008). Table 8.3 shows preventive dose reduction or treatment discontinuation in patients with different grades of thalidomide or bortezomib-induced PNP, and

Table 8.3 Strategies for PNP symptom control and recommendations for dose reduction or treatment discontinuation (Becker 2011; Briani et al. 2013; Ludwig et al. 2014)

Prevention of progression of PNP: dose modification of anti-myeloma drugs	
Bortezomib	
Grade 1 with pain	If IV → switch to SC
	BWD dosing → reduce dose or switch to QW
	QW dosing → reduce dose
Grade 2	If IV → switch to SC
	BWD dosing → reduce dose or switch to QW
	QW dosing → reduce dose or temporary discontinuation
	If PNP resolves to grade ≤1, QW bortezomib at reduced dose may be restarted
Grade 2 plus pain, grade 3 or 4	Discontinue Bortezomib
Thalidomide	
Grade 1	Reduce dose by 50%
Grade 2	Discontinue Thalidomide
	If PNP resolves to grade ≤1, thalidomide may be restarted at 50% dose reduction
Grade 3 or 4	Discontinue Thalidomide
PNP symptom control	
Opioids	μ Opioid receptor antagonists: Morphine, Hydromorphone, Dihydrocodeine, Tapentadol, Tramadol, Fentanyl plaster κ Opioid receptor antagonists: Oxycodone, Nalbuphine
Muscle relaxants	Tolperisone, Baclofen
Ca-antagonists	Nifedipine
Anticonvulsive agents	Gabapentin, Pregabalin, Carbamazepine
Antidepressants	Tricyclic: Amitriptyline, Nortriptyline
	Reuptake inhibitors: Paroxetine (SSRI), Duloxetine (SSNRI), Bupropion (NDRI) Tetracyclic: Maprotiline
Topic therapies	EMLA (1:1 EMLA of Lidocaine and Prilocaine), Lidocaine 5%, Capsaicin

BWD twice a week, *EMLA* eutectic mixture of local anesthetic, *IV* intravenous administration, *NDRI* noradrenalin dopamine reuptake inhibitor, *PNP* peripheral neuropathy, *QW* once weekly, *SC* subcutaneous administration, *SSRI* selective serotonin reuptake inhibitor, *SSNRI* selective serotonin noradrenalin reuptake inhibitor general measures recommended to control PNP symptoms. Most important is timely dose reduction or discontinuation of therapy, depending on the severity of PNP. Bortezomib should be administered s.c in all patients and in those with preexistent or emerging PNP in weekly instead of biweekly intervals.

Symptomatic treatment options are suboptimal at best. Drug classes commonly used are opioids, muscle relaxants, Ca-antagonists, anticonvulsive agents, antidepressants, and topic therapies with lidocaine, capsaicin crèmes, or plasters.

8.5 Coagulation Disorders

8.5.1 Epidemiology

A variety of disease- and treatment-related factors affect the coagulation system in patients with multiple myeloma, leading to an increased risk of bleeding and thrombotic complications (Boyle et al. 2012). Overt bleeding is relatively rare in multiple myeloma, whereas venous thromboembolism (VTE) is more frequent with a reported incidence of 8–22/1000 person-years (De Stefano et al. 2014). VTE incidence may increase to up to 70% with IMiDs in combination with dexamethasone or chemotherapeutic agents in the absence of anticoagulation (Kristinsson 2010). The risk

for VTE is highest within the first months after start of therapy and decreases thereafter. Interestingly, the risk for arterial thrombosis (myocardial infarction, transient ischemic attack, ischemic stroke, and angina) is increased as well (Palumbo et al. 2008) (Fig. 8.3).

8.5.2 Pathophysiology

Interactions between paraproteins (especially in case of hyperviscosity), coagulation factors, platelets, and vessels can interfere with physiological hemostasis and may result in bleeding. Rarely, acquired von Willebrand syndrome may lead to increased bleeding tendency as well. In a number of patients, bleeding is due to uncommon hemostatic defects, which are not detectable with routine coagulation tests (Boyle et al. 2012).

The increased risk for thromboembolic complications was also associated with the interaction of paraproteins with platelets, which may result in enhanced platelet adhesion and aggregation. In addition, an increase of fibrin protofibrils, enhanced fibrin assembling, increased expression of factor VIII, von Willebrand factor, and incidence of protein C resistance were proposed as likely procoagulant mechanisms contributing to the heightened VTE risk in multiple myeloma (De Stefano et al. 2014). Furthermore, several patient- and treatment-related risk factors

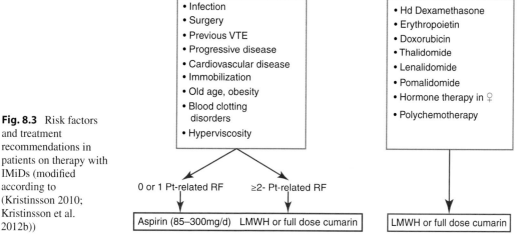

Fig. 8.3 Risk factors and treatment recommendations in patients on therapy with IMiDs (modified according to (Kristinsson 2010; Kristinsson et al. 2012b))

predispose patients to VTE: High age, immobility, infections, surgery, progressive disease, previous VTE, cardiovascular disease, renal insufficiency, diabetes, obesity, and inherited thrombophilia account for the former and treatment with IMiDs, high-dose dexamethasone, anthracycline, ESAs, and hormone substitution in females for the latter category (Kristinsson 2010). Inherited thrombophilic abnormalities such as factor V Leiden, prothrombin G20210A mutation, protein C or protein S deficiency, and antithrombin deficiency are likely found in the same frequency as in the normal population and may also increase the risk for VTE (Palumbo et al. 2008).

8.5.3 Treatment

Management of clinically significant bleeding is often challenging because of the multiple mechanisms involved. Plasmapheresis is very effective when hyperviscosity is the major cause of symptoms. Cytoreductive treatment may be started simultaneously, whereas RBCTs should be delayed when possible, to avoid further increase of blood viscosity. The prevalence of hyperviscosity, however, has become relatively rare with earlier diagnosis and more effective therapy being available nowadays. Therapy depends on the underlying pathology. In case of deficiency of specific coagulation factors, substitution of these factors should be considered, and supplementation with recombinant activated factor VII (rFVIIa) could be considered in patients with severe hemorrhages (Boyle et al. 2012).

VTE prophylaxis should be used in all patients starting treatment with an IMiD (Kristinsson 2010; Musallam et al. 2009; Palumbo et al. 2010). In those with low risk for a VTE, namely, in patients with no or one of the abovementioned risk factors, aspirin (100 mg/day) during anti-myeloma treatment and until 30 days posttreatment is recommended (Boyle et al. 2012). Patients already receiving anticoagulation before diagnosis of multiple myeloma should remain on their current medication, providing it is appropriate. In high-risk patients with more than one patient- or treatment-related risk factor, prophylactic dose of low-molecular-weight-heparin (LMWH) or coumarin is recommended. This recommendation is supported by the reduced incidence of VTE (2.25% vs. 1.2%) and pulmonary embolism (1.7% vs. 0%) in patients on LMWH prophylaxis compared to those on aspirin prophylaxis in patients on lenalidomide-based therapy (Palumbo et al. 2011). In contrast, no significant differences in VTE rate have been noted in patients on a thalidomide-based regimen between prophylaxis with aspirin, LMWH, or warfarin (6.4% vs. 5.0% vs. 8.2%, respectively) (Larocca et al. 2012). Evidence-based data on the optimal duration of anti-VTE prophylaxis are not available, but given the ease and tolerability of aspirin, continuation of prophylaxis after achievement of tumor response and during maintenance therapy seems to be a reasonable choice. For patients who started with LMWH or coumarin, discontinuation of therapy or switching to aspirin may be considered in patients with excellent tumor control or on maintenance therapy. Presently, it is unknown whether thromboprophylaxis might also reduce the risk of arterial events (Boyle et al. 2012; Palumbo et al. 2011). If VTE occurs despite the use of prophylaxis, the responsible anti-myeloma drug should be discontinued, the VTE be treated (Zangari et al. 2010), and anti-myeloma therapy should be reinstated only upon full resolution of the VTE event. A retrospective analysis of the lenalidomide-dexamethasone vs high-dose dexamethasone studies (MM09 and MM10) did not reveal a negative impact of the occurrence of a VTE on OS (Kristinsson et al. 2012b), which is different to the occurrence of arterial thromboembolic complications, which are associated with shortened survival in multiple myeloma.

References

Anaissie E (2011) Infection prophylaxis including vaccination for MM patients. International Myeloma Workshop (IMW), Paris

Arvin A, Campadelli-Fiume G, Mocarski E et al (2007) Human herpesviruses: biology, therapy, and immunoprophylaxis. Cambridge University Press, Cambridge

Badros AZ, Vij R, Martin T et al (2013) Carfilzomib in multiple myeloma patients with renal impairment: pharmacokinetics and safety. Leukemia 27(8):1707–1714

Bahlis NJ, Lazarus HM (2006) Multiple myeloma-associated AL amyloidosis: is a distinctive therapeutic approach warranted? Bone Marrow Transplant 38(1):7–15

Becker PS (2011) Genetic predisposition for chemotherapy-induced neuropathy in multiple myeloma. J Clin Oncol 29(7):783–786

Beguin Y, Yerna M, Loo M et al (1992) Erythropoiesis in multiple myeloma: defective red cell production due to inappropriate erythropoietin production. Br J Haematol 82(4):648–653

Beguin Y, Maertens J, De Prijck B et al (2013) Darbepoetin-alfa and intravenous iron administration after autologous hematopoietic stem cell transplantation: a prospective multicenter randomized trial. Am J Hematol 88(12):990–996

Birgegard G, Gascon P, Ludwig H (2006) Evaluation of anaemia in patients with multiple myeloma and lymphoma: findings of the European CANCER ANAEMIA SURVEY. Eur J Haematol 77(5):378–386

Blade J, Sonneveld P, San Miguel JF et al (2008) Pegylated liposomal doxorubicin plus bortezomib in relapsed or refractory multiple myeloma: efficacy and safety in patients with renal function impairment. Clin Lymphoma Myeloma 8(6):352–355

Blimark C, Holmberg E, Mellqvist UH et al (2015) Multiple myeloma and infections: a population-based study on 9253 multiple myeloma patients. Haematologica 100(1):107–113

Boyle EM, Fouquet G, Manier S et al (2012) Immunomodulator drug-based therapy in myeloma and the occurrence of thrombosis. Expert Rev Hematol 5(6):617–626

Briani C, Torre CD, Campagnolo M et al (2013) Lenalidomide in patients with chemotherapy-induced polyneuropathy and relapsed or refractory multiple myeloma: results from a single-centre prospective study. J Peripher Nerv Syst 18(1):19–24

Bridoux F, Leung N, Hutchison CA et al (2015) Diagnosis of monoclonal gammopathy of renal significance. Kidney Int 87:698–711

Bridoux F, Carron P-L, Pegourie B et al (2017) Effect of high-cutoff hemodialysis vs conventional hemodialysis on hemodialysis independence among patients with myeloma cast nephropathy: a randomized clinical trial. JAMA 318(21):2099–2110. https://doi.org/10.1001/jama.2017.17924

Burnette BL, Leung N, Rajkumar SV (2011) Renal improvement in myeloma with bortezomib plus plasma exchange. N Engl J Med 364(24):2365–2366

Chapel HM, Lee M, Hargreaves R et al (1994) Randomised trial of intravenous immunoglobulin as prophylaxis against infection in plateau-phase multiple myeloma. The UK Group for Immunoglobulin Replacement Therapy in Multiple Myeloma. Lancet 343(8905):1059–1063

Cook M, Hutchison C, Fifer L et al (2016) High cut-off haemodialysis (HCO-HD) does not improve outcomes in myeloma cast nephropathy: results of European trial of free light chain removal by extended haemodialysis in cast nephropathy (EULITE). Annual congress of the European Hematology Association, Abstract 270 https://learningcenter.ehaweb.org/eha/2016/21st/133257/mark.cook.high.cut-off.haemodialysis.28hcohd29.does.not.improve.outcomes.in.html?f=m3

Coppola A, Tufano A, Di Capua M et al (2011) Bleeding and thrombosis in multiple myeloma and related plasma cell disorders. Semin Thromb Hemost 37(8):929–945

Dammacco F, Castoldi G, Rodjer S (2001) Efficacy of epoetin alfa in the treatment of anaemia of multiple myeloma. Br J Haematol 113(1):172–179

De Stefano V, Za T, Rossi E (2014) Venous thromboembolism in multiple myeloma. Semin Thromb Hemost 40(3):338–347

Delforge M, Blade J, Dimopoulos MA et al (2010) Treatment-related peripheral neuropathy in multiple myeloma: the challenge continues. Lancet Oncol 11(11):1086–1095

Dimopoulos M, Alegre A, Stadtmauer EA et al (2010) The efficacy and safety of lenalidomide plus dexamethasone in relapsed and/or refractory multiple myeloma patients with impaired renal function. Cancer 116(16):3807–3814

Dimopoulos MA, Kastritis E, Rosinol L et al (2008) Pathogenesis and treatment of renal failure in multiple myeloma. Leukemia 22(8):1485–1493

Dimopoulos MA, Richardson PG, Schlag R et al (2009a) VMP (Bortezomib, Melphalan, and Prednisone) is active and well tolerated in newly diagnosed patients with multiple myeloma with moderately impaired renal function, and results in reversal of renal impairment: cohort analysis of the phase III VISTA study. J Clin Oncol 27(36):6086–6093

Dimopoulos MA, Roussou M, Gavriatopoulou M et al (2009b) Reversibility of renal impairment in patients with multiple myeloma treated with bortezomib-based regimens: identification of predictive factors. Clin Lymphoma Myeloma 9(4):302–306

Dimopoulos MA, Chen C, Spencer A et al (2009c) Long-term follow-up on overall survival from the MM-009 and MM-010 phase III trials of lenalidomide plus dexamethasone in patients with relapsed or refractory multiple myeloma. Leukemia 23(11):2147–2152

Dimopoulos MA, Palumbo A, Attal M et al (2011) Optimizing the use of lenalidomide in relapsed or refractory multiple myeloma: consensus statement. Leukemia 25(5):749–760

Dimopoulos MA, Roussou M, Gkotzamanidou M et al (2013) The role of novel agents on the reversibility of renal impairment in newly diagnosed symptomatic patients with multiple myeloma. Leukemia 27(2):423–429

Dimopoulos MA, Delimpasi S, Katodritou E et al (2014a) Significant improvement in the survival of patients with multiple myeloma presenting with severe renal impairment after the introduction of novel agents. Ann Oncol 25(1):195–200

Dimopoulos MA, Leleu X, Palumbo A et al (2014b) Expert panel consensus statement on the optimal use of pomalidomide in relapsed and refractory multiple myeloma. Leukemia 28(8):1573–1585

Dimopoulos MA, Sonneveld P, Leung N et al (2016a) International myeloma working group recommendations for the diagnosis and management of myeloma-related renal impairment. J Clin Oncol 34(13):1544–1557

Dimopoulos MA, Moreau P, Palumbo A et al (2016b) Carfilzomib and dexamethasone versus bortezomib and dexamethasone for patients with relapsed or refractory multiple myeloma (ENDEAVOR): a randomised, phase 3, open-label, multicentre study. Lancet Oncol 17(1):27–38

Eleutherakis-Papaiakovou V, Bamias A, Gika D et al (2007) Renal failure in multiple myeloma: incidence, correlations, and prognostic significance. Leuk Lymphoma 48(2):337–341

Fakhouri F, Guerraoui H, Presne C et al (2004) Thalidomide in patients with multiple myeloma and renal failure. Br J Haematol 125(1):96–97

Fermand JP, Bridoux F, Kyle RA et al (2013) How I treat monoclonal gammopathy of renal significance (MGRS). Blood 122:3583–3590

Gordon DS, Hearn EB, Spira TJ et al (1984) Phase I study of intravenous gamma globulin in multiple myeloma. Am J Med 76(3A):111–116

Gorson KC, Ropper AH (1997) Axonal neuropathy associated with monoclonal gammopathy of undetermined significance. J Neurol Neurosurg Psychiatry 63(2):163–168

Hainz N, Thomas S, Neubert K et al (2012) The proteasome inhibitor bortezomib prevents lupus nephritis in the NZB/W F1 mouse model by preservation of glomerular and tubulointerstitial architecture. Nephron Exp Nephrol 120(2):e47–e58

Hammond SP, Gagne LS, Stock SR et al (2012) Respiratory virus detection in immunocompromised patients with FilmArray respiratory panel compared to conventional methods. Clin Microbiol 50(10):3216–3221

Hargreaves RM, Lea JR, Griffiths H et al (1995) Immunological factors and risk of infection in plateau phase myeloma. J Clin Pathol 48(3):260–266

Hedenus M, Adriansson M, San Miguel J et al (2003) Efficacy and safety of darbepoetin alfa in anaemic patients with lymphoproliferative malignancies: a randomized, double-blind, placebo-controlled study. Br J Haematol 122(3):394–403

Hutchison CA, Batuman V, Behrens J et al (2011) The pathogenesis and diagnosis of acute kidney injury in multiple myeloma. International Kidney and Monoclonal Gammopathy Research Group. Nat Rev Nephrol 8(1):43–51

Jagannath S, Barlogie B, Berenson JR et al (2005) Bortezomib in recurrent and/or refractory multiple myeloma. Initial clinical experience in patients with impaired renal function. Cancer 103(6):1195–1200

Jhaveri KD, Wanchoo R (2015) Carfilzomib-induced nephrotoxicity. Kidney Int 88(1):199–200

Johnson WJ, Kyle RA, Pineda AA et al (1990) Treatment of renal failure associated with multiple myeloma. Plasmapheresis, hemodialysis, and chemotherapy. Arch Intern Med 150(4):863–869

Kastritis E, Anagnostopoulos A, Roussou M et al (2007) Reversibility of renal failure in newly diagnosed multiple myeloma patients treated with high dose dexamethasone-containing regimens and the impact of novel agents. Haematologica 92(4):546–549

Kastritis E, Terpos E, Dimopoulos MA (2013) Current treatments for renal failure due to multiple myeloma. Expert Opin Pharmacother 14(11):1477–1495

Khalafallah A, Maiwald M, Cox A et al (2010) Effect of immunoglobulin therapy on the rate of infections in multiple myeloma patients undergoing autologous stem cell transplantation or treated with immunomodulatory agents. Mediterr J Hematol Infect Dis 2(1):e2010005

Knudsen LM, Hippe E, Hjorth M et al (1994) Renal function in newly diagnosed multiple myeloma--a demographic study of 1353 patients. The Nordic Myeloma Study Group. Eur J Haematol 53(4):207–212

Kristinsson SY (2010) Thrombosis in multiple myeloma. Hematology Am Soc Hematol Educ Program 2010:437–444

Kristinsson SY, Tang M, Pfeiffer RM et al (2012a) Monoclonal gammopathy of undetermined significance and risk of infections: a population-based study. Haematologica 97(6):854–858

Kristinsson SY, Pfeiffer RM, Björkholm M et al (2012b) Thrombosis is associated with inferior survival in multiple myeloma. Haematologica 97(10):1603–1607. https://doi.org/10.3324/haematol.2012.064444

Kyle RA, Gertz MA, Witzig TE et al (2003) Review of 1027 patients with newly diagnosed multiple myeloma. Mayo Clin Proc 78(1):21–33

Larocca A, Cavallo F, Bringhen S et al (2012) Aspirin or enoxaparin thromboprophylaxis for patients with newly diagnosed multiple myeloma treated with lenalidomide. Blood 119(4):933–939

Lebouleux M, Lelongt B, Mougenot B et al (1995) Protease resistance and binding of Ig light chains in myeloma-associated tubulopathies. Kidney Int 48(1):72–79

Leung N, Bridoux F, Hutchison CA, Nasr SH, Cockwell P, Fermand JP, Dispenzieri A, Song KW, Kyle RA (2012) Monoclonal gammopathy of renal significance: when MGUS is no longer undetermined or insignificant; International Kidney and Monoclonal Gammopathy Research Group. Blood 120(22):4292–4295

Ludwig H, Fritz E, Kotzmann H, Höcker P et al (1990) Erythropoietin treatment of anemia associated with multiple myeloma. N Engl J Med 322(24):1693–1699

Ludwig H, Adam Z, Hajek R et al (2010) Light chain-induced acute renal failure can be reversed by bortezomib-doxorubicin-dexamethasone in multiple myeloma: results of a phase II study. J Clin Oncol 28(30):4635–4641

Ludwig H, Miguel JS, Dimopoulos MA, Palumbo A, Garcia Sanz R, Powles R, Lentzsch S, Ming Chen W, Hou J, Jurczyszyn A, Romeril K, Hajek R, Terpos E, Shimizu K, Joshua D, Hungria V, Rodriguez Morales A, Ben-Yehuda D, Sondergeld P, Zamagni E, Durie B (2014) International Myeloma Working Group recommendations for global myeloma care. Leukemia 28(5):981–992

Ludwig H, Rauch E, Kuehr T et al (2015) Lenalidomide and dexamethasone for acute light chain-induced renal failure: a phase II study. Haematologica 100(3):385–391

Ma CX, Lacy MQ, Rompala JF et al (2004) Acquired Fanconi syndrome is an indolent disorder in the absence of overt multiple myeloma. Blood 104(1):40–42

Magrangeas F, Kuiper R, Avet-Loiseau H et al (2016) A genome-wide association study identifies a novel locus for bortezomib-induced peripheral neuropathy in European multiple myeloma patients. Clin Cancer Res 22(17):4350–4355

Martin TG (2013) Peripheral neuropathy experience in patients with relapsed and/or refractory multiple myeloma treated with carfilzomib. Oncology (Williston Park) 27(Suppl 3):4–10

Morabito F, Gentile M, Ciolli S et al (2010) Safety and efficacy of bortezomib-based regimens for multiple myeloma patients with renal impairment: a retrospective study of Italian Myeloma Network GIMEMA. Eur J Haematol 84(3):223–228

Moreau P, Pylypenko H, Grosicki S et al (2011) Subcutaneous versus intravenous administration of bortezomib in patients with relapsed multiple myeloma: a randomised, phase 3, non-inferiority study. Lancet Oncol 12(5):431–440

Moreau P, Masszi T, Grzasko N et al (2016) Oral ixazomib, lenalidomide, and dexamethasone for multiple myeloma. N Engl J Med 374(17):1621–1634

Musallam KM, Dahdaleh FS, Shamseddine AI et al (2009) Incidence and prophylaxis of venous thromboembolic events in multiple myeloma patients receiving immunomodulatory therapy. Thromb Res 123(5):679–686

Myatt EA, Westholm FA, Weiss DT et al (1994) Pathogenic potential of human monoclonal immunoglobulin light chains: relationship of in vitro aggregation to in vivo organ deposition. Proc Natl Acad Sci U S A 91(8):3034–3038

Nucci M, Anaissie E (2009) Infections in patients with multiple myeloma in the era of high-dose therapy and novel agents. Clin Infect Dis 49(8):1211–1225

Osterborg A, Brandberg Y, Molostova V et al (2002) Randomized, double-blind, placebo-controlled trial of recombinant human erythropoietin, epoetin Beta, in hematologic malignancies. J Clin Oncol 20(10):2486–2494

Palumbo A, Rajkumar SV, Dimopoulos MA et al (2008) Prevention of thalidomide- and lenalidomide-associated thrombosis in myeloma. Leukemia 22(2):414–423

Palumbo A, Davies F, Kropff M et al (2010) Consensus guidelines for the optimal management of adverse events in newly diagnosed, transplant-ineligible patients receiving melphalan and prednisone in combination with thalidomide (MPT) for the treatment of multiple myeloma. Ann Hematol 89(8):803–811

Palumbo A, Cavo M, Bringhen S et al (2011) Aspirin, warfarin, or enoxaparin thromboprophylaxis in patients with multiple myeloma treated with thalidomide: a phase III, open-label, randomized trial. J Clin Oncol 29(8):986–993

Palumbo A, Rajkumar SV, San Miguel JF et al (2014) International Myeloma Working Group consensus statement for the management, treatment, and supportive care of patients with myeloma not eligible for standard autologous stem-cell transplantation. J Clin Oncol 32(6):587–600

Pirani CL, Valeri A, D'Agati V et al (1987) Renal toxicity of nonsteroidal anti-inflammatory drugs. Contrib Nephrol 55:159–175

Ponisch W, Moll B, Bourgeois M et al (2013) Bendamustine and prednisone in combination with bortezomib (BPV) in the treatment of patients with relapsed or refractory multiple myeloma and light chain-induced renal failure. J Cancer Res Clin Oncol 139(11):1937–1946

Rajkumar SV, Dimopoulos MA, Palumbo A et al (2014) International Myeloma Working Group updated criteria for the diagnosis of multiple myeloma. Lancet Oncol 15(12):e538–e548

Richardson PG, Delforge M, Beksac M et al (2012) Management of treatment-emergent peripheral neuropathy in multiple myeloma. Leukemia 26(4):595–608

Rizzo JD, Brouwers M, Hurley P et al (2010) American Society of Clinical Oncology/American Society of Hematology clinical practice guideline update on the use of epoetin and darbepoetin in adult patients with cancer. J Clin Oncol 28(33):4996–5010

Robertson JD, Nagesh K, Jowitt SN et al (2000) Immunogenicity of vaccination against influenza, Streptococcus pneumoniae and Haemophilus influenzae type B in patients with multiple myeloma. Br J Cancer 82(7):1261–1265

Salonen J, Nikoskelainen J (1993) Lethal infections in patients with hematological malignancies. Eur J Haematol 51(2):102–108

Sanders PW, Herrera GA, Kirk KA et al (1991) Spectrum of glomerular and tubulointerstitial renal lesions associated with monotypical immunoglobulin light chain deposition. Lab Invest 64(4):527–537

San-Miguel JF, Richardson PG, Sonneveld P et al (2008) Efficacy and safety of bortezomib in patients with renal impairment: results from the APEX phase 3 study. Leukemia 22(4):842–849

Scheid C, Sonneveld P, Schmidt-Wolf IG et al (2014) Bortezomib before and after autologous stem cell transplantation overcomes the negative prognostic impact of renal impairment in newly diagnosed multiple myeloma: a subgroup analysis from the HOVON-65/GMMG-HD4 trial. Haematologica 99(1):148–154

Schrijvers D (2011) Management of anemia in cancer patients: transfusions. Oncologist 16(Suppl 3):12–18

Silvestris F, Cafforio P, Tucci M et al (2002) Negative regulation of erythroblast maturation by Fas-L(+)/TRAIL(+) highly malignant plasma cells: a major pathogenetic mechanism of anemia in multiple myeloma. Blood 99(4):1305–1313

Taylor C, Navarrete C, Contreras M (2008) Immunological complications of blood transfusion. Transfus Altern Transfus Med 10(3):112–126

Teh BW, Harrison SJ, Worth LJ, Spelman T, Thursky KA, Slavin MA (2015) Risks, severity and timing of infections in patients with multiple myeloma: a longitudinal cohort study in the era of immunomodulatory drug therapy. Br J Haematol 171:100–108

Terpos E, Kleber M, Engelhardt M et al (2015) European Myeloma Network guidelines for the management of multiple myeloma-related complications. Haematologica 100(10):1254–1266

Tonia T, Mettler A, Robert N et al (2012) Erythropoietin or darbepoetin for patients with cancer. Cochrane Database Syst Rev 12:CD003407

Torra R, Blade J, Cases A et al (1995) Patients with multiple myeloma requiring long-term dialysis: presenting features, response to therapy, and outcome in a series of 20 cases. Br J Haematol 91(4):854–859

Tosi P, Zamagni E, Cellini C et al (2004) Thalidomide alone or in combination with dexamethasone in patients with advanced, relapsed or refractory multiple myeloma and renal failure. Eur J Haematol 73(2):98–103

Weinstein DA, Roy CN, Fleming MD et al (2002) Inappropriate expression of hepcidin is associated with iron refractory anemia: implications for the anemia of chronic disease. Blood 100(10):3776–3781

Wolf S, Barton D, Kottschade L et al (2008) Chemotherapy-induced peripheral neuropathy: prevention and treatment strategies. Eur J Cancer 44(11):1507–1515

Zangari M, Tricot G, Polavaram L et al (2010) Survival effect of venous thromboembolism in patients with multiple myeloma treated with lenalidomide and high-dose dexamethasone. J Clin Oncol 28(1):132–135

Plasma Cell Leukemia and Extramedullary Plasmacytoma

9

Morie A. Gertz, Laura Rosinol, and Joan Bladé

9.1 Plasma Cell Leukemia

Plasma cell leukemia represents a unique subset of patients with multiple myeloma. The current operational definition requires that either: (1) for a blood leukocyte count of >10,000/μL, at least 2000/μL are circulating plasma cells or (2) for a peripheral blood white count of <10,000/μL, 20% of the circulating cells must be plasma cells. The leukemia is classified as primary when this is the patient's initial presentation of multiple myeloma or secondary when it is in the context of relapsing disease.

The reason why plasma cell leukemia is considered an independent entity is because plasma cell leukemia defines a high-risk population of patients, with genetics that are distinctly different from multiple myeloma. The clinical course, the median survival, and the effectiveness of various therapies are also different, which justifies the consideration of plasma cell leukemia as a distinct subset of multiple myeloma. In primary plasma cell leukemia, a constellation of adverse

biologic and prognostic factors are already present at diagnosis, similar to patients presenting with advanced aggressive disease. Primary plasma cell leukemia has a more aggressive clinical presentation than multiple myeloma, with a higher frequency of extramedullary involvement, anemia, thrombocytopenia, hypercalcemia, and renal failure, many of which are defined as adverse prognostic factors in patients with multiple myeloma (Blade and Kyle 1999).

The definition of plasma cell leukemia alluded to above, however, has no biologic basis. The definition of >20% plasma cells circulating or >2000 absolute is an arbitrary definition that was created based on the available tools at the time and does not have a sound biologic underpinning to justify its use. Newer techniques for the identification of plasma cells in the blood are likely to redefine this entity going forward. Sensitive multiparameter flow cytometry allows assessment of circulating plasma cells in myeloma and provides a greater understanding of this entity. Six-color multiparameter flow cytometry was used to examine samples with a target of detecting 150,000 events. Plasma cells were selectively analyzed using the light scatter properties of CD38 and CD138. Normal plasma cells were then separated from clonal plasma cells based on the differential expression of CD45, CD19, and polytypic immunoglobulin light chains. Among 158 consecutive newly diagnosed multiple myeloma patients, the 2-year overall survival for

M. A. Gertz (✉)
Division of Hematology, Department of Medicine, Mayo Clinic, Rochester, MN, USA
e-mail: gertz.morie@mayo.edu

L. Rosinol • J. Bladé
Hematology Department, IDIBAPS, Hospital Clinic, Barcelona, Spain

© Springer International Publishing Switzerland 2018
M. A. Dimopoulos et al. (eds.), *Multiple Myeloma and Other Plasma Cell Neoplasms*, Hematologic Malignancies, https://doi.org/10.1007/978-3-319-25586-6_9

patients with any number of circulating plasma cells by flow was 76% compared with 91% that had no circulating plasma cells. However, using a receiver-operator analysis, the ideal cut point for predicting mortality at 1 and 2 years was 435 and 376 plasma cells, respectively. When reanalyzing this patient population using 400 events as a cut-off, the time to next treatment was 14 months compared to 26 months for those with <400 events. The median overall survival was 32 months for patients with >400 events compared to not reached. Independent analysis showed that patients with >400 circulating plasma cells had a higher international stage, serum creatinine, LDH, and bone marrow plasma cells. In a univariate analysis, only circulating plasma cells were prognostic for overall survival. Therefore, it is conceivable that flow will replace peripheral blood estimations for defining plasma cell leukemia in the future. The proposal of >400 clonal events per 150,000 mononuclear events will need to be validated by other groups (Gonsalves et al. 2014a, b).

Looking at a cohort of patients with ultrahigh-risk multiple myeloma, secondary plasma cell leukemia was seen in 14.3% compared to none of the patients that did not have ultrahigh-risk disease, reflecting the powerful correlation between the presence of plasma cell leukemia and risk. The median survival of patients with ultrahigh-risk myeloma was 5 months (Zhuang et al. 2014).

Other groups have investigated whether alternate thresholds for circulating plasma cells can be used instead of the classic criteria. A Spanish group reported on 370 patients and classified patients into three groups: those that had <5% circulating cells, 5–20%, and then the classic >20%; 1.1% of patients fulfilled classic plasma cell leukemia criteria, but an additional 2.4% had 5–20% circulating plasma cells or an absolute plasma cell count in the peripheral blood of over 500. The group that had an intermediate percentage of plasma cells had a shorter survival than those with classically defined plasma cell leukemia, 7 vs. 12 months. The authors concluded that the criteria for plasma cell leukemia could be relaxed to include patients with >5% circulating plasma cells or an absolute plasma cell count in

the peripheral blood of >500. This definition of plasma cell leukemia has not been adopted by the Multiple Myeloma Working Group (Granell et al. 2015). When the presence of circulating plasma cells was defined as >2% compared with the traditional definition of 20%, there was little difference in median progression-free or overall survival, 12 and 15 months, respectively. Again, although the number of circulating plasma cells did not rise to the level for the classical diagnosis of plasma cell leukemia, the survival was comparable and suggests that the definition currently is too strict (An et al. 2015).

It is easy to overlook the diagnosis of plasma cell leukemia when analysis is not done by flow. In one report, a patient with 89% large atypical blasts was initially thought to have acute myeloblastic leukemia when protein studies demonstrated myeloma (Pavlovic et al. 2012). The United Kingdom has a Leukocyte Immunophenotyping Quality Committee that sent slides from two patients with plasma cell leukemia; and a significant number of laboratories failed to make the correct diagnosis, suggesting that standard morphologic techniques in the absence of immunophenotyping and flow could overlook patients with plasma cell leukemia. The definition of plasma cell leukemia introduced 40 years ago may not be appropriate with current technologies (van Veen et al. 2004).

The detection of plasma cells in the peripheral blood of a patient with multiple myeloma is not straightforward. There is significant variability in the flow characteristics between mature and immature plasma cells, and they can appear as distinct populations in a flow scatter plot. Experience is required to accurately detect peripheral blood plasma cells by flow, necessary in recognizing plasma cell leukemia (Marionneaux et al. 2006).

One hundred and four patients were evaluated for circulating plasma cells by flow, and the optimal cutoff of circulating plasma cells for defining a poor prognosis was 41. In a multivariable analysis, the presence of circulating plasma cells >41 and age adversely affected progression-free survival. Redefining plasma cell leukemia using a flow cutoff of 41 events provides important prognostic information that predicts high-risk and poor outcome. The median survival of patients with >41 plasma cells in the peripheral blood was approximately 24 months with a hazard ratio of 2.63 compared to those with <41 plasma cells (Vagnoni et al. 2015).

The frequency with which plasma cell leukemia occurs varies by reporting group. In a group of 148 patients treated with bortezomib-based therapy, plasma cell leukemia was seen in two (1.4%) (Ahn et al. 2014). Sweden has a population-based registry and had clinical data available for 2494 patients diagnosed between 2008 and 2011. Plasma cell leukemia was reported in 1% (Blimark et al. 2013). At the Arkansas Cancer Research Center, 27 out of 1474 patients (1.8%) were diagnosed as primary plasma cell leukemia. These patients had low hemoglobin, high β2 microglobulin, and high LDH, and were classified as high risk. The median overall survival was 1.8 years with a progression-free survival of 0.8 years and was a highly significant independent adverse feature. The incidence of plasma cell leukemia ranges between 1 and 2%. A report by the International Myeloma Working Group has also suggested that the thresholds for diagnosis of multiple myeloma be reexamined because the criteria for diagnosis have not been evaluated prospectively. Lower values of circulating plasma cells may have the same prognostic impact as higher values (Fernandez de Larrea et al. 2013).

9.2 Biologic Features of Plasma Cell Leukemia

Plasma cell leukemia is acknowledged to have a high proliferative index; and although tumor lysis syndrome is quite unusual in multiple myeloma, it is a recognized complication of induction therapy in patients who have plasma cell leukemia. Tumor lysis syndrome was first reported after bortezomib therapy in 2005 (Jaskiewicz et al. 2005). In an observational study from 1976 to 1994, 6 patients with primary plasma cell leukemia out of 512 myeloma patients (1.2%) showed a mean survival of 14 months for primary plasma cell leukemia and 6.8 months for secondary plasma cell leukemia, reflecting the high-risk nature of the disease (Pasqualetti et al. 1996).

Our own group has reported on the natural history of plasma cell leukemia by reviewing the surveillance epidemiology and end-results database, detecting 445 patients with primary plasma cell leukemia. The median overall survival was 5, 6, 4, and 12 months for those diagnosed from 1973 to 1995, 1996 to 2000, 2001 to 2005, and 2006 to 2009, respectively. Survival is improving but remains far below that expected with other myeloma patients (Gonsalves et al. 2014a). A report of patients with plasma cell leukemia was compared with multiple myeloma. The median survival of primary plasma cell leukemia, secondary plasma cell leukemia, and multiple myeloma were 22.2, 1.3, and 36.4 months, respectively (Cha et al. 2007). A recent review of *How I Treat Plasma Cell Leukemia* has been published (van de Donk et al. 2012) and acknowledges that patients with plasma cell leukemia more often have extramedullary involvement, anemia, thrombocytopenia, hypercalcemia, elevated β2 microglobulin, and LDH. A retrospective report on the natural history of 31 patients with plasma cell leukemia from China, 22 primary and 9 secondary, reported 17 of 21 plasma cell leukemia patients had abnormal karyotypes with a survival of primary plasma cell leukemia, secondary plasma cell leukemia, and multiple myeloma of 14, 2, and 37 months, respectively (Peijing et al. 2009).

A SEER analysis of survival outcomes of plasma cell leukemia reviewed 74,826 patients with myeloma, of whom 479 had plasma cell leukemia, representing 0.6%. The median overall survival was 6 months, with a 2-year overall survival of only 20%, compared with myeloma that had a median survival of just over 2 years (Ravipati et al. 2013). Another SEER database report covering 1973–2004 reported 291 patients with plasma cell leukemia among 49,106 (0.6%). The median overall survival was 4 months with 1-year overall survival at 27.8%. Patients under the age of 60 had a better survival (7 vs. 3 months) (Ramsingh et al. 2009).

Plasma cell leukemia has been recognized to be a multiclonal disease. FISH analysis for aneuploid patterns in plasma cell leukemia has been reported in 75%. Moreover, the incidence of two or more plasma cell clones was reported in 15% of patients. The aneuploid clones seen in patients with plasma cell leukemia were different from those in MGUS (Rasillo et al. 2003).

One of the mechanisms hypothesized for the development of plasma cell leukemia was the loss of adhesion receptors that tie the plasma cell to bone marrow stroma and prevent egress into the circulating blood. Forty percent of all CD56-negative malignant plasma cell patients developed a leukemic phase vs. only 15% of CD56-positive patients. This supported the hypothesis that the lack or weak expression of CD56 is a characteristic feature of plasma cell leukemia (Pellat-Deceunynck et al. 1998). Others have also reported the aberrant expression profiles of plasma cell leukemia, particularly emphasizing the decrease in expression of CD40 (Perez-Andres et al. 2005).

Routine karyotyping of 126 plasma cell leukemia patients identified whole chromosome losses and immunoglobulin heavy chain rearrangements. Most plasma cell leukemia patients had 10 abnormalities at diagnosis. It is hypothesized that the accumulation of abnormalities such as 17p13 and 1p losses triggers some of the extramedullary growth features of plasma cell leukemia (Jimenez-Zepeda et al. 2011). The flow cytometric and immunophenotypic characteristics of 36 plasma cell leukemia patients were reported, and one-third expressed CD56, CD71, and CD117 (Kraj et al. 2011a). Impaired expression of adhesion molecules such as CD11A/CD18 or CD56 was felt to explain hematologic dissemination of plasma cells into the peripheral blood.

9.3 Case Series of Plasma Cell Leukemia

There have been a number of reported case series on outcomes in plasma cell leukemia. One series reported 10 patients with a median age of 58 (78% female) with primary plasma cell leukemia in 8, secondary plasma cell leukemia in 2. Interestingly, there was a 20% incidence of venous thrombosis. The mean survival was 5.9 months, ranging 2–17 months. Secondary plasma cell leukemia had a median survival of 2 months (Jimenez-Zepeda and Dominguez 2006).

A single-center experience with 30 patients with primary plasma cell leukemia has been reported. These 30 patients were identified among 934 consecutive patients (3.1%). There was a strong male preponderance (22 out of 30); extramedullary involvement in 18 of 30 (60%); 21 patients had cytogenetic studies; 6 were normal; 6 showed complex hypodiploidy, 5 pseudodiploidy, and 4 hyperdiploidy. Median survival was 4.5 months. LDH, performance status, and platelet count were independent predictors of survival (Colovic et al. 2008). In a clinical series of 63 patients (37 primary leukemia, 26 secondary leukemia), one-third of patients expressed CD56, CD71, and CD117. A complete response was achieved in only 17% of primary plasma cell leukemia patients, with a median progression-free survival of 6 months and a median overall survival of 9 months. In secondary plasma cell leukemia, time from diagnosis to the development of secondary leukemia was 21 months, and subsequent median survival was 2 months (Kraj et al. 2011b).

9.4 Genetics of Plasma Cell Leukemia

Data on the genetics of this disorder has evolved rapidly. Fifteen years ago, using allele-specific amplification, N-RAS and/or K-RAS mutations were found in 54.5% of myeloma patients and 50% of primary plasma cell leukemia. These mutations are very uncommon in indolent multiple myeloma. K-RAS mutations were more frequent than N-RAS mutations and were thought to help define higher-risk patients (Bezieau et al. 2001). One of the first FISH analyses of multiple myeloma was published in 2001. Plasma cell leukemia was found in 40 of 240 newly diagnosed patients with stage 3 multiple myeloma. Cytogenetic abnormalities were found in 23 of 34, usually complex hypodiploidy. Patients commonly had rearrangements of 14q32 and t (14;16) (13%). The hypodiploid karyotypes were thought to explain, in part, the poor prognosis of primary plasma cell leukemia (Avet-Loiseau et al. 2001). In a second series, 71% of plasma cell leukemia patients displayed chromosomal abnormalities (Lloveras et al. 2004). A series of 14 patients (5 with primary and 9 with secondary plasma cell leukemia) reported chromosomal abnormalities in all, with deletions of 13q14 in 78% and deletions of 17p13 in 43%. There was no association among the genetic abnormalities. This frequency of genetic changes was greater than that seen in multiple myeloma (Chang et al. 2005). The same group reported on a series of 26 plasma cell leukemia patients. CKS1B was absent in MGUS but was detected in 62% of plasma cell leukemia patients, raising a hypothesis that CKS1B amplification was associated with progression to plasma cell leukemia (Chang et al. 2006).

Our group reported on genetic aberrations and survival in plasma cell leukemia. Eighty patients with primary or secondary plasma cell leukemia were compared with 439 cases of multiple myeloma. Primary plasma cell leukemia patients presented 10 years earlier than secondary plasma cell leukemia (55 vs. 65 years) and had a median survival of 11.1 vs. 1.3 months; 14q32 translocations were present in both forms of leukemia (82 and 87%); and in primary plasma cell leukemia, the IgH translocations involved 11q13, whereas, in secondary plasma cell leukemia, multiple partner chromosome abnormalities were found. Both showed a high incidence of −17p (56% and 83%, respectively, in primary and secondary leukemia) and frequent N-RAS and K-RAS mutations. Survival was consistently short (Tiedemann et al. 2008). A series of 41 plasma cell leukemia patients reported Del(13q), t(4;14), 1q21 amplification, and del(1p21) to be more common in plasma cell leukemia and patients with t(4;14) and del(1p21) having shorter overall survivals (Chang et al. 2009). Frequent upregulation of MYC in plasma cell leukemia has been reported. In 8 of 12 patients, abnormalities directly targeted or close to MYC were found. Only four were detected by FISH analysis. Quantitative RT PCR demonstrated that these abnormalities were associated with increased levels of MYC mRNA, and MYC dysregulation is an important molecular event in the development of plasma cell leukemia (Chiecchio et al. 2009).

Twenty-one Chinese patients with plasma cell leukemia were reported, showing cytogenetic aberrations in 18. Four patients simultaneously had 13q14, illegitimate IgH translocations and 1q abnormalities. Most plasma cell leukemia patients had chromosomal abnormalities, rearrangements, and deletions (Xu et al. 2009). A series of 34 patients with plasma cell leukemia reported at least one chromosomal abnormality in 100%. Patients with plasma cell leukemia had deletion 12p13 in 64.7% and had the highest frequency of chromosome 1 alterations. Their immunophenotype showed a higher expression of CD117 and CD19.

Poor-risk genetic abnormalities were more common in plasma cell leukemia than MGUS or myeloma (Ruggeri et al. 2010). Sixteen untreated plasma cell leukemia patients and six secondary plasma cell leukemia patients had their genomic profiles investigated by integrative microarray; 237 differentially expressed genes in plasma cell leukemia vs. myeloma, of which 155 positively modulated genes were enriched in cytoskeleton organization, cell adhesion, and migration categories. Compared to primary plasma cell leukemia, secondary plasma cell leukemia overexpressed transcripts; 30 upregulated and 21 downregulated miRNAs were identified in primary plasma cell leukemia. Genotyping analysis and FISH detected 13q deletion in 77%, 17p deletion in 58%, and 1q gain in 61.5%. Twenty-three miRNAs, mostly mapping to chromosome 1p (22%), were reported. This highlights a wide gene-dosage effect, suggesting that genomic abnormalities in primary plasma cell leukemia reflect expression imbalances (Lionetti et al. 2011). Results were subsequently updated to 17 untreated patients; 13q and 17p deletions were seen in 12 and 8, respectively; t(11;14), t(4;14), and MAF translocations were found in 4, 1, and 8 patients, respectively; 199 probes whose expression level strongly correlated with the occurrence of allelic imbalances were identified; 23 miRNAs mapping to 1p13 and 19 were found to be positively correlated (Mosca et al. 2011).

Gene and miRNA expression profiles in 16 primary plasma cell leukemia patients and 6 secondary plasma cell leukemia patients were reported. Unsupervised gene and miRNA expression analyses grouped most of plasma cell leukemias in two distinct branches according to IgH chromosomal translocations. The comparison of plasma cell leukemia forms revealed, in secondary plasma cell leukemia, overexpression of transcripts concerning mitosis, spindle organization, and chromosome segregation. Transcriptomic analyses of plasma cell leukemia patients can identify molecular alterations characterizing this aggressive disorder (Todoerti et al. 2011). Analysis of the transcriptome and genomic profiles was performed in association with a prospective series of newly diagnosed patients receiving lenalidomide and dexamethasone. There were 23 such patients, and all but 3 had either t(4;14), t(11;14), or MAF-associated translocation. However, none of these alterations predicted overall survival or response. A 27-gene model was able to dissect the plasma cell leukemia patients into two groups; one contained six patients with a poor outcome. The 27-gene model was independent of cytogenic abnormalities as well as independent of autologous stem cell transplant therapy. Two miRNAs reached a significant correlation with overall survival miR-92a and miR-330-3p (Agnelli et al. 2012).

Affymetrix gene chip mapping in primary plasma cell leukemia demonstrated alterations of chromosome 8 in 10 of 17. In particular, 8p deletions were observed in six. Eight genes were found downregulated in primary plasma cell leukemia with 8p loss, two of which mapped to 12q and six to 8p. A gene-dosage effect associated to 8p loss provided novel candidate disease-associated genes (Barbieri et al. 2012). A multicenter study of 21 previously untreated primary plasma cell leukemia patients had transcriptional profiling. Grouping was driven by major IgH chromosomal translocations. Comparing primary plasma cell leukemia with myeloma identified 366 upregulated and 137 downregulated genes. A 38-gene signature, which clustered patients with the poorest prognosis, was developed, and this gene signature can discriminate high-risk primary plasma cell leukemia (Todoerti et al. 2012).

An Eastern European analysis of seven plasma cell leukemia samples revealed early phases of cell cycle (G1 and G1/S) to be affected. In plasma cell leukemia samples, co-expression changes were associated with late phases of cell cycle (G2/M, S, and M) with severe alteration in early phases. Oncogenic stress was evidenced in the progression from myeloma to plasma cell leukemia (Kryukov et al. 2013). miRNA expression signatures were reported in plasma cell leukemia from 18 patients. Results were integrated with gene expression profiles. There were 42 upregulated and 41 downregulated miRNAs compared to myeloma. All four miRNAs (miR-497, miR-106b, miR-181a, and miR-181b) had expression levels that correlated with treatment response and four additional with clinical outcome. The contribution of miRNAs in the pathogenesis of primary plasma cell leukemia suggests potential future therapeutic targets (Lionetti et al. 2013). A genome-wide analysis of primary plasma cell leukemia identified IgH translocations in 87%, with a prevalence of t(11;14) of 40% and t(14;16) of 30.5%. Mutations of p53 were identified in four. Gene expression profiling data showed a significant dosage effect of genes involved in transcription, translation, methyltransferase activity, and apoptosis (Mosca et al. 2013). Of 33 patients with primary plasma cell leukemia, 16 were hypodiploid, 13 were pseudodiploid, and 4 were hyperdiploid; 33% had p53 deletion, 73% had RB1 deletion, and 3 of 7 had CCND1 rearrangement. The overall median survival was 106 weeks. The genetic changes did not impact survival (Muzzafar et al. 2013).

Transcriptional characterization of 21 newly diagnosed primary plasma cell leukemia patients showed immunoglobulin heavy chain locus translocation in all but one; 503-gene signature distinguished primary plasma cell leukemia from myeloma; 27-gene signature was associated with overall survival independently. Gene expression profiling may be of great value in plasma cell leukemia. 17p deletion was seen in 8 of 44 plasma cell leukemia patients at diagnosis (18%), nearly three times the risk in newly diagnosed myeloma (Parmar et al. 2014). Among 23 primary plasma cell leukemia and 11 secondary plasma cell leukemia patients, variable genes on the plasma cell leukemia cases distinguished secondary from primary. All secondary plasma cell leukemia cases were grouped with the HMCL. Primary plasma cell leukemia cases were in a separate cluster. Upregulated miRNAs promoted proliferation, angiogenesis, and cell survival. Downregulated miRNAs mimic the effect of translocations on specific oncogenic targets. Specific gene and miRNA expression profiles help to elucidate the molecular alterations discriminating the two forms of plasma cell leukemia (Todoerti et al. 2014). Whole-exome sequencing of primary plasma cell leukemia has been performed. In 12 primary plasma cell leukemia patients, 166 variants per sample were seen. Only a few were recurrent in two or more samples. Fourteen candidate cancer driver genes were identified, but there was remarkable genetic heterogeneity of mutational patterns (Cifola et al. 2015).

9.5   Therapy of Plasma Cell Leukemia

In the pre-novel agent era, the prognosis of patients with plasma cell leukemia was poor; 18 patients were reported in the era before the introduction of novel agents and were treated with anthracycline regimens such as VAD; 6 of 18 had no response, and there was only 1 complete response. Median survival was 7 months (Costello et al. 2001). The first meaningful benefit was achieved with the introduction of bortezomib. A decade ago, the Spanish group reported on four patients with plasma cell leukemia; the result was normalization of peripheral blood counts and transfusion independence. Bortezomib induced procaspase-3 and poly (ADP-ribose) polymerase cleavage and decreased the amount of Erk1/2 (Esparis-Ogando et al. 2005).

Twelve patients with plasma cell leukemia received bortezomib, five partial responses, four very good partial responses, and two complete responses were seen with a median progression-free and overall survival of 8 and 12 months, respectively. Bortezomib's effectiveness was recognized early for plasma cell leukemia (Musto et al. 2007). Twenty-nine patients with primary plasma cell leukemia received bortezomib in combination with dexamethasone, thalidomide, doxorubicin, melphalan, prednisone, vincristine, and cyclophosphamide. The overall response rate was 79%, 38% VGPR. At 24 months, 16 patients were alive, 12 in remission, and 4 relapses (D'Arena et al. 2012). At the Moffitt Cancer Center, 25 patients with plasma cell leukemia were identified; 18 received a bortezomib-based regimen. The median overall survival for all patients was 23.6 months, and bortezomib-treated patients had a median survival of 28.4 months, significantly higher than non-bortezomib-treated patients (Lebovic et al. 2011). In a CIBMTR database review of plasma cell leukemia, 28 patients were identified, representing 1.6% of patients in the database. Median progression-free survival was 66% at 3 years with an overall survival of 73% at 4 years. In the secondary plasma cell leukemia subset, the median progression-free survival was 3 months, and median overall survival was 3 months; but cytoreduction with bortezomib-based regimens followed by early stem cell transplant and then RVD maintenance delivered superior and sustained response rates and prevented early relapse in primary plasma cell leukemia (Nooka et al. 2012).

Twelve patients with primary plasma cell leukemia and five with secondary plasma cell leukemia were reported from the Penn State Cancer Center. Median overall survival was 18 months, 21 for primary plasma cell leukemia, and 4 months for secondary plasma cell leukemia. However, their overall survival was improved with the use of novel agents that modestly improved outcomes (Talamo et al. 2012).

The Greek Myeloma Study Group reported on treatment with bortezomib in patients with plasma cell leukemia. Forty-two consecutive plasma cell leukemia patients (25 primary, 17 secondary) were reported. Serum calcium was significantly higher in primary plasma cell leukemia, LDH was higher in secondary plasma cell leukemia, and 64% had high-risk cytogenetics. A bortezomib-based regimen was given to 29 of 42 patients. An objective response was obtained in 57% of patients, 80% primary plasma cell leukemia, and 23.6% secondary plasma cell leukemia. Time to progression and overall survival was 13 and 14 months, respectively, for primary plasma cell leukemia and 2 and 5 months, respectively, for secondary plasma cell leukemia. Treatment with a bortezomib-based regimen predicted for overall survival from the diagnosis of plasma cell leukemia and was felt to prolong overall survival (Katodritou et al. 2013). The Japanese Myeloma Society reported 38 consecutive patients. The incidence of primary plasma cell leukemia was 1.1%. The median survival data of all patients was 2.85 years, those treated with novel agents, 2.85 years, vs. those not treated with novel agents, 1.16 years. This improved survival reflects the high level utilization of bortezomib (Iriuchishima et al. 2014).

Lenalidomide-based therapy has also been used in the treatment of plasma cell leukemia. A multicenter Italian trial of the first-line therapy with lenalidomide and dexamethasone in primary plasma cell leukemia was first reported in 2010. After a median follow-up of 9 months, 12 patients were alive (85.7%), 9 that had responsive disease (Musto et al. 2010). This was updated when 20 patients were enrolled; and on an intention to treat, 11 of 18 evaluable patients completing four cycles achieved a PR (61.1%, 39% VGPR). The interim analysis suggested that lenalidomide-dexamethasone was promising (Musto et al. 2011a). Final results of this study included 23 patients, including those with renal failure, elevated LDH, and extramedullary disease in 39%, 44%, and 13% of patients, respectively. On an intention to treat, 14 of the 23 completed four cycles of Rd. The overall response rate was 61%. VGPR or better was 35% with a median follow-up 15 months. Overall and progression-free survival at 2 years was 65% and 52%, respectively (Musto et al. 2011b). Two subsequent updates have been published on this

trial. At a median follow-up of 23 months, median-overall and progression-free survival in the intention-to-treat population were not reached at 22 months, respectively. Median overall survival was 12 months in 11 patients that did not receive stem cell transplant. Stem cell transplant was positively correlated to both overall and progression-free survival (Musto et al. 2012). Final publication on this series demonstrated an overall response rate of 74%, 39% VGPR, progression-free and overall survivals of 14 and 28 months, respectively, but progression-free survival in the transplanted patients was 27 months. Stem cell transplant after response to Ld impacted progression-free survival. Overall survival was influenced only by stem cell transplant. t(14;16) was found in 31% of patients, TP53 in 4 of 17. First-line lenalidomide-dexamethasone followed by autologous stem cell transplant is capable of prolonging survival in patients with primary plasma cell leukemia (Musto et al. 2013).

The National Intergroup Trial for the treatment of high-risk myeloma is a comparison of elotuzumab, lenalidomide, bortezomib, dexamethasone vs. lenalidomide, bortezomib, and dexamethasone. In the first report of accrual, three primary plasma cell leukemia patients were enrolled as part of the phase 1 MTD dose escalation. Patients received eight cycles of RVD with elotuzumab, with lenalidomide at 25 mg, 14 of 21 days; bortezomib 1.3 mg/m² subcutaneously days 1, 4, 8, 11; dexamethasone the day of and the day after bortezomib; and elotuzumab 10 mg/kg day 1, 8, 15 for the first two cycles and then days 1 and 11 cycles 3 to 8. Stem cell transplant was not planned as part of initial therapy on this trial. The MTD was determined, safety was established, and the randomized phase 2 portion of this trial is accruing (Usmani et al. 2014).

Lenalidomide, bortezomib, dexamethasone (RVD) has been reported for the treatment of secondary plasma cell leukemia. The median overall survival for the entire group was 5.1 months with median overall survival longer for patients achieving an objective response (7.9 vs. 2.9 months) (Jimenez Zepeda et al. 2013).

9.6   Stem Cell Transplantation in the Treatment of Plasma Cell Leukemia

Planned autologous stem cell transplant in the management of plasma cell leukemia has been reported. In an evaluation of the EBMT database, 272 patients with plasma cell leukemia were identified and were transplanted within 6 months of diagnosis. Those patients were more likely to enter complete remission after transplantation with a median overall survival of 25.7 months. This is the largest number of plasma cell leukemia patients reported, suggesting autologous transplantation can improve outcome, although its benefit remains inferior to those patients with standard-risk multiple myeloma (Drake et al. 2010). One hundred twenty-eight plasma cell leukemia, 73 primary, were reported; and patients receiving autologous stem cell transplant had both a longer overall survival and duration of response, 38.1 and 25.8 months, respectively, compared with non-transplanted patients that had an overall survival and duration of response of 9.1 and 7.3 months, respectively. Response duration is favorably influenced by stem cell transplantation, which increased overall survival and duration of response by 69% and 88%, respectively (Pagano et al. 2011). The group at the Princess Margaret Hospital reported on induction therapy with cyclophosphamide, bortezomib, dexamethasone (CYBOR-D) followed by planned autologous stem cell transplant. Ten newly diagnosed patients with primary plasma cell leukemia received this therapy with an overall response rate of 100%, a VGPR of 50%, and a CR in 20%. Patients were given maintenance therapy after transplant, including thalidomide and lenalidomide. The median progression-free survival for all patients was 18 months, with seven patients alive after a median follow-up of 25 months. Disease progression was common and occurred early, but CYBOR-D followed by autologous stem cell transplant can provide longer-term disease control (Reece et al. 2013).

A prospective phase 2 trial of primary plasma cell leukemia treated with either bortezomib-cyclophosphamide-dexamethasone or bortezomib-doxorubicin-dexamethasone followed by high-dose melphalan has been reported. After induction therapy, 17 of 27 responded (63%). Of 17 responding patients, 16 went to autologous stem cell transplant. Median progression-free survival was reported at 17.8 months, with three deaths due to sepsis. The feasibility of planned induction followed by autologous stem cell transplant in plasma cell leukemia was demonstrated, including high response rates (Royer et al. 2013).

Allogeneic transplant has also been reported for the treatment of plasma cell leukemia. Five years ago, a haploidentical stem cell transplant for the treatment of plasma cell leukemia, using stem cells from a daughter, was used. Complete donor chimerism was established by day 34, and this patient has been disease-free for 56 months, following stem cell transplantation without graft vs. host disease (Guifang et al. 2010). Seventeen patients receiving stem cell transplant have been reported. A 31-year-old male who presented with extramedullary disease underwent allogeneic bone marrow transplant from an HLA-identical sister and survived 7 years after diagnosis. Allogeneic transplant is feasible for high-risk patients and can provide durable responses, although it does not appear to be curative (Saccaro et al. 2005). A review of results from the CIBMTR identified 147 patients with primary plasma cell leukemia, 97 autologous transplants, and 50 allogeneic transplants within 18 months of diagnosis. Progression-free survival at 3 years was 34% in the autologous group and 20% in the allogenic group. Relapse at 3 years was 61% in the autologous group and 38% in the allogeneic group; and overall survival at 3 years was 64% in the autologous group and 39% in the allogeneic group. The encouraging overall survival after autologous transplant establishes the safety and feasibility of this for plasma cell leukemia. Allogeneic transplant, however, carried a much higher risk of non-relapse mortality, 41%, at 3 years without overall survival benefit (Mahindra et al. 2012).

A prospective trial of allotransplant for 17 patients has been reported. Six patients developed acute graft vs. host disease. At day 100, 16 patients were evaluable, 76% VGPR, 12% PR, 12% died. Three patients received donor lymphocyte infusions. They had a median follow-up of 22 months, 6 of 17 relapsed, and 5 of them died. One-year post diagnosis, overall survival was 87%, and the progression-free survival was 86% and 65%, respectively. The prospect of allogeneic transplant should not be unilaterally abandoned for this high-risk group (Charbonnier et al. 2014). Seven patients with primary plasma cell leukemia and two patients with refractory myeloma underwent a Mel-100 TBI allogeneic transplant at the University of Pennsylvania. Three of nine patients, however, died before day 100. The median event-free survival was 28.2 months with a median overall survival not reached. Consolidation with a Mel-TBI allotransplant can result in long-term survival without severe toxicity (Landsburg et al. 2014).

9.6.1 Extramedullary Plasmacytomas

9.6.2 Localized Plasmacytomas

Localized plasmacytomas are plasma cell tumors, histologically indistinguishable from multiple myeloma that develop as single tumors, either in bone (solitary plasmacytoma of bobe – SPB-) or in soft tissues (extramedyllary _EMP-). Both are uncommon disorders accounting for less than 5% of all plasma cell malignancies. SPB has been developed in Chap. 2 of this book; in consequence among localized plasmacytomas only, the extramedullary will be reviewed in this chapter.

9.6.3 Localized Extramedullary Plasmacytoma

Extramedullary plasmacytoma is an uncommon plasma cell disorder consisting of a plasma cell soft tissue tumor. EMP may originate in many anatomical sites, although more than 90%

developed in the head or neck area, particularly in the upper respiratory structures (Wiltshaw 1976; Woodruff et al. 1979; Knowling et al. 1983).

9.6.3.1 Clinical Findings and Diagnostic Criteria

The incidence of EMP is about 3% of all plasma cell malignancies. It is more frequent in males than in females (2:1) and the median age at diagnosis is 60 years (Wiltshaw 1976; Woodruff et al. 1979; Knowling et al. 1983). The clinical features depend on the site and organ involved. Considering the frequent locations in the upper respiratory tract, patients usually present with symptoms such as nasal obstruction or discharge, epistaxis, hoarseness, or hemoptysis. Pain and tenderness at the plasmacytoma site may occur. EMP can occur in any organ including gastrointestinal tract, brain, thyroid, breasts, testes, or lymph nodes (Wiltshaw 1976; Woodruff et al. 1979; Knowling et al. 1983; Meiss et al. 1987). There is a predominance of IgA immunoglobulin type. The diagnosis is based on the finding of a plasma cell proliferation in an extramedullary site and the absence of MM.

9.6.3.2 Treatment and Outcome

As in the SPB the treatment consists of tumoricidal radiation at the dose of 40–50 Gys over 4–5 weeks (Wiltshaw 1976; Knowling et al. 1983; Meiss et al. 1987; Mayr et al. 1990). Radiation therapy on local lymph nodes may be considered since up to 25% of patients with EMP of the head and neck may develop lymph node involvement. EMP localized in the upper respiratory tract have a better outcome than those arising outside the head and neck area. Involvement of the adjacent bone has been reported as an adverse factor. Local relapses, including lymph nodes involvement, occur in up to 15% of cases (Knowling et al. 1983; Mayr et al. 1990; Tong et al. 1980). Progression to MM is uncommon with a frequency ranging from 8 to 23% (Wiltshaw 1976; Woodruff et al. 1979; Knowling et al. 1983; Mayr et al. 1990; Tong et al. 1980; Corwin and Lindberg 1979; Chak et al. 1987; Dores et al. 2008; Katodritou et al. 2014).

9.6.4 Soft Tissue Plasmacytomas in Multiple Myeloma

9.6.4.1 Bone Marrow Homing in Multiple Myeloma

Multiple myeloma is characterized by a plasma cell proliferation with a strong dependence on the bone marrow (BM) microenvironment (Tong et al. 1980). However, up to one-third of patients with MM can develop soft tissue plasmacytomas, which can be the most prominent disease features (Bladé et al. 2011).These soft tissue masses can have two different origins: (1) direct growth from skeletal lesions by disrupting the bone cortical and (2) resulting from hematogenous spread with no contact with bone. The mechanisms involved in the extramedullary myeloma dissemination are poorly understood; however, some hypotheses are (1) decreased expression of adhesion molecules, (2) low expression of cytokine receptors, or (3) increased angiogenesis. It is likely that the physiopathological mechanisms involved in the hematogenous dissemination and direct growth from lytic lesions are different (Bladé et al. 2011).

9.6.4.2 Incidence

In autopsy studies an extraskeletal involvement up to 70% was recognized. Pasmantier and Azar (1969) reported the findings in 57 consecutive autopsy cases and proposed a classification in three stages: stage I or intraskeletal were the disease was confined to the bone marrow or bone, stage II or paraskeletal with tumor masses arising from bones, and stage III or extraskeletal resulting from hematogenous spread. However, the definition of extramedullary disease in MM has not been uniform. Some authors consider EMD only when it results from hematogenous spread, while others also include the soft tissue masses originated directly from bones (Wu et al. 2009; Varettoni et al. 2009; Pour et al. 2014; Varga et al. 2015; Usmani et al. 2012; Short et al. 2011; Weinstock et al. 2015). In this regard, the international Myeloma Working Group (IMWG) is working on a Consensus Statement on the definition of extramedullary involvement in MM.

Data on the incidence of EM involvement in MM are only observational. The rate of plasmacytomas arising from bone lesions at diagnosis ranges from 7 to 34%, this incidence remaining similar ranging from 6 to 34% at the time of relapse while the incidence of EMD resulting from hematogenous spread at diagnosis is from 2 to 5% increasing up to 5–10% at the time of relapse. To note, about 50% of patients with plasmacytomas at diagnosis develop plasmacytomas at the time of relapse (Wu et al. 2009; Papanikolaou et al. 2013). The reported incidence of extramedullary involvement after allogeneic transplantation is between 20 and 37%, and it has been suggested that patients undergoing allogeneic transplantation with reduced intensity conditioning (Allo-RIC) have a higher incidence of extramedullary relapse (Pérez Simón et al. 2006; Minnema et al. 2004; Zeiser et al. 2004). In fact, the reported incidence after autologous stem cell transplantation (ASCT) ranges from 9 to 24%. The reasons for the discrepancy between the incidence of plasmacytomas after ASCT and Allo-RIC are unclear. In a recent report on 663 patients who underwent stem cell transplantation (SCT) biopsy proven extramedullary disease was reported in 8.3% and the authors suggested that there was no increase after SCT (Weinstock et al. 2015). In this study there is no information on the incidence of extramedullary involvement in patients relapsing from ASCT or from an allogeneic procedure. It has been claimed that soft tissue involvement in patients relapsing after novel agents exposure is increased. However, in several studies the risk of plasmacytomas was not increased by the use of front-line regimens incorporating thalidomide, bortezomib or lenalidomide (Varga et al. 2015; Bladé et al. 2015). However, the data is still limited and better control of medullary disease with novel drugs can lead to a survival prolongation resulting in a higher risk of plasmacytomas at the time of relapse/progression.

The most common locations of plasmacytomas arising from bones are the vertebrae, ribs, sternum, skull, and pelvis. The hematogenous or metastatic spread can consist of (1) single or multiple highly vascularized large subcutaneous nodules with a red-purple appearance, (2) multiple small nodules located at any organ, particularly skin, liver, breast, or kidney, (3) pleura, (4) lymph nodes, and 5 central nervous system (CNS). Skin is the most common location at diagnosis, being the most frequent locations at relapse liver, pleura, and CNS. The CNS involvement will be developed later in this chapter. Plasmacytomas can develop on scars of surgical procedures performed during the course of the disease or even years before MM is diagnosed. They can arise from laparotomy scars, bone surgery, or catheter insertions and can precede systemic relapses (Muchtar et al. 2014; Rosiñol et al. 2014).

9.6.4.3 Plasma Cell Characteristics at Extramedullary Sites

Plasma cells from hematogenous spread usually show plasmablastic morphology, while myeloma cells from plasmacytomas arising from focal bone lesions usually show a plasmacytic morphology. CD56 tends to be downregulated in plasma cells at extramedullary locations. However, more data are needed to definitively establish the role of CD56 in the extramedullary myeloma progression. The frequency of 17p deletion and GEP-defined high-risk MM is more frequent in patients with extramedullary dissemination.

9.6.4.4 Assessment of Plasmacytomas

In some patients plasmacytomas consist of palpable masses and can be assessed by physical examination. However, in most of the cases, radiographic imaging techniques are required. Magnetic resonance imaging (MRI) is useful in patients with suspicion of spinal cord or nerve root compression and is also mandatory when CNS involvement is suspected (Dimopoulos et al. 2015). Fluorodeoxyglucose (FDG) positron emission combined with computed tomography (PET/CT) is the most useful whole body technique in patients in whom soft tissue involvement is suspected (Nanni et al. 2016; Zamagni and Cavo 2012; Zamagni et al. 2014). A limitation of PET/CT is that it is not standardized and the possible lack of interobserver reproducibility. In any event, a PET/CT should be done when soft tissue involvement is suspected based on clinical data or in high-risk

patients, such as those with high LDH serum levels as well as at the time of relapse in patients with previous history of plasmacytomas, considering the high frequency of plasmacytomas at relapse in this population.

Concerning response evaluation, the IMWG criteria requires the disappearance of plasmacytomas for CR and a decrease equal or higher than 50% for PR. Progression is defined as the recurrence of a plasmacytoma that had disappeared with treatment, the appearance of new soft tissue involvement or the increase in at least 25% of pre-existing lesions (Mesguish et al. 2014). The same imaging technique should be used at baseline and during follow-up assessment (Durie et al. 2016).

9.6.4.5 Prognosis

The Pavia group, using a time-dependent statistical methodology, showed that the presence of extramedullary involvement at any time during the course of the disease was associated to a poorer prognosis (Varettoni et al. 2009). In other study, patients with extramedullary plasmacytomas had worse prognosis when treated with conventional chemotherapy (Wu et al. 2009). However, in both studies, patients who underwent ASCT had similar outcome, irrespective of the presence or absence of extramedullary involvement, suggesting that high-dose therapy can overcome the negative impact of the presence of extramedullary disease. A more recent study showed similar results (Wu et al. 2009; Varettoni et al. 2009). In a PETHEMA transplantation trial, there were no significant differences in PFS between patients with or without extramedullary involvement, while the OS was shorter in those with plasmacytomas (Rosiñol et al. 2012). The Arkansas group reported that patients with extramedullary hematogenous spread had a significantly poorer PFS and OS even in the era of novel agents (Usmani et al. 2012). Pour et al. (2014) reported that in the relapse setting the survival of patients with extramedullary disease was poorer than in patients with no plasmacytomas. In addition the survival of those with hematogenous spread was significantly shorter when compared with that of patients with plasmacytomas arising from lytic bone lesions (Pour et al. 2014).

9.6.4.6 Treatment

In the up-front setting, alkylating agents, particularly high-dose melphalan are of benefit in patients with plasmacytomas arising from bones, while the efficacy is more doubtful in patients with hematogenous extramedullary disease. Bortezomib seems to be of benefit in patients with soft tissue masses adjacent to bones with less evidence for hematogenous dissemination (Patriarca et al. 2005; Rosiñol et al. 2006). The efficacy of other proteasome inhibitors such as carfilzomib or ixazomib is unknown. The efficacy of IMiDs is limited. Thus, thalidomide is not effective on extramedullary myeloma involvement (Rosiñol et al. 2004; Avigdor et al. 2001; Juliusson et al. 2000; Myers et al. 2001; Anagnostopoulos et al. 2004). There are no published data on the efficacy of lenalidomide on plasmacytomas. The Mayo group reported that 4 of 13 (31%) patients responded to pomalidomide plus low-dose dexamethasone. Of interest, a dissociation between medullary and extramedullary response to thalidomide and bortezomib has been reported (Short et al. 2011). In any event, the small sample size and the absence of controlled studies are important limitations in the assessment of the efficacy of bortezomib and IMiDs on soft tissue involvement in MM. In the front line, a bortezomib- and alkylating-based regimen such as MPV would be the treatment of choice for patients non-eligible for ASCT (San Miguel et al. 2008). For younger patients a triple induction regimen such as VTD or VRD or VTD/PACE followed by ASCT would be the initial treatment of choice (Sonneveld et al. 2013; Barlogie et al. 2007; Moreau et al. 2014). In patients relapsing with extramedullary disease, the most effective treatment consists of a lymphoma-like regimen such as PACE, Dexa-BEAM, or HyperCVAD (Srikanth et al. 2008; Rasche et al. 2014). With these regimens the response rate is about 50%; however, the response only last for a median of 4 months. In consequence, the treatment with the above chemotherapy regimen should be followed by high-dose therapy/stem cell transplantation whenever possible.

9.6.5 Neurological Complications

Spinal cord compression resulting from plasmacytomas arising vertebrae is the most frequent and severe neurological complication which occurs in up to 10% of patients (Bladé and Rosiñol 2007). The dorsal spine is the most commonly involved. The clinical picture is usually back pain and paraparesis that may evolve in a matter of hours or days. Paraparesis is usually accompanied by a sensory level. This complication is a medical emergency which requires confirmation through an immediate MRI. Treatment with high-dose dexamethasone with a loading dose of 100 mg followed by 25 mg every 6 h with subsequent progressive tapering plus radiation therapy should be immediately started (Posner 1987). If the spinal cord compression is caused by a vertebral collapse rather than from a vertebral plasmacytoma, which is extremely rare, urgent surgical decompression with a prosthesis insertion is required.

Lumbar vertebral involvement can be the cause of cauda equine syndrome, with low back radicular pain and legs weakness. Treatment with dexamethasone and radiation therapy can quickly relieve the symptoms.

Intracranial plasmacytomas are very uncommon despite the frequent skull involvement. Occasionally, myeloma skull extension can result in a subdural plasmacytoma, direct leptomeningeal involvement, or in a brain plasmacytoma. Parenchymal brain plasmacytomas not associated with bone structures are exceedingly rare (Husain et al. 1987). Myeloma involvement of skull base can extend into the orbits causing orbital pain, exophthalmos, and diplopia (Woodruff and Ireton 1982). When orbital involvement is suspected, the radiological imaging with CT scan or MRI should be extended to explore the orbital area in order that potential lesions are not missed.

Leptomeningeal or CNS involvement occurs in about 1% (Fassas et al. 2004; Nieuwenhuizen and Biesma 2007; Schluteman et al. 2004; Chamberlain and Glanz 2008; Gozzetti et al. 2012; Jurczyszyn et al. 2016). The more frequent presenting features are confusion, paraparesis, and cranial nerve palsies. The cerebrospinal fluid (CSF) shows increased protein levels and a positive immunofixation for the myeloma M-protein as well as plasma cells usually with plasmablastic morphology. The MRI may show a diffuse leptomeningeal enhancement. Leptomeningeal involvement can result in spastic paraparesis, with MRI suggesting a parasagittal meningioma. CNS involvement is associated with poor prognostic features such as high-risk cytogenetics, plasma cell leukemia, high LDH serum levels, and additional extramedullary plasmacytoma involvement. In a recent report, eight of the nine patients with CNS involvement harvested 17p deletion. Leptomeningeal involvement can present as an isolated relapse in patients in complete remission. It is likely that, in these cases, myeloma viable cells are seeded in the active phase of the disease and remained dormant at the CNS sanctuary until the time of relapse. The prognosis is particularly poor with a median survival of less than 3 months, even when novel agents are used (Fassas et al. 2004; Nieuwenhuizen and Biesma 2007; Gozzetti et al. 2012; Jurczyszyn et al. 2016; Katadritou et al. 2015). The treatment of myeloma CNS involvement with intrathecal therapy with methotrexate, hydrocortisone, and cytosine arabinoside as well as cranial radiation is unsatisfactory. Craniospinal radiation can be considered. It has recently been reported that local plus systemic therapy can improve the outcome (Jurczyszyn et al. 2016).

References

Agnelli L, Musto P, Todoerti K et al (2012) Analysis of transcriptome, mirnome and genomic profiles in association with clinical outcome in a prospective series of primary plasma cell leukemia. Blood 120(21):3938

Ahn JS, Jung SH, Yang DH et al (2014) Patterns of relapse or progression after bortezomib-based salvage therapy in patients with relapsed/refractory multiple myeloma. Clin Lymphoma Myeloma Leuk 14(5):389–394. https://doi.org/10.1016/j.clml.2014.02.004

An G, Qin X, Acharya C et al (2015) Multiple myeloma patients with low proportion of circulating plasma cells had similar survival with primary plasma cell leukemia patients. Ann Hematol 94(2):257–264. https://doi.org/10.1007/s00277-014-2211-0

Anagnostopoulos A, Gika D, Hamilos G et al (2004) Treatment of relapse refractory multiple myeloma with thalidomide-based regimens: identification of prognostic factors. Leuk Lymphoma 45:2275–2279

Avet-Loiseau H, Daviet A, Brigaudeau C et al (2001) Cytogenetic, interphase, and multicolor fluorescence in situ hybridization analyses in primary plasma cell leukemia: a study of 40 patients at diagnosis, on behalf of the Intergroupe Francophone du Myelome and the Groupe Francais de Cytogenetique Hematologique. Blood 97(3):822–825

Avigdor A, Raanani P, Levi I et al (2001) Extramedullary progression despite a good response in the bone marrow in patients treated with thalidomide for multiple myeloma. Leuk Lymphoma 42:683–687

Barbieri M, Mosca L, Musto P et al (2012) Genome-wide approach identify recurrent 8p21.2 loss in more aggressive form of primary plasma-cell leukemia. Haematologica 97:S46

Barlogie B, Anaissie E, Rhee F et al (2007) The Arkansas approach to therapy in patients with multiple myeloma. Best Pract Res 20:761–781

Bezieau S, Devilder MC, Avet-Loiseau H et al (2001) High incidence of N and K-Ras activating mutations in multiple myeloma and primary plasma cell leukemia at diagnosis. Hum Mutat 18(3):212–224

Blade J, Kyle RA (1999) Nonsecretory myeloma, immunoglobulin D myeloma, and plasma cell leukemia. Hematol Oncol Clin North Am 13(6):1259–1272

Bladé J, Rosiñol L (2007) Complications of multiple myeloma. Hematol Oncol Clin North Am 21:1231–1246

Bladé J, Fernández de Larrea C, Rosiñol L, Cibeira MT, Jiménez R, Ponles R (2011) Soft-tissue plasmacytomas in multiple myeloma: incidence, mechanisms of extramedullary spread, and treatment approach. J Clin Oncol 29:3805–3812

Bladé J, Fernández de Larrrea C, Rosiñol L (2015) Extramedullary disease in multiple myeloma in the era of novel agents. Br J Haematol 169:763–765

Blimark C, Holmberg E, Juliusson G et al (2013) Real world data in myeloma: experiences from the swedish population-based registry on 2494 myeloma patients diagnosed 2008–2011. Blood 122(21):1972

Cha CH, Park CJ, Huh JR, Chi HS, Suh CW, Kang YK (2007) Significantly better prognosis for patients with primary plasma cell leukemia than for patients with secondary plasma cell leukemia. Acta Haematol 118(3):178–182

Chak LY, Cox RS, Bostwick DG, Hoppe RT (1987) Solitary plasmacytoma of bone: treatment, progression and survival. J Clin Oncol 5:1811–1815

Chamberlain MC, Glanz M (2008) Myelomatous meningitis. Cancer 112:1562–1567

Chang H, Sloan S, Li D, Patterson B (2005) Genomic aberrations in plasma cell leukemia shown by interphase fluorescence in situ hybridization. Cancer Genet Cytogenet 156(2):150–153

Chang H, Yeung J, Xu W, Ning Y, Patterson B (2006) Significant increase of CKS1B amplification from monoclonal gammopathy of undetermined significance to multiple myeloma and plasma cell leukaemia as demonstrated by interphase fluorescence in situ hybridisation. Br J Haematol 134(6):613–615

Chang H, Qi X, Yeung J, Reece D, Xu W, Patterson B (2009) Genetic aberrations including chromosome 1 abnormalities and clinical features of plasma cell leukemia. Leuk Res 33(2):259–262. https://doi.org/10.1016/j.leukres.2008.06.027

Charbonnier A, Michalet M, Xhaard A et al (2014) Allogeneic hematopoietic stem cell transplantation (ALLOHSCT) for primary plasma cell leukemia (PPCL): a prospective study of IFM group. Haematologica 99:165

Chiecchio L, Dagrada GP, White HE et al (2009) Frequent upregulation of MYC in plasma cell leukemia. Genes Chromosomes Cancer 48(7):624–636. https://doi.org/10.1002/gcc.20670.

Cifola I, Lionetti M, Pinatel E et al (2015) Whole-exome sequencing of primary plasma cell leukemia discloses heterogeneous mutational patterns. Oncotarget 6(19):17543–17558

Colovic M, Jankovic G, Suvajdzic N, Milic N, Dordevic V, Jankovic S (2008) Thirty patients with primary plasma cell leukemia: a single center experience. Med Oncol 25(2):154–160. https://doi.org/10.1007/s12032-007-9011-5

Corwin J, Lindberg RD (1979) Solitary plasmacytoma of bone vs. extramedullary plasmacytoma and their relationship to multiple myeloma. Cancer 45:1007–1013

Costello R, Sainty D, Bouabdallah R et al (2001) Primary plasma cell leukaemia: a report of 18 cases. Leuk Res 25(2):103–107

D'Arena G, Valentini CG, Pietrantuono G et al (2012) Frontline chemotherapy with bortezomib-containing combinations improves response rate and survival in primary plasma cell leukemia: a retrospective study from GIMEMA Multiple Myeloma Working Party. Ann Oncol 23(6):1499–1502. https://doi.org/10.1093/annonc/mdr480

Dimopoulos MA, Hillengas H, Usmani S et al (2015) Role of magnetic resonance imaging in the management of multiple myeloma: a consensus statement. J Clin Oncol 33:657–664

van de Donk NW, Lokhorst HM, Anderson KC, Richardson PG (2012) How I treat plasma cell leukemia. Blood 120(12):2376–2389

Dores GM, Landgren O, McGlynn KA et al (2008) Plasmacytoma of bone, extramedullary plasmacytoma, and multiple myeloma: incidence and survival in the United States, 1992-2004. Br J Haematol 144:86–94

Drake MB, Iacobelli S, van Biezen A et al (2010) Primary plasma cell leukemia and autologous stem cell trans-plantation. Haematologica 95(5):804–809. https://doi.org/10.3324/haematol.2009.013334

Durie BGM, Harouseau JL, San Miguel JF et al (2016) International uniform response criteria for multiple myeloma. Leukemia 20:1467–1473

Esparis-Ogando A, Alegre A, Aguado B et al (2005) Bortezomib is an efficient agent in plasma cell leukemias. Int J Cancer 114(4):665–667

Fassas AB, Ward S, Muwalla F et al (2004) Myeloma of the central nervous system: strong association with unfavourable chromosomal abnormalities and other high-risk disease features. Leuk Lymphoma 45:291–300

Fernandez de Larrea C, Kyle RA, Durie BG et al (2013) Plasma cell leukemia: consensus statement on diagnostic requirements, response criteria and treatment recommendations by the International Myeloma Working Group. Leukemia 27(4):780–791. https://doi.org/10.1038/leu.2012.336.

Gonsalves WI, Rajkumar SV, Go RS et al (2014a) Trends in survival of patients with primary plasma cell leukemia: a population-based analysis. Blood 124(6):907–912. https://doi.org/10.1182/blood-2014-03-565051

Gonsalves WI, Rajkumar V, Go RS et al (2014b) Trends in survival of patients with primary plasma cell leukemia: a population-based analysis from 1973 to 2010. J Clin Oncol 32(15 Suppl 1):8608

Gozzetti A, Cesare A, Lotti F et al (2012) Extramedullary intracranial localization of multiple myeloma and treatment with novel agents: a retrospective survey of 50 patients. Cancer 118:1574–1584

Granell M, Calvo X, Garcia A et al (2015) Prognostic impact of circulating plasma cells on survival of patients with multiple myeloma. Haematologica 100:517

Guifang O, Huiling Z, Yongwei H et al (2010) Haploidentical stem cell transplantation used in treating primary plasma cell leukemia: a case report. J Med Coll PLA 25(1):54–57. https://doi.org/10.1016/S1000-1948%2810%2960018-4

Husain MM, Metzer WS, Bider EF (1987) Multiple intra-parenchymal brain plasmacytomas with spontaneous intratumoral hemorrhage. Neurology 20:619–623

Iriuchishima H, Murakami H, Ozaki S et al (2014) Primary plasma cell leukemia in the era of novel agent: report of multicenter study from Japanese society of myeloma. Blood 124(21):2008

Jaskiewicz AD, Herrington JD, Wong L (2005) Tumor lysis syndrome after bortezomib therapy for plasma cell leukemia. Pharmacotherapy 25(12):1820–1825

Jimenez Zepeda VH, Reece DE, Trudel S, Chen CI, Tiedemann RE, Kukreti V (2013) Lenalidomide (revlimid), bortezomib (velcade) and dexamethasone (RVD) for the treatment of secondary plasma cell leukaemia. Blood 122(21):5398

Jimenez-Zepeda VH, Dominguez VJ (2006) Plasma cell leukemia: a rare condition. Ann Hematol 85(4):263–267

Jimenez-Zepeda VH, Neme-Yunes Y, Braggio E (2011) Chromosome abnormalities defined by conventional cytogenetics in plasma cell leukemia: what have we learned about its biology? Eur J Haematol 87(1):20–27. https://doi.org/10.1111/j.1600-0609.2011.01629.x

Juliusson G, Celsing F, Turesson I et al (2000) Frequent good partial remissions from thalidomide including best response ever in patients with advamced refractory and relapsed myeloma. Br J Haematol 109:89–96

Jurczyszyn A, Grzasko N, Gozzetti A et al (2016) Central nervous system involvement by multiple myeloma: a multi-institutional retrospective study of 172 patients in daily clinical practice. Am J Hematol 91(6):575–580

Katadritou E, Terpos E, Kastritis E et al (2015) Lack of survival improvement with novel anti-myeloma agents for patients with multiple myeloma and central nervous system involvement: the Greek Myeloma Study Group experience. Ann Hematol 94:2033–2042

Katodritou E, Terpos E, Kelaidi C et al (2013) Treatment with bortezomib-based regimens improves overall response and predicts for survival in patients with primary or secondary plasma cell leukemia: analysis of the greek myeloma study group. Haematologica 98:331

Katodritou E, Terpos E, Symeonidis AS et al (2014) Clinical features, outcome, and prognostic factors for survival and evolution to multiple myeloma of solitary plasmacytomas : a report of the Greek myeloms study group in 97 patients. Am J Hematol 89:803–808

Knowling MA, Harwwd AR, Bergsagel DE (1983) Comparing extramedullary plasmacytomas with solitary and multiple plasma cell tumours of bone. J Clin Oncol 1:255–262

Kraj M, Kopec-Szlezak J, Poglod R, Kruk B (2011a) Flow cytometric immunophenotypic characteristics of 36 cases of plasma cell leukemia. Leuk Res 35(2):169–176. https://doi.org/10.1016/j.leukres.2010.04.021

Kraj M, Poglod R, Kopec-Szlezak J, Kruk B, Letowska M (2011b) Clinical and immunophenotypic characteristics of 63 plasma cell leukemia (PCL) cases. Haematologica 96:S67

Kryukov F, Ihnatova I, Nemec P et al (2013) Cell cycle gene sets coordination in multiple myeloma and plasma cell leukemia. Blood 122(21):1901

Landsburg DJ, Vogl DT, Plastaras JP, Stadtmauer EA (2014) Melphalan/total body irradiation-conditioned myeloablative allogeneic hematopoietic cell transplantation for patients with primary plasma cell leukemia. Clin Lymphoma Myeloma Leuk 14(6):e225–e228. https://doi.org/10.1016/j.clml.2014.07.012

Lebovic D, Zhang L, Alsina M et al (2011) Clinical outcomes of patients with plasma cell leukemia in the era of novel therapies and hematopoietic stem cell transplantation strategies: a single-institution experience. Clin Lymphoma Myeloma Leuk 11(6):507–511. https://doi.org/10.1016/j.clml.2011.06.010

Lionetti M, Musto P, Todoerti K et al (2011) The investigation of genomic profiles in plasma cell leukemias by means of an integrative microarray approach. Haematologica 96:194

Lionetti M, Musto P, Di Martino MT et al (2013) Biological and clinical relevance of miRNA expres-sion signatures in primary plasma cell leukemia. Clin Cancer Res 19(12):3130–3142. https://doi.org/10.1158/1078-0432.CCR-12-2043

Lloveras E, Granada I, Zamora L et al (2004) Cytogenetic and fluorescence in situ hybridization studies in 60 patients with multiple myeloma and plasma cell leukemia. Cancer Genet Cytogenet 148(1):71–76

Mahindra A, Kalaycio ME, Vela-Ojeda J et al (2012) Hematopoietic cell transplantation for primary plasma cell leukemia: results from the Center for International Blood and Marrow Transplant Research. Leukemia 26(5):1091–1097. https://doi.org/10.1038/leu.2011.312

Marionneaux S, Monsalve B, Plante N, Shulman S, Vega AM (2006) The application of Beckman Coulter VCS technology at a major cancer center, with emphasis on the detection of circulating immature plasma cells in plasma cell leukemia. Lab Hematol 12(4):210–216

Mayr NA, Wen BC, Hussey DH et al (1990) The role of radiation therapy in the treatment of solitary plasmacytomas. Radiother Oncol 17:293–303

Meiss JM, Butler JJ, Osborne BM, Ordoñez NG (1987) Solitary plasmacytoma of bone and extramedullary plasmacytoma. A clinicopathologic and immunohistochemical study. Cancer 59:1475–1485

Mesguish C, Fardanesh R, Tanenbaum L et al (2014) State of the art imaging of multiple myeloma: comparative review of FDG PET/CT imaging in various clinical settings. Eur J Radiol 83:2203–2223

Minnema MC, van de Donk NW, Zweegman S et al (2004) Extramedullary relapses after allogeneic non-myeloablative stem cell transplantation in multiple myeloma patients do not negativaly affect treament outcome. Bone Marrow Transplant 34:1057–1065

Moreau P, Cavo M, Sonneveld P et al (2014) Combination of international scoring system 3, high lactate dehidrogenase, and t(4;14) or del (17p) identifies patients with multiple myeloma (MM) treated with front-line autologous stem-cell transplantation at high risk of early MM progression-related death. J Clin Oncol 32:2173–2180

Mosca L, Musto P, Fabris S et al (2011) Integrative genomic analysis of primary plasma cell leukemia reveals strong gene and microRNA dosage effect. Haematologica 96:S54

Mosca L, Musto P, Todoerti K et al (2013) Genome-wide analysis of primary plasma cell leukemia identifies recurrent imbalances associated with changes in transcriptional profiles. Am J Hematol 88(1):16–23. https://doi.org/10.1002/ajh.23339

Muchtar E, Raanani P, Yeshurum M, Shpilberg O, Magen-Nativ H (2014) Myeloma in scar tissue – an underrepresented phenomenon or an emerging entity in the novel agents`era? A single center series. Acta Haematol 132:39–54

Musto P, Rossini F, Gay F et al (2007) Efficacy and safety of bortezomib in patients with plasma cell leukemia. Cancer 109(11):2285–2290

Musto P, D'Auria F, Petrucci MT et al (2010) First line therapy with lenalidomide and dexamethasone in primary plasma cell leukemia. Haematologica 95:S43

Musto P, D'Auria F, Petrucci MT et al (2011a) Efficacy and safety of lenalidomide in combination with low dose dexamethasone (LD) as first line treatment of primary plasma cell leukemia (PPCL). Haematologica 96:126

Musto P, D'Auria F, Petrucci MT et al (2011b) Final results of a phase II study evaluating lenalidomide in combination with low dose dexamethasone as first line therapy for primary plasma cell leukemia. Blood 118(21):2925

Musto P, Fraticelli VL, Mansueto G et al (2012) Bendamustine as salvage therapy in multiple myeloma: a retrospective, multicenter study from the italian compassionate use program in 78 heavily pretreated patients. Blood 120(21):2971

Musto P, Neri A, Simeon V et al (2013) Conclusive analysis of clinical and molecular results. From RV-PCL-PI-350 trial, the first prospective study of a novel agent (lenalidomide) in primary plasma cell leukemia. Haematologica 98:10–11

Muzzafar T, Kaul S, Gonzalez-Berjon JM, Shah J (2013) Plasma cell leukemia: impact of cytogenetic profile on prognosis. Lab Investig 93:350A. https://doi.org/10.1038/labinvest.2013.24

Myers B, Grimley C, Crouch D et al (2001) Lack of response to thalidomide in plasmacytomas. Br J Haematol 115:324

Nanni C, Zamagni E, Versari A et al (2016) Image interpretation criteria fod FDG PET/CT in multiple myeloma; a new proposal from an Italian expert panel. IMPeTUs (Italian Myeloma criteria for PET USe). Eur J Nucl Med Mol Imaging 43(3):414–421

Nieuwenhuizen L, Biesma DH (2007) Central nervous system myelomatosis: review of the literature. Eur J Haematol 80:1–9

Nooka A, Kaufman J, Muppidi S et al (2012) Plasma cell leukemia: sustained responses are possible with innovative treatment strategies. Haematologica 97:601

Pagano L, Valentini CG, De Stefano V et al (2011) Primary plasma cell leukemia: a retrospective multicenter study of 73 patients. Ann Oncol 22(7):1628–1635. https://doi.org/10.1093/annonc/mdq646

Papanikolaou X, Repousis P, Tzenou T et al (2013) Incidence, clinical features, laboratory findings and outcome of patients with multiple myeloma presenting with extramedullary relapse. Leuk Lymphoma 54:1459–1464

Parmar G, Masih-khan E, Atenafu EG et al (2014) Outcome of 17p deleted multiple myeloma (MM) in the era of novel agents and tandem transplantation: a single centre experience. Blood 124(21):4756

Pasmantier MW, Azar HA (1969) Extraskeletal spread in multiple plasma cell myeloma: a review of 57 autopsied cases. Cancer 23:167–174

Pasqualetti P, Festuccia V, Collacciani A, Acitelli P, Casale R (1996) Plasma cell leukemia. A report on 11 patients and review of the literature. Panminerva Med 38(3):179–184

Patriarca F, Prosdocimo S, Tomadini V et al (2005) Efficacy of bortezomib therapy for extramedullary relapse of myeloma after autologous and non-myeloablative allogeneic transplantation. Haematologica 90:278–279

Pavlovic A, Radic-Kristo D, Ostojic Kolonic S et al (2012) Atypical blast morphology of primary plasma cell leukemia with renal involvement and plasmablasts in urine. Cytopathology 23:79. https://doi.org/10.1111/cyt.12004

Peijing Q, Yan X, Yafei W et al (2009) A retrospective analysis of thirty-one cases of plasma cell leukemia from a single center in China. Acta Haematol 121(1):47–51. https://doi.org/10.1159/000210555

Pellat-Deceunynck C, Barille S, Jego G et al (1998) The absence of CD56 (NCAM) on malignant plasma cells is a hallmark of plasma cell leukemia and of a special subset of multiple myeloma. Leukemia 12(12):1977–1982

Pérez Simón JA, Sureda A, Fernández- Avilés F et al (2006) Reduce-intensity conditioning allogeneic transplantation is associated with a high incidence of extramedullary relapse in multiple myeloma patients. Leukemia 20:542–545

Perez-Andres M, Almeida J, Martin-Ayuso M et al (2005) Clonal plasma cells from monoclonal gammopathy of undetermined significance, multiple myeloma and plasma cell leukemia show different expression profiles of molecules involved in the interaction with the immunological bone marrow microenvironment. Leukemia 19(3):449–455

Posner JB (1987) Back pain and epidural spinal cord compression. Med Clin North Am 71:185–201

Pour L, Sevcikova S, Greslikova H et al (2014) Soft-tissue extramedullary multiple myeloma prognosis is significantly worse in comparison to bone-related extramedullary relapse. Haematologica 99:360–364

Ramsingh G, Mehan P, Luo J, Vij R, Morgensztern D (2009) Primary plasma cell leukemia: a surveillance, epidemiology, and end results database analysis between 1973 and 2004. Cancer 115(24):5734–5739. https://doi.org/10.1002/cncr.24700

Rasche L, Strifler S, Duell J et al (2014) The lymphoma-like polychemotherapy regimen "Dexa-BEAM" in advanced and extramedullary multiple myeloma. Ann Hematol 93:1207–1214

Rasillo A, Tabernero MD, Sanchez ML et al (2003) Fluorescence in situ hybridization analysis of aneuploidization patterns in monoclonal gammopathy of undetermined significance versus multiple myeloma and plasma cell leukemia. Cancer 97(3):601–609

Ravipati HP, Kaufman JL, Langston AA et al (2013) Survival outcomes of plasma cell leukemia (PCL) in the United States: A SEER analysis. J Clin Oncol 31(15 Suppl 1):8609

Reece DE, Phillips M, Chen CI et al (2013) Induction therapy with cyclophosphamide, bortezomib dexamethasone (cybord) for primary plasma cell leukemia (PPCL). Blood 122(21):5378

Rosiñol L, Cibeira MT, Bladé J et al (2004) Extramedullary multiple myeloma escapes the effect of thalidomide. Haematologica 89:832–836

Rosiñol L, Cibeira MT, Bladé J et al (2006) Bortezomib: an effective agent in extramedullary disease in multiple myeloma. Eur J Haematol 76:405–408

Rosiñol L, Oriol A, Teruel AI et al (2012) Superiority of bortezomib, thalidomide and dexamethasone (VTD) as induction pre-transplantation therapy in multiple myeloma: results of a randomized phase III PETHEMA/GEM study. Blood 120:1589–1596

Rosiñol L, Fernández de Larrea C, Bladé J (2014) Extramedullary myeloma spread triggered by surgical procedures: an emerging entity? Acta Haematol 132:36–38

Royer B, Merlusca L, Lioure B et al (2013) Bortezomib-doxorubicine-dex/bortezomibcyclophosphamide-dex for primary plasma cell leukemia: a phase 2 study by the IFM. Clin Lymphoma Myeloma Leuk 13:S116–S117

Ruggeri M, Caltagirone S, Gilestro M et al (2010) 12p, 1p, 1q, 5q, 11q abnormalities and immunophenotype in monoclonal gammopathy of undetermined significance, multiple myeloma and plasma cell leukemia. Haematologica 95:S68–S69

Saccaro S, Fonseca R, Veillon DM et al (2005) Primary plasma cell leukemia: report of 17 new cases treated with autologous or allogeneic stem-cell transplantation and review of the literature. Am J Hematol 78(4):288–294

San Miguel JF, Schlag R, Khuageva NK et al (2008) Bortezomib plus melphalan and prednisone for initial treatment of multiple myeloma. N Engl J Med 359:906–917

Schluteman KO, Fassas AB, Van Hemert RL et al (2004) Multiple myeloma invasion of the central nervous system. Arch Neurol 61:1423–1429

Short KD, Rajkumar SV, Larson D et al (2011) Incidence of extramedullary disease in patients with multiple myeloma in the era of novel therapy and the activity of pomalidomide in extramedullary myeloma. Leukemia 25:906–908

Sonneveld P, Goldschmith H, Rosiñol L et al (2013) Bortezomib-based versus non-bortezomib-based induction treatment before autologous stem-cell transplantation in patients with previously untreated multiple myeloma: a meta-analysis of phase III randomized, controlled trials. J Clin Oncol 31:3279–3287

Srikanth M, Davies FE, Wu P et al (2008) Survival and outcome of blastoid variant myeloma following treatment with the novel thalidomide containing regimen DT-PACE. Eur J Haemtol 81:432–436

Talamo G, Dolloff NG, Sharma K, Zhu J, Malysz J (2012) Clinical features and outcomes of plasma cell leukemia: a single-institution experience in the era of novel agents. Rare Tumors 4(3):e39. https://doi.org/10.4081/rt.2012.e39

Tiedemann RE, Gonzalez-Paz N, Kyle RA et al (2008) Genetic aberrations and survival in plasma cell leukemia. Leukemia 22(5):1044–1052. https://doi.org/10.1038/leu.2008.4

Todoerti K, Musto P, Lionetti M et al (2011) Gene and miRNA expression profiles in plasma cell leukemias. Haematologica 96:S54

Todoerti K, Musto P, Agnelli L et al (2012) Transcriptome analysis of primary plasma cell leukemia tumors from a multicenter prospective gimema study: biological and clinical implications. Haematologica 97:S49

Todoerti K, Manzoni M, Fabris S et al (2014) Different gene and mirna expression profiles in primary and secondary plasma cell leukemia by high-resolution microarray analyses. Haematologica 99:S39

Tong D, Griffin TW, Laramore GE et al (1980) Solitary plasmacytoma of bone and soft tissues. Radiology 135:195–198

Usmani SZ, Heuck C, Mitchell A et al (2012) Extramedullary disease portends poor prognosis in multiple myeloma and is overrepresented in high-risk disease even in the era of novel agents. Haematologica 97:4761–4767

Usmani SZ, Sexton R, Ailawadhi S et al (2014) Swog 1211: initial report on phase I trial of RVD-elotuzumab for newly diagnosed high risk multiple myeloma (HRMM). Blood 124(21):4762

Vagnoni D, Travaglini F, Pezzoni V et al (2015) Circulating plasma cells in newly diagnosed symptomatic multiple myeloma as a possible prognostic marker for patients with standard-risk cytogenetics. Br J Haematol 170(4):523–531. https://doi.org/10.1111/bjh.13484.

Varettoni M, Corso A, Pica G et al (2009) Incidence, presenting features and outcome of extramedullary disease in multiple myeloma: a longitudinal study on 1,003 consecutive patients. Ann Oncol 21:325–330

Varga C, Xie W, Laubach J et al (2015) Development of extramedullary myeloma in the era of novel agents: no evidence of increased risk with lenalidomide-bortezomib combinations. Br J Haematol 169:843–850

van Veen JJ, Reilly JT, Richards SJ et al (2004) Diagnosis of plasma cell leukaemia: findings of the UK NEQAS for Leucocyte Immunophenotyping scheme. Clin Lab Haematol 26(1):37–42

Weinstock M, Aljawai Y, Morgan EA et al (2015) Incidence and clinical features of extramedullary multiple myeloma in patients who underwent stem cell transplantation. Br J Haematol 169:851–858

Wiltshaw E (1976) The natural history of extramedullary plasmacytoma and its relation to solitary myeloma of bone and myelomatosis. Medicine 55:217–237

Woodruff RK, Ireton HJC (1982) Multiple nerve palsies as the presenting features of meningeal myelomatosis. Cancer 49:1710–1712

Woodruff RK, Whittle JM, Malpas JS (1979) Solitary plasmacytoma. I. Extramedullary soft-tissue plasmacytoma. Cancer 43:2340–2343

Wu P, Davies F, Boyd K et al (2009) The impact of extramedullary disease at presentation on the outcome of myeloma. Leuk Lymphoma 50:230–235

Xu W, Li JY, Fan L et al (2009) Molecular cytogenetic aberrations in 21 Chinese patients with plasma cell leukemia. Int J Lab Hematol 31(3):338–343. https:// doi.org/10.1111/j.1751-553X.2008.01037.x

Zamagni E, Cavo M (2012) The role of imaging techniques in the management of multiple myeloma. Br J Haematol 159:499–513

Zamagni E, Nanni C, Tachetti P et al (2014) Positron emission tomography with computed tomography-based diagnosis of massive extramedullary progression in a patient with high-risk multiple myeloma. Clin Lymphoma Myeloma Leuk 14:101–104

Zeiser R, Deaschler B, Bertz H et al (2004) Extramedullary vs. Medullary relapse after autologous or allogeneic hematopoietic stem cell transplantation (HSCT) in multiple myeloma (MM) and its correlation to clinical outcome. Bone Marrow Transplant 34:1057–1065

Zhuang J, Da Y, Li H et al (2014) Cytogenetic and clinical risk factors for assessment of ultra high-risk multiple myeloma. Leuk Res 38(2):188–193. https://doi.org/10.1016/j.leukres.2013.11.010

POEMS Syndrome

10

Dimitrios C. Ziogas, Angela Dispenzieri, and Evangelos Terpos

10.1 Definition and Incidence

POEMS syndrome, less frequently known as osteosclerotic myeloma, Takatsuki syndrome, or Crow-Fukase syndrome, is a rare paraneoplastic syndrome due to an underlying plasma cell disorder (Dispenzieri 2015; Warsame et al. 2017). In 1980, Bardwick defined initially the acronym describing some of the features of the syndrome: polyneuropathy, organomegaly, endocrinopathy, monoclonal plasma cell disorder, and skin changes (Bardwick et al. 1980). Notably, not all of the features within the acronym are required to make the diagnosis, while other important features are not labeled in the POEMS acronym, including papilledema, extravascular volume overload, sclerotic bone lesions, thrombocytosis/erythrocytosis (P.E.S.T.), elevated VEGF levels, a predisposition toward thrombosis, and abnormal pulmonary function tests. Furthermore, there is a Castleman variant of POEMS that may not be driven by a clonal plasma cell disorder (Dispenzieri 2008).

Based on early reports from Japan, the disorder was firstly believed to be more common in Japanese cases (Takatsuki and Sanada 1983; Nakanishi et al. 1984), and a recent national survey showed a prevalence of 0.3 per 100,000 in Japan (Nasu et al. 2012). However, over the years, multiple series have also been reported from around the world (France, the United States, China, and India) (Nasu et al. 2012; Zhang et al. 2010; Li et al. 2011a; Kulkarni et al. 2011).

10.2 Theories of Pathogenesis

In order to elucidate the pathogenesis of this syndrome, two theories have been developed. The first theory correlates the disease activity with the increased production of cytokines and mainly high levels of VEGF (D'Souza et al. 2011; Scarlato et al. 2005; Watanabe et al. 1996; Nishi et al. 1999; Soubrier et al. 1998, 1999; Nobile-Orazio et al. 2009). VEGF, acting on endothelial cells, induces angiogenesis and reversible vascular permeability, contributing to polyneuropathy (D'Souza et al. 2011; Scarlato et al. 2005; Watanabe et al. 1996; Nishi et al. 1999; Soubrier et al. 1998, 1999; Nobile-Orazio et al. 2009). This cytokine is expressed in the majority of implicated cells in the syndrome, such as osteoblasts, macrophages, plasma cells (Soubrier et al. 1997; Nakano et al. 2001), and megakaryocytes/platelets (Koga et al. 2002). Unfortunately,

D. C. Ziogas • E. Terpos (✉)
Department of Clinical Therapeutics, National and Kapodistrian University of Athens, School of Medicine, Athens, Greece
e-mail: eterpos@med.uoa.gr

A. Dispenzieri
Division of Hematology, Department of Medicine, Mayo Clinic, Rochester, MN, USA

studies that targeted the VEGF inhibition with drugs such as bevacizumab never achieved to confirm successfully this hypothesis, concluding that VEGF pathway may be only one component of a much more complex cytokine process (Badros et al. 2005; Samaras et al. 2007; Sekiguchi et al. 2013; Kanai et al. 2007). Among the other cytokines, IL-1b and IL-6 have been shown to stimulate VEGF production (Soubrier et al. 1997), while IL-12 has also been found to be correlated with disease activity (Kanai et al. 2012). The second theory is based on the fact that the plasma cells in POEMS syndrome produced in more than 95% of the time lambda light chains with restricted immunoglobulin light chain variable gene usage (IGLV1) (Dispenzieri 2015; Warsame et al. 2017). There is a predilection for the genetic aberrations: $V\lambda$1-44*01 (75% of the cases) and $V\lambda$-40*01 (25% of the cases) seen in the vast majority (95%) of the cases (Abe et al. 2008). Translocations and deletion of chromosome 13 have been described, but hyperdiploidy is not seen (Kang et al. 2013; Bryce et al. 2008).

Summarizing the two theories, a genetically mutated B/plasma cells clone, which will produce excess cytokines and primarily, VEGF, could potentially trigger the cataract of clinical manifestations in POEMS.

10.3   Diagnosis of POEMS

The identification of POEMS is quite difficult, as this condition, except for its rarity, is also characterized by a wide spectrum of nonspecific presenting signs and symptoms that lead to frequent misdiagnoses and delays in diagnosis. Reasonably, the median time from onset of symptoms to diagnosis of POEMS extends to more than 1 year (13–18 months) (Li et al. 2011a; Dispenzieri et al. 2003).

In order to overcome the challenge of diagnosis, a comprehensive approach of a patient with a suspected POEMS syndrome is needed. This includes a detailed history and physical examination followed by skeletal imaging (Shi et al. 2016), monoclonal protein studies (serum and urine 24 h protein electrophoresis,

immunofixation, and serum-free light chains), measurement of VEGF levels (D'Souza et al. 2011; Scarlato et al. 2005; Watanabe et al. 1996; Nobile-Orazio et al. 2009), electromyography (EMG), and careful analysis of bone marrow biopsy (Dao et al. 2011). The diagnosis of POEMS syndrome relies on the fulfillment of certain clinical and laboratory criteria. By definition, all patients must have a peripheral neuropathy, usually demyelinating, and a monoclonal plasma cell disorder. In addition, the patient must have at least one of the other major criteria (Castleman disease, sclerotic bone lesions, or VEGF elevation) and one of the six minor criteria (organomegaly, extravascular volume overload, endocrinopathy, skin changes, papilledema, thrombocytosis/polycythemia).

Given the highly heterogeneous clinical picture of syndrome, it is critical to suspect the disorder in any patient with a combination of peripheral neuropathy and monoclonal protein, particularly a lambda-restricted monoclonal gammopathy. Table 10.1 presents the clinical characteristics, the diagnostic criteria, the estimated frequencies of findings, and the recommended tests for POEMS syndrome. The most crucial symptom is the peripheral neuropathy. It is ascending, symmetrical, and could affect both sensation and motor function (Kelly et al. 1983) while in significant proportion of patients could coexist with pain (Nasu et al. 2012; Koike et al. 2008). Nerve conduction studies in patients with POEMS syndrome show slowing of nerve conduction in the intermediate than distal nerve segments as compared to chronic inflammatory demyelinating polyneuropathy (CIDP), more predominantly in the lower than upper limbs (Nasu et al. 2012; Mauermann et al. 2012; Min et al. 2005). Additionally, in approximately 95% of patients, osteosclerotic lesions are recognized but can be confused with benign bone islands, aneurysmal bone cysts, non-ossifying fibromas, and fibrous dysplasia (Dispenzieri 2015; Nakanishi et al. 1984; Dispenzieri et al. 2003). Bone windows of CT imaging, FDG uptake, and the whole body CT scan—using in multiple myeloma (MM)—could be very helpful in the detection of such lesions. Among the other

Table 10.1 Characteristics, diagnostic criteria, frequencies of findings, and recommended tests for POEMS syndrome

Characteristics	Criteria for the diagnosis	Frequencies of findings (based on large retrospective series)	Recommended testing
Polyneuropathy • Peripheral, ascending, and symmetrical • Initially, sensory, progresses to motor, with features similar to CIDP, although conduction block is rare and axonal loss is greater • Painful in 10–15% of patients • Typically demyelinating with distal symmetric, progressive, and gradual proximal spread • Areflexia, with step-page/foot-drop gait, is common	Mandatory major criteria	100%	• Detailed neurologic history (numbness, pain, weakness, balance, orthostasis) and examination (including funduscopic exam) • Electrophysiologic study (nerve conduction studies) • Sural nerve biopsy
Monoclonal plasma cell proliferative disorder (almost always lambda) • M protein (IgAλ or IgGλ) on serum protein electrophoresis • Inclusion of immunofixation and serum FLC is necessary • Monoclonal proteins can also be seen on BM and osteosclerotic bone lesions • Clonal λ plasma cells are evident on biopsy in patients without an M-spike	Mandatory major criteria	100% (24–54%)	• Serum protein electrophoresis and immunofixation • Affected quantitative immunoglobulin • Complete blood count (hemoglobin, platelet) • 24-h urine total protein, electrophoresis, and immunofixation • Bone marrow aspirate and biopsy (test for kappa/lambda by IHC)
Castleman disease (CD) • POEMS patients with coexisting CD have shorter OS • Patients with CD without peripheral neuropathy and a plasma cell clone can be classified as a Castleman disease variant of POEMS if they have other features consistent with POEMS syndrome	Other major criteria (one required)	11–25%	
VEGF elevation • The ideal method of assay requires the use of serum. Plasma assay can be used (sensitivity 68%, specificity 95%) • VEGF levels are independent of the M protein size	Other major criteria (one required)		• VEGF levels
Osteosclerotic lesions (OSL)	Other major criteria (one required)	27–97%	• Skeletal radiographs, bone windows of CT images, and/or PET/CT
Organomegaly • Splenomegaly • Hepatomegaly • Lymphadenopathy	Minor criteria	45–85% 24–78% 22–70% 26–74%	• Physical exam and CT scan documenting lymphadenopathy, organomegaly, ascites, pleural effusions, and edema
Extravascular volume overload • Peripheral edema • Ascites • Pleural effusion • Pericardial effusion	Minor criteria	29–87% 24–89% 7–54% 3–43% 1–64%	

(continued)

Table 10.1 (continued)

Characteristics	Criteria for the diagnosis	Frequencies of findings (based on large retrospective series)	Recommended testing
Endocrinopathy • Hypogonadism • Hypothyroidism • Pituitary-adrenal axis (Endocrinopathies can improve with treatment directed against the plasma cell clone)		85% 55–89% 9-67% 16–33%	• History regarding menstrual and sexual function • Testosterone, estradiol, fasting glucose, glycosylated hemoglobin, thyroid-stimulating hormone, parathyroid hormone, prolactin, serum cortisol, luteinizing hormone, follicle-stimulating hormone, and adrenocorticotropin hormone • Cortrosyn stimulation test
Skin changes • Hyperpigmentation • Acrocyanosis and plethora • Hemangioma/telangiectasia • Hypertrichosis • Thickening (Treatment for POEMS leads to improvement in the skin changes)		68–89% 46–93% 19% 9–35% 26–74% 5–43%	• History and physical with attention to skin pigment, thickening and texture, body hair quantity and texture, color of distal extremities, and development of cherry angiomata
Papilledema • Blurred vision, diplopia, and ocular pain • CSF protein is increased above normal levels • Unfavorable prognostic feature		29–64%	
Thrombocytosis/polycythemia	Other symptoms and signs	54–88% 12–19%	
Pulmonary hypertension/restrictive lung disease	Other symptoms and signs		• Pulmonary function tests • Echocardiography to assess right ventricular systolic and pulmonary artery pressures
Clubbing, weight loss, hyperhidrosis, thrombotic diatheses, diarrhea, low vitamin B12 values	Other symptoms and signs		

BM bone marrow, *IHC* immunohistochemistry, *OS* overall survival

clinical symptoms, papilledema is present in at least one-third of patients (Cui et al. 2014; Kaushik et al. 2011), while skin manifestations including hyperpigmentation, hemangioma, hypertrichosis, acrocyanosis, white nails, sclerodermoid changes, facial atrophy, flushing, or clubbing (Dispenzieri 2015; Warsame et al. 2017; Kulkarni et al. 2011; Singh et al. 2003; Barete et al. 2010) and pulmonary/respiratory complaints including pulmonary hypertension (in 27% of unselected patients with POEMS), restrictive lung disease, impaired neuromuscular respiratory function, and impaired DLCO have also been documented (Allam et al. 2008; Lesprit et al. 1998). Nearly 20% of patients experience one arterial and/or venous thrombosis (Dispenzieri 2007, 2015; Lesprit et al. 1996), and 10% patients present with a cerebrovascular event, most commonly embolic or vessel dissection and stenosis (Dupont et al. 2009). Extravascular overload most commonly manifests as peripheral edema, but pleural effusion, ascites, and pericardial effusions are also common (Dispenzieri 2015; Warsame et al. 2017). Endocrinopathy is a central but poorly understood feature of POEMS, with hypogonadism being the most common abnormality, followed by thyroid abnormalities, glucose metabolism abnormalities, and lastly by adrenal insufficiency (Gandhi et al. 2007). The majority of patients have evidence of multiple endocrinopathies in the four major endocrine axes (gonadal, thyroid, glucose, and adrenal) (Gandhi et al. 2007).

Bone marrow (BM) is infiltrated by clonal plasma cells in the two-thirds of patients with POEMS syndrome (91% clonal lambda), while those without BM infiltration have a solitary or multiple plasmacytomas. BM biopsy reveals megakaryocyte hyperplasia and megakaryocyte clustering in 54 and 93% of cases, respectively (Dao et al. 2011). These megakaryocytes declare the presence of a myeloproliferative disorder but without JAK2V617F mutation. In patients with POEMS, VEGF levels are markedly elevated in plasma and serum and are correlated with the disease activity (D'Souza et al. 2011; Scarlato et al. 2005; Watanabe et al. 1996; Nishi et al. 1999; Soubrier et al. 1998, 1999; Nobile-Orazio et al. 2009). Focusing further on this finding, the higher level observed in serum is coming from the release of VEGF by the platelets in vitro during serum processing. Because plasma is a product of an anticoagulated sample, there is less platelet activation and therefore less platelet VEGF contributing to the plasma measurement than the serum sample. Thus, VEGF levels for diagnosis of POEMS syndrome were recognized over 200 pg/mL in plasma (with a specificity of 95% and a sensitivity of 68%) (D'Souza et al. 2011) and over 1920 pg/mL in serum (with a specificity of 98% and a sensitivity of 73%) (Wang et al. 2014). A novel marker was added by Wang et al. (2014), when they found that the best cutoff of N-terminal propeptide of type I collagen to diagnose POEMS syndrome is 70 ng/mL with a specificity of 91.5% and a sensitivity of 80%.

In clinical practice, the differential diagnosis of POEMS syndrome includes CIDP, light chain amyloid neuropathy (AL neuropathy), MGUS neuropathy, MM, cryoglobulinemia, and Waldenstrom macroglobulinemia (WM). Any patient who carries a diagnosis of CIDP refractory to intravenous immunoglobulin therapy should be considered as a possible POEMS syndrome patient. Both CIDP and POEMS are demyelinating neuropathies, but the electromyography (EMG) in patients with POEMS syndrome demonstrates greater axonal loss and slowing of intermediate nerve segments (Nasu et al. 2012; Mauermann et al. 2012). To distinguish the two entities, platelet count could be helpful. Approximately half of POEMS patients present with thrombocytosis (54%), while CIDP rarely shows concurrent increase of platelet count (1.5%) (Naddaf et al. 2015). Peripheral neuropathy in AL is mixed sensory and motor, and light chain component is lambda-restricted. In AL, the diagnosis is based on BM infiltration and presence of amyloid in organ targets (Congo Red positive staining). Instead of POEMS, MGUS neuropathy is frequently associated with an antibody against myelin-associated glycoprotein (anti-MAG antibodies) and neural antigens and typically does not demonstrate any of the other features of the syndrome (Dispenzieri 2015; Warsame et al. 2017). From MM, POEMS syndrome is differentiated due to the following distinctive characteristics: (1) dominant symptoms are typically neuropathy, endocrine dysfunction, and volume overload; (2) these dominant symptoms have nothing to do with bone pain, extremely high infiltration of BM by plasma cells, or renal failure; (3) high VEGF levels; (4) sclerotic bone lesions in the majority of cases; (5) superior overall survival; and (6) mainly lambda clones (Dispenzieri 2007). Cryoglobulinemia can sometimes mimic POEMS with its neuropathy, skin changes, and paraproteinemia; however, the underlying disorders such as hepatitis C, autoimmune diseases, or lymphomas and the presence of serum will definitively differentiate between the two conditions. WM may also share some common clinical characteristics including papilledema (caused by hyperviscosity), neuropathy, and a monoclonal protein with POEMS syndrome. However, a BM biopsy is distinguishing, with a lymphocytic infiltration and the presence of MYD88-L256P mutation in the vast majority of patients with WM (Kapoor et al. 2017). The specific BM histopathology in POEMS syndrome with the plasma cell rimming around lymphoid aggregates in the BM of nearly 50% of patients can help distinguish it from other plasma cell disorders (Dao et al. 2011).

10.4 Castleman Variant of POEMS

As already reported, there is a Castleman variant of POEMS syndrome that does not have a clonal plasma cell proliferative disorder underlying, but a lymphoproliferative disease with many clinical features indicative of POEMS syndrome (Dispenzieri 2008, 2015; Warsame et al. 2017). The percentage of POEMS with Castleman ranges from 11 to 25% (Nakanishi et al. 1984; Li et al. 2011a; Kulkarni et al. 2011; Dispenzieri et al. 2003). Instead of POEMS syndrome, the predominantly elevated cytokine is IL-6 and not VEGF (Scarlato et al. 2005). The therapeutic approach to Castleman variant of POEMS in the presence of bone lesions or monoclonal protein is similar to the classical POEMS. However, in the absence of these features, the use of a monoclonal antibody (rituximab or siltuximab) alone may be justified (Dispenzieri 2008). Two series have separately demonstrated that patients of POEMS with coexisting Castleman disease may have an inferior overall survival (OS) (Li et al. 2011a; Dispenzieri et al. 2003).

10.5 Risk Stratification

Before the incorporation of autologous stem cell transplant for POEMS syndrome and the renaissance of therapeutic options for patients with multiple myeloma, median survivals were nearly 14 years (Dispenzieri et al. 2003; Allam et al. 2008). Patients treated with ASCT have a 10-year OS of approximately 90% (Kourelis et al. 2016a).

Risk stratification is limited to clinical phenotype rather than specific molecular and genetic risk markers. The number of clinical criteria

does not affect survival (Dispenzieri 2007; Soubrier et al. 1994), but the extent of the plasma cell disorder is prognostic. Some of the clinical manifestations of the syndrome have been identified to be associated with a significantly shorter OS such as clubbing, extravascular volume overload—effusions, edema, and ascites (Dispenzieri et al. 2003)—respiratory symptoms (Allam et al. 2008), pulmonary hypertension (Li et al. 2013), impaired DLCO, and papilledema (Kaushik et al. 2011). Candidate patients for local radiation therapy with negative BM aspiration have a better OS (Dispenzieri et al. 2003). Patients with coexisting Castleman disease may have an inferior OS as compared to patients without (Li et al. 2011a; Dispenzieri et al. 2003). In a series of 11 patients, lower VEGF levels predicted for better response to therapy, with resolution of the skin changes, improvement of the neuropathic disturbances, and reduction of all the features assumed to be related to increased permeability, like papilledema and organomegaly (Scarlato et al. 2005). Wang and colleagues have developed a prognostic nomogram that includes age greater than 50, pulmonary hypertension, pleural effusion, and eGFR <30 mL/min/1.73 m^2 (Wang et al. 2017). The Mayo group identified young age, albumin greater than 3.2 g/dL, and attainment of complete hematologic response as favorable prognostic factors in their series of 291 patients (Kourelis et al. 2016a). Thrombocytosis and increased bone marrow infiltration are associated with risk for cerebrovascular accidents (Dupont et al. 2009).

10.6 Therapy of POEMS

Therapy for POEMS is divided into the treatment of the underlying aberrant B/plasma cell clone(s), and the management of the organ-specific symptomatology. Initial BM infiltration plays a key role in the therapeutic approach. Patients without clonal plasma cells on BM biopsy and with an isolated bone lesion or a dominant sclerotic plasmacytoma are candidates for local radiation therapy; those with a more extensive disease will be candidates for systemic therapy.

10.7 Therapy of Localized POEMS Syndrome Without BM Infiltration

The radiation (usual doses between 30 and 50 Gy) in localized disease improves the symptoms of POEMS syndrome for a time duration of 3–36 months and can achieve the eradication of the aberrant clone with clinical response rates in 47% to 75% of cases and hematologic response rates in 45% to 50% of cases (Suh et al. 2014; Humeniuk et al. 2013). More specifically, Mayo clinic presented a series of 35 patients with POEMS syndrome that were radiated as primary therapy and reached to a 4-year OS of 97% (Humeniuk et al. 2013). In this retrospective study, a high 4-year failure-free survival of 52% was observed with more than half the "failures" occurred within 12 months of radiation (Humeniuk et al. 2013). Another recent study from South Korea included six patients who had radiotherapy as primary therapy—two of whom had multiple lesions but were deemed too sick for chemotherapy—and seven patients received consolidative radiotherapy for persistent M-spike and/or persistent clinical symptoms (Suh et al. 2014). For radiation alone, the response rates were comparable to that of the Mayo clinic, but both OS and PFS were inferior, largely due to the fact that these patients were sicker at time of treatment (Suh et al. 2014). Successful outcomes have been associated with directing therapy at the underlying clonal plasma cell disorder.

10.8 Systemic Therapy for POEMS Syndrome with Disseminated BM Involvement

Systemic therapies for POEMS are borrowed from other plasma cell disorders (MM and AL amyloidosis) and generally include either high-dose melphalan (140 or 200 mg/m^2) followed by ASCT, or therapeutic combinations of melphalan, thalidomide, bortezomib, or lenalidomide with dexamethasone. Two recent reviews on therapy for POEMS syndrome recapped the published evidence noticing the absence of randomized controlled studies (Dispenzieri 2015; Warsame et al. 2017). Table 10.2 has a summary of large studies that included more than 30 patients with POEMS and the outcomes of various treatments.

10.8.1 Transplantation in POEMS

Multiple series have documented improvement in many of the features associated with POEMS including the neuropathy, the papilledema, and the extravascular overload after ASCT (Barete et al. 2010; Kuwabara et al. 2006; Soubrier et al. 2002; Peggs et al. 2002; Hogan et al. 2001; Cook et al. 2017). Patients usually do not require induction chemotherapy since the plasma cell burden is typically low, unless a delay in transplant is anticipated for logistical issues or the patients are too ill to proceed with this approach (Dispenzieri 2012). The updated Mayo Clinic series had 83 (29%) patients undergoing an ASCT, and the 10-year survival was significantly superior to radiation and chemotherapy alone, respectively (90 vs. 70 vs. 46%, $p < 0.0001$) (Kourelis et al. 2016a). However, the outstanding outcomes may not be entirely attributable to transplant, and selection bias must be taken into account since transplant-eligible patients are fitter and generally have less advanced disease. There has been one report of tandem transplant, but no additional benefit was demonstrated with the second transplant (Kojima et al. 2006). Splenomegaly at baseline has been reported to be predictive of peri-transplant complications such as engraftment syndrome that is characterized by fever, diarrhea, rash, weight gain, and dyspnea between 7 and 15 days post stem cell infusion. Patients with splenomegaly have delayed neutrophil engraftment (median 16 vs. 12 days) and longer time to platelet recovery (median 19.5 vs. 14 days) (Schmitz et al. 1996; Dispenzieri et al. 2008). Treatment responses from ASCT are durable with a 5-year survival rate quoted at 94%; however, late relapses have been reported (D'Souza et al. 2012; Imai et al. 2009). Usually, those relapses are clinically asymptomatic with

Table 10.2 Large studies (>30 cases) focusing on patients with POEMS syndrome and/or prospective studies

Author, year	Sample size	Therapy	Median PFS	Median OS	Response and toxicity
Suh et al. (2014)	33	Radiation ($n = 6$) Chemotherapy ($n = 16$) Melphalan and prednisolone Vincristine, doxorubicin, and dexamethasone ASCT Radiation + chemotherapy (9)	51 months	65 months	CRR 75%/HRR 50% CRR 50%/HRR 81% CRR 66%/HRR 66%
Humeniuk et al. (2013) Kourelis and Dispenzieri (2017) Kourelis et al. (2016b) Kourelis et al. (2016a)[a]	38	Radiation	52% at 4 years	97% at 4 years	CRR 47% HRR 45% PET RR 22%
Dispenzieri et al. (2008)	30	ASCT			CRR 100% HRR 82.5%
D'Souza et al. (2012)	59	ASCT	75% at 5 years	94% at 5 years	HRR 79% CRR 92% PET RR 35%
Kourelis and Dispenzieri (2017) Kourelis et al. (2016b) Kourelis et al. (2016a) Cook et al. (2017)[a]	291	ASCT ($n = 83$) Radiation ($n = 91$) Chemotherapy ($n = 94$)	72% at 5 years 62% at 5 years 45% at 5 years	89% at 10 years 75% at 10 years 50% at 10 years	HRR 60%
Li et al. (2011b)[b]	31	Melphalan and dexamethasone		NR	Neurologic RR 100% HRR 82%
Cook et al. (2017)	127	ASCT	74% at 5 years	89% at 5 years	HRR 69%
Kuwabara et al. (1997)	51	Lenalidomide-based therapy as first line 28.6% As second line 47.6%	93.9% at 12 months 41.7% at 24 months	No deaths	VEGF reduction—all evaluable patients Neuropathy improvement 92%; stabilized 8% Hematological CR 18.6%; VGPR 39.5%; PR 37.2%

HRR hematologic response rate according to revised hematologic criteria for multiple myeloma, *CRR* clinical response rate of POEMS symptoms (e.g., neuropathy), patients can have significant clinical benefit without a hematologic response, *ASCT* autologous stem cell therapy, *VGPR* very good partial response, *PR* partial response, *CR* complete response, *RR* response rate
[a]Mayo clinic experience is described by all these references, including the same patients
[b]Prospective study

either VEGF increase or radiographic changes and amenable to salvage chemotherapy treatment (D'Souza et al. 2012).

10.8.2 Alkylators

Alkylating agents have been the backbone of treatment when transplant is not an option. In the first prospective study for POEMS syndrome evaluated the use of melphalan and dexamethasone for 12 cycles on 31 patients, 81% of patients had a hematologic response, while all patients had a VEGF response and reported some improvement in neuropathy, although follow-up was short at 21 months (Li et al. 2011b). In a retrospective study by Dispenzieri et al., 48 patients were managed with the combination of melphalan and prednisone; an improvement in symptoms was noted in only 44%, with a 2-year survival rate of 78% (Dispenzieri et al. 2003). The clinical benefit of melphalan use was also recognized in other smaller cohorts of six and eight patients, with the 2-year survival of 100% (Kuwabara et al. 2006; Kuwabara et al. 1997). Melphalan-based induction regimens are not recommended in patients who are considered candidates for ASCT due to the stem cell toxicity of melphalan, and a short course of a cyclophosphamide-based regimen is followed for patients if ASCT is delayed for logistical reasons or due to patients' disease-related disabilities/comorbidities at diagnosis.

10.8.3 Immunomodulatory Drugs (IMiDs)

Similarly to other plasma cell dyscrasias, IMiDs in POEMS syndrome are used for patients with disseminated disease who are transplant ineligible or relapse post-ASCT or have refractory disease. IMiDs (thalidomide, lenalidomide, and pomalidomide) are known to have anti-VEGF property. Despite their off-label use over a decade now, no randomized controlled trial proves their efficacy was available until recently (Zagouri et al. 2014; Cai et al. 2015). The J-POST study was the first landmark double-blind placebo-controlled trial, was conducted in Japan, and came to clearly support the role of thalidomide. The use of dexamethasone in combination with thalidomide showed significant VEGF reduction and improvement in motor function and certain relevant clinical/laboratory parameters as well as in some measures of quality of life compared to dexamethasone plus placebo (Katayama et al. 2015; Misawa et al. 2016). This study has several limitations such as the small sample size ($n = 25$), the selection of primary end point of VEGF reduction, and finally the only marginal benefits in the clinical scores, which did not necessarily translate into functional improvement, although the results were statistically significant. Patients on the thalidomide arm experienced bradycardia more frequently. The authors did not document

worsening neuropathy, a well-known adverse effect of thalidomide, on this trial (Jaccard and Magy 2016), but the small fiber neuropathy caused by thalidomide is not easily quantifiable by routine measures. In parallel, Cai et al. have shown the efficacy of daily low-dose lenalidomide (10 mg) with weekly dexamethasone (40 mg) in relapsed/refractory settings in a cohort of 12 patients. The estimated 2-year OS and PFS were 92%, respectively, without treatment-related mortality or ≥ 3 grade toxicities (Cai et al. 2015). A pooled analysis of patients with POEMS syndrome who received lenalidomide ($n = 51$) showed similar results with a 1-year PFS of 93.9%, VEGF reduction in all patients, and improvement in neuropathy in 92% of the patients (Zagouri et al. 2014).

10.8.4 Proteasome Inhibitors (PI)

Bortezomib is a first-generation proteasome inhibitor (PI) presenting anti-VEGF and anti-TNF properties (Roccaro et al. 2006). Several case reports have highlighted the successful use of bortezomib in POEMS (Warsame et al. 2012; Li et al. 2012; Ohguchi et al. 2011; Kaygusuz et al. 2010; He et al. 2017) resulting in significant improvement of ascites and fluid overload without exacerbation of peripheral neuropathy. It has been used both as a single agent and in combination with dexamethasone, cyclophosphamide, and/or thalidomide. Bortezomib should be used with caution, especially when it is used in combination with thalidomide due to the increased risk for exacerbation of peripheral neuropathy.

10.8.5 Experimental Therapies

As described previously in the theories of pathogenesis, studies that targeted the VEGF inhibition with drugs such as bevacizumab never achieved to reach to strong results, concluding that VEGF pathway may be only one component of a much more complex cytokine process (Badros et al. 2005; Samaras et al. 2007; Sekiguchi et al. 2013; Kanai et al. 2007). The role of IVIG is controversial in the management of POEMS, with evidence of reduction in the VEGF levels but without simultaneous clinical responses. Thus, the use of IVIG has not included yet in clinical routine (Dispenzieri 2015; Terracciano et al. 2010). Investigators have also used agents such as tamoxifen, ticlopidine, all-trans-retinoic acid (ATRA), and interferon-α in the management of POEMS but with limited success (Dispenzieri 2007, 2015; Authier et al. 1996). Autologous cytokine-induced killer (CIK) cells in combination with cyclophosphamide have been studied in five patients with POEMS syndrome. CIK infusion was well tolerated and was associated with marginally improved symptoms and quality of life, with decrease in serum VEGF levels and increase in lymphocyte counts (Ma et al. 2016). Returning back to the pathogenesis theories, CIK infusion seems to interrupt the pro-inflammatory background of POEMS syndrome associated with increased cytokines, presenting as a novel and promising treatment approach. Additional studies are needed before its generalized use. Ixazomib, a neuropathy-sparing oral PI, is also currently being evaluated in POEMS treatment.

10.9   Management of the Organ-Specific Symptom Complex Supportive Care

In clinical practice, the management of individual clinical symptoms is very important because therapies such as radiation, ASCT, and chemotherapy help in only decreasing the clonal plasma cell load, with no direct benefit to the clinical symptoms. As described previously, the organ response can delay by months to years after administration of plasma cell-directed therapeutic approaches. Endocrinopathies require a close follow-up by an endocrinologist and extraneous replacement of the deficient hormones. Neuropathic pain is needed to be effectively controlled with gabapentin and tricyclic antidepressants like nortriptyline, duloxetine, and pregabalin (Dispenzieri 2015; Warsame et al. 2017). However, neuropathy could progress despite

these medications. Patients should be actively monitored for the development of any subtle signs of depression. The use of orthopedic tools (such as ankle and foot braces) and physiotherapy are recommended in order to improve mobility and functional capabilities. In addition, diuretics may be used to manage extravascular fluid overload. In some case with severe neuromuscular weakness, continuous positive airway pressure (CPAP) may be required to improve oxygenation.

Conclusions

In summary, POEMS syndrome is a rare paraneoplastic disorder associated with a clonal plasma cell neoplasm and likely caused by a pro-inflammatory cytokines-based background. Reaching to the diagnosis can be a challenge, but a comprehensive approach of the patient, followed by appropriate testing, can differentiate this syndrome from other conditions like CIDP, AL, MM, and MGUS neuropathy. Patients with limited disease should be treated with primary radiation, while those with widespread disease and BM involvement should receive systemic therapy which is preferred. ASCT is the up-front treatment of choice in patients that are eligible; otherwise, systemic therapies are active in MM.

Either in active treatment or in supportive care, regular monitoring of the relevant laboratory parameters such as VEGF and periodic assessment of the clinical symptoms are critical for the long-term management of the syndrome.

References

Abe D, Nakaseko C, Takeuchi M et al (2008) Restrictive usage of monoclonal immunoglobulin lambda light chain germline in POEMS syndrome. Blood 112:836–839

Allam JS, Kennedy CC, Aksamit TR, Dispenzieri A (2008) Pulmonary manifestations in patients with POEMS syndrome: a retrospective review of 137 patients. Chest 133:969–974

Authier FJ, Belec L, Levy Y et al (1996) All-trans-retinoic acid in POEMS syndrome. Therapeutic effect associated with decreased circulating levels of proinflammatory cytokines. Arthritis Rheum 39:1423–1426

Badros A, Porter N, Zimrin A (2005) Bevacizumab therapy for POEMS syndrome. Blood 106:1135

Bardwick PA, Zvaifler NJ, Gill GN, Newman D, Greenway GD, Resnick DL (1980) Plasma cell dyscrasia with polyneuropathy, organomegaly, endocrinopathy, M protein, and skin changes: the POEMS syndrome. Report on two cases and a review of the literature. Medicine 59:311–322

Barete S, Mouawad R, Choquet S et al (2010) Skin manifestations and vascular endothelial growth factor levels in POEMS syndrome: impact of autologous hematopoietic stem cell transplantation. Arch Dermatol 146:615–623

Bryce AH, Ketterling RP, Gertz MA et al (2008) A novel report of cig-FISH and cytogenetics in POEMS syndrome. Am J Hematol 83:840–841

Cai QQ, Wang C, Cao XX, Cai H, Zhou DB, Li J (2015) Efficacy and safety of low-dose lenalidomide plus dexamethasone in patients with relapsed or refractory POEMS syndrome. Eur J Haematol 95:325–330

Cook G, Iacobelli S, van Biezen A et al (2017) High-dose therapy and autologous stem cell transplantation in patients with POEMS syndrome: a retrospective study of the Plasma Cell Disorder sub-committee of the Chronic Malignancy Working Party of the European Society for Blood & Marrow Transplantation. Haematologica 102:160–167

Cui R, Yu S, Huang X, Zhang J, Tian C, Pu C (2014) Papilloedema is an independent prognostic factor for POEMS syndrome. J Neurol 261:60–65

Dao LN, Hanson CA, Dispenzieri A, Morice WG, Kurtin PJ, Hoyer JD (2011) Bone marrow histopathology in POEMS syndrome: a distinctive combination of plasma cell, lymphoid, and myeloid findings in 87 patients. Blood 117:6438–6444

Dispenzieri A (2007) POEMS syndrome. Blood Rev 21:285–299

Dispenzieri A (2008) Castleman disease. Cancer Treat Res 142:293–330

Dispenzieri A (2012) How I treat POEMS syndrome. Blood 119:5650–5658

Dispenzieri A (2015) POEMS syndrome: update on diagnosis, risk-stratification, and management. Am J Hematol 90:951–962

Dispenzieri A, Kyle RA, Lacy MQ et al (2003) POEMS syndrome: definitions and long-term outcome. Blood 101:2496–2506

Dispenzieri A, Lacy MQ, Hayman SR et al (2008) Peripheral blood stem cell transplant for POEMS syndrome is associated with high rates of engraftment syndrome. Eur J Haematol 80:397–406

D'Souza A, Hayman SR, Buadi F et al (2011) The utility of plasma vascular endothelial growth factor levels in the diagnosis and follow-up of patients with POEMS syndrome. Blood 118:4663–4665

D'Souza A, Lacy M, Gertz M et al (2012) Long-term outcomes after autologous stem cell transplantation for patients with POEMS syndrome (osteosclerotic myeloma): a single-center experience. Blood 120:56–62

Dupont SA, Dispenzieri A, Mauermann ML, Rabinstein AA, Brown RD Jr (2009) Cerebral infarction in POEMS syndrome: incidence, risk factors, and imaging characteristics. Neurology 73:1308–1312

Gandhi GY, Basu R, Dispenzieri A, Basu A, Montori VM, Brennan MD (2007) Endocrinopathy in POEMS syndrome: the Mayo Clinic experience. Mayo Clin Proc 82:836–842

He H, Fu W, Du J, Jiang H, Hou J (2017) Successful treatment of newly diagnosed POEMS syndrome with reduced-dose bortezomib based regimen. Br J Haematol. doi:10.1111/bjh.14497. [Epub ahead of print] PubMed PMID: 28146276

Hogan WJ, Lacy MQ, Wiseman GA, Fealey RD, Dispenzieri A, Gertz MA (2001) Successful treatment of POEMS syndrome with autologous hematopoietic progenitor cell transplantation. Bone Marrow Transplant 28:305–309

Humeniuk MS, Gertz MA, Lacy MQ et al (2013) Outcomes of patients with POEMS syndrome treated initially with radiation. Blood 122:68–73

Imai N, Taguchi J, Yagi N, Konishi T, Serizawa M, Kobari M (2009) Relapse of polyneuropathy, organomegaly, endocrinopathy, M-protein, and skin changes (POEMS) syndrome without increased level of vascular endothelial growth factor following successful autologous peripheral blood stem cell transplantation. Neuromuscul Disord 19:363–365

Jaccard A, Magy L (2016) Thalidomide and POEMS syndrome: a cautious step forward. Lancet Neurol 15:1104–1105

Kanai K, Kuwabara S, Misawa S, Hattori T (2007) Failure of treatment with anti-VEGF monoclonal antibody for long-standing POEMS syndrome. Intern Med 46:311–313

Kanai K, Sawai S, Sogawa K et al (2012) Markedly upregulated serum interleukin-12 as a novel biomarker in POEMS syndrome. Neurology 79:575–582

Kang WY, Shen KN, Duan MH et al (2013) 14q32 translocations and 13q14 deletions are common cytogenetic abnormalities in POEMS syndrome. Eur J Haematol 91:490–496

Kapoor P, Ansell SM, Fonseca R et al (2017) Diagnosis and management of waldenstrom macroglobulinemia: mayo stratification of macroglobulinemia and risk-adapted therapy (mSMART) guidelines 2016. JAMA Oncol 3(9):1257–1265

Katayama K, Misawa S, Sato Y et al (2015) Japanese POEMS syndrome with Thalidomide (J-POST) Trial: study protocol for a phase II/III multicentre, randomised, double-blind, placebo-controlled trial. BMJ Open 5:e007330

Kaushik M, Pulido JS, Abreu R, Amselem L, Dispenzieri A (2011) Ocular findings in patients with polyneuropathy, organomegaly, endocrinopathy, monoclonal gammopathy, and skin changes syndrome. Ophthalmology 118:778–782

Kaygusuz I, Tezcan H, Cetiner M, Kocakaya O, Uzay A, Bayik M (2010) Bortezomib: a new therapeutic option for POEMS syndrome. Eur J Haematol 84:175–177

Kelly JJ Jr, Kyle RA, Miles JM, Dyck PJ (1983) Osteosclerotic myeloma and peripheral neuropathy. Neurology 33:202–210

Koga H, Tokunaga Y, Hisamoto T et al (2002) Ratio of serum vascular endothelial growth factor to platelet count correlates with disease activity in a patient with POEMS syndrome. Eur J Intern Med 13:70–74

Koike H, Iijima M, Mori K et al (2008) Neuropathic pain correlates with myelinated fibre loss and cytokine profile in POEMS syndrome. J Neurol Neurosurg Psychiatry 79:1171–1179

Kojima H, Katsuoka Y, Katsura Y et al (2006) Successful treatment of a patient with POEMS syndrome by tandem high-dose chemotherapy with autologous CD34+ purged stem cell rescue. Int J Hematol 84:182–185

Kourelis TV, Dispenzieri A (2017) Validation of a prognostic score for patients with POEMS syndrome: a mayo clinic cohort. Leukemia 31:1251

Kourelis TV, Buadi FK, Kumar SK et al (2016a) Long-term outcome of patients with POEMS syndrome: an update of the Mayo Clinic experience. Am J Hematol 91:585–589

Kourelis TV, Buadi FK, Gertz MA et al (2016b) Risk factors for and outcomes of patients with POEMS syndrome who experience progression after first-line treatment. Leukemia 30:1079–1085

Kulkarni GB, Mahadevan A, Taly AB et al (2011) Clinicopathological profile of polyneuropathy, organomegaly, endocrinopathy, M protein and skin changes (POEMS) syndrome. J Clin Neurosci 18:356–360

Kuwabara S, Hattori T, Shimoe Y, Kamitsukasa I (1997) Long term melphalan-prednisolone chemotherapy for POEMS syndrome. J Neurol Neurosurg Psychiatry 63:385–387

Kuwabara S, Misawa S, Kanai K et al (2006) Autologous peripheral blood stem cell transplantation for POEMS syndrome. Neurology 66:105–107

Lesprit P, Authier FJ, Gherardi R et al (1996) Acute arterial obliteration: a new feature of the POEMS syndrome? Medicine 75:226–232

Lesprit P, Godeau B, Authier FJ et al (1998) Pulmonary hypertension in POEMS syndrome: a new feature mediated by cytokines. Am J Respir Crit Care Med 157:907–911

Li J, Zhou DB, Huang Z et al (2011a) Clinical characteristics and long-term outcome of patients with POEMS syndrome in China. Ann Hematol 90:819–826

Li J, Zhang W, Jiao L et al (2011b) Combination of melphalan and dexamethasone for patients with newly diagnosed POEMS syndrome. Blood 117:6445–6449

Li J, Zhang W, Kang WY, Cao XX, Duan MH, Zhou DB (2012) Bortezomib and dexamethasone as first-line therapy for a patient with newly diagnosed polyneuropathy, organomegaly, endocrinopathy, M protein and skin changes syndrome complicated by renal failure. Leuk Lymphoma 53:2527–2529

Li J, Tian Z, Zheng HY et al (2013) Pulmonary hypertension in POEMS syndrome. Haematologica 98:393–398

Ma L, Wang Y, Bo J et al (2016) Autologous cytokine-induced killer (CIK) cell immunotherapy combined with cyclophosphamide in five patients with POEMS syndrome. Clin Exp Immunol 184:83–89

Mauermann ML, Sorenson EJ, Dispenzieri A et al (2012) Uniform demyelination and more severe axonal loss distinguish POEMS syndrome from CIDP. J Neurol Neurosurg Psychiatry 83:480–486

Min JH, Hong YH, Lee KW (2005) Electrophysiological features of patients with POEMS syndrome. Clin Neurophysiol 116:965–968

Misawa S, Sato Y, Katayama K et al (2016) Safety and efficacy of thalidomide in patients with POEMS syndrome: a multicentre, randomised, double-blind, placebo-controlled trial. Lancet Neurol 15:1129–1137

Naddaf E, Dispenzieri A, Mandrekar J, Mauermann ML (2015) Thrombocytosis distinguishes POEMS syndrome from chronic inflammatory demyelinating polyneuropathy. Muscle Nerve 52:658–659

Nakanishi T, Sobue I, Toyokura Y et al (1984) The Crow-Fukase syndrome: a study of 102 cases in Japan. Neurology 34:712–720

Nakano A, Mitsui T, Endo I, Takeda Y, Ozaki S, Matsumoto T (2001) Solitary plasmacytoma with VEGF overproduction: report of a patient with polyneuropathy. Neurology 56:818–819

Nasu S, Misawa S, Sekiguchi Y et al (2012) Different neurological and physiological profiles in POEMS syndrome and chronic inflammatory demyelinating polyneuropathy. J Neurol Neurosurg Psychiatry 83:476–479

Nishi J, Arimura K, Utsunomiya A et al (1999) Expression of vascular endothelial growth factor in sera and lymph nodes of the plasma cell type of Castleman's disease. Br J Haematol 104:482–485

Nobile-Orazio E, Terenghi F, Giannotta C, Gallia F, Nozza A (2009) Serum VEGF levels in POEMS syndrome and in immune-mediated neuropathies. Neurology 72:1024–1026

Ohguchi H, Ohba R, Onishi Y et al (2011) Successful treatment with bortezomib and thalidomide for POEMS syndrome. Ann Hematol 90:1113–1114

Peggs KS, Paneesha S, Kottaridis PD et al (2002) Peripheral blood stem cell transplantation for POEMS syndrome. Bone Marrow Transplant 30:401–404

Roccaro AM, Hideshima T, Raje N et al (2006) Bortezomib mediates antiangiogenesis in multiple myeloma via direct and indirect effects on endothelial cells. Cancer Res 66:184–191

Samaras P, Bauer S, Stenner-Liewen F et al (2007) Treatment of POEMS syndrome with bevacizumab. Haematologica 92:1438–1439

Scarlato M, Previtali SC, Carpo M et al (2005) Polyneuropathy in POEMS syndrome: role of angiogenic factors in the pathogenesis. Brain 128:1911–1920

Schmitz N, Linch DC, Dreger P et al (1996) Randomised trial of filgrastim-mobilised peripheral blood progenitor cell transplantation versus autologous bone-marrow transplantation in lymphoma patients. Lancet 347:353–357

Sekiguchi Y, Misawa S, Shibuya K et al (2013) Ambiguous effects of anti-VEGF monoclonal antibody (bevacizumab) for POEMS syndrome. J Neurol Neurosurg Psychiatry 84:1346–1348

Shi X, Hu S, Luo X et al (2016) CT characteristics in 24 patients with POEMS syndrome. Acta Radiol 57:51–57

Singh D, Wadhwa J, Kumar L, Raina V, Agarwal A, Kochupillai V (2003) POEMS syndrome: experience with fourteen cases. Leuk Lymphoma 44:1749–1752

Soubrier MJ, Dubost JJ, Sauvezie BJ (1994) POEMS syndrome: a study of 25 cases and a review of the literature. French Study Group on POEMS syndrome. Am J Med 97:543–553

Soubrier M, Dubost JJ, Serre AF et al (1997) Growth factors in POEMS syndrome: evidence for a marked increase in circulating vascular endothelial growth factor. Arthritis Rheum 40:786–787

Soubrier M, Guillon R, Dubost JJ et al (1998) Arterial obliteration in POEMS syndrome: possible role of vascular endothelial growth factor. J Rheumatol 25:813–815

Soubrier M, Sauron C, Souweine B et al (1999) Growth factors and proinflammatory cytokines in the renal involvement of POEMS syndrome. Am J Kidney Dis 34:633–638

Soubrier M, Ruivard M, Dubost JJ, Sauvezie B, Philippe P (2002) Successful use of autologous bone marrow transplantation in treating a patient with POEMS syndrome. Bone Marrow Transplant 30:61–62

Suh YG, Kim YS, Suh CO et al (2014) The role of radiotherapy in the management of POEMS syndrome. Radiat Oncol 9:265

Takatsuki K, Sanada I (1983) Plasma cell dyscrasia with polyneuropathy and endocrine disorder: clinical and laboratory features of 109 reported cases. Jpn J Clin Oncol 13:543–555

Terracciano C, Fiore S, Doldo E et al (2010) Inverse correlation between VEGF and soluble VEGF receptor 2 in POEMS with AIDP responsive to intravenous immunoglobulin. Muscle Nerve 42:445–448

Wang C, Zhou YL, Cai H et al (2014) Markedly elevated serum total N-terminal propeptide of type I collagen is a novel marker for the diagnosis and follow up of patients with POEMS syndrome. Haematologica 99:e78–e80

Wang C, Huang XF, Cai QQ et al (2017) Prognostic study for overall survival in patients with newly diagnosed POEMS syndrome. Leukemia 31:100–106

Warsame R, Kohut IE, Dispenzieri A (2012) Successful use of cyclophosphamide, bortezomib, and dexamethasone to treat a case of relapsed POEMS. Eur J Haematol 88:549–550

Warsame R, Yanamandra U, Kapoor P (2017) POEMS syndrome: an enigma. Curr Hematol Malig Rep 12(2):85–95

Watanabe O, Arimura K, Kitajima I, Osame M, Maruyama I (1996) Greatly raised vascular endothelial growth factor (VEGF) in POEMS syndrome. Lancet 347:702

Zagouri F, Kastritis E, Gavriatopoulou M et al (2014) Lenalidomide in patients with POEMS syndrome: a systematic review and pooled analysis. Leuk Lymphoma 55:2018–2023

Zhang B, Song X, Liang B et al (2010) The clinical study of POEMS syndrome in China. Neuro Endocrinol Lett 31:229–237

Waldenström's Macroglobulinemia

Steven P. Treon, Giampaolo Merlini, and Meletios A. Dimopoulos

11.1 Epidemiology

The age-adjusted incidence rate of WM is 3.4 per 1 million among males and 1.7 per 1 million among females in the United States. It increases in incidence geometrically with age (Groves et al. 1998; Herrinton and Weiss 1993). The incidence rate is higher among Americans of European descent. African American descendants represent approximately 5% of all patients.

Genetic factors play a role in the pathogenesis of WM. Approximately 20% of WM patients are of Ashkenazi-Jewish ethnic background (Hanzis et al. 2011). Familial disease has been reported commonly, including multigenerational clustering of WM and other B-cell lymphoproliferative diseases (Hanzis et al. 2011; Bjornsson et al. 1978; Renier et al. 1989; Ogmundsdottir et al. 1999). Approximately 28% of 924 sequential patients with WM presenting to a tertiary referral center had a first- or second-degree relative with either WM or another B-cell disorder (Hanzis et al. 2011). Familial clustering of WM with other immunologic disorders, including hypogammaglobulinemia and hypergammaglobulinemia (particularly polyclonal IgM), autoantibody production (particularly to the thyroid), and manifestation of hyperactive B cells has also been reported in relatives without WM (Hanzis et al. 2011; Ogmundsdottir et al. 1999). Increased expression of the *BCL-2* gene with enhanced survival has been observed in B cells from familial patients and their family members (Ogmundsdottir et al. 1999).

The role of environmental factors is uncertain, but chronic antigenic stimulation from infections and certain drug or chemical exposures have been considered but have not reached a level of scientific certainty. Hepatitis C virus (HCV) infection was implicated in WM causality in some series, but in a study of 100 consecutive WM patients in whom serologic and molecular diagnostic studies for HCV infection were performed no association was found (Santini et al. 1993; Silvestri et al. 1996; Leleu et al. 2007).

S. P. Treon (✉)
Bing Center for Waldenström's Macroglobulinemia, Dana-Farber Cancer Institute, Harvard Medical School, Boston, MA, USA
e-mail: steven_treon@dfci.harvard.edu

G. Merlini
Department of Molecular Medicine, Amyloidosis Research and Treatment Center, Foundation Istituto di Ricovero e Cura a Carattere Scientifico (IRCCS) Policlinico San Matteo, University of Pavia, Pavia, Italy

M. A. Dimopoulos
Department of Clinical Therapeutics, National and Kapodistrian University of Athens, School of Medicine, Athens, Greece

© Springer International Publishing Switzerland 2018
M. A. Dimopoulos et al. (eds.), *Multiple Myeloma and Other Plasma Cell Neoplasms*, Hematologic Malignancies, https://doi.org/10.1007/978-3-319-25586-6_11

11.2 Pathogenesis

11.2.1 Nature of the WM Clone

Examination of the B-cell clone(s) found in the bone marrow of WM patients reveals a range of differentiation from small lymphocytes with large focal deposits of surface immunoglobulins to lymphoplasmacytic cells and to mature plasma cells that contain intracytoplasmic IgM (Fig. 11.1) (Swerdlow et al. 2008). Circulating clonal B cells are often detectable in patients with WM, though lymphocytosis is uncommon (Smith et al. 1983; Treon 2009). WM cells express the monoclonal IgM, and some clonal cells also express surface IgD (Preud'homme and Seligmann 1972). The characteristic immunophenotypic profile of WM lymphoplasmacytic cells includes the expression of the pan B-cell markers CD19, CD20 (including FMC7), CD22, and CD79 (Preud'homme and Seligmann 1972; San Miguel et al. 2003). Expression of CD5, CD10, and CD23 can be present in 10–20% of cases, and their presence does not exclude the diagnosis of WM (Hunter et al. 2005). In addition, multiparameter flow cytometric analysis has also identified CD25 and CD27 as being characteristic of the WM clone and that a CD22^{dim}/CD25$^+$/CD27$^+$/IgM$^+$ population can be observed

among clonal B lymphocytes in IgM MGUS patients who ultimately progressed to WM (Paiva et al. 2013).

Somatic mutations in immunoglobulin genes are present with increased frequency of nonsynonymous versus silent mutations in compliment determining regions along with somatic hypermutation thereby supporting a post-germinal center derivation for the WM B-cell clone in most patients (Wagner et al. 1994; Aoki et al. 1995). A strong preferential usage of VH3/JH4 gene families without intraclonal variation and without evidence for any isotype-switched transcripts has also been shown (Shiokawa et al. 2001; Sahota et al. 2002). Taken together, these data support an IgM$^+$ and/or IgM$^+$IgD$^+$ memory B-cell origin for most cases of WM.

In contrast to myeloma plasma cells, no recurrent translocations have been described in WM, which can help to distinguish IgM myeloma cases that often exhibit $t(11;14)$ translocations from WM (Ackroyd et al. 2005; Avet-Loiseau et al. 2003). Despite the absence of IgH translocations, recurrent chromosomal abnormalities are present in WM cells. These include deletions in chromosome 6q21-23 in 40–60% of WM patients, with concordant gains in 6p in 41% of 6q deleted patients (Braggio et al. 2009a; Schop et al. 2002; Hunter et al. 2014; Nguyen-Khac

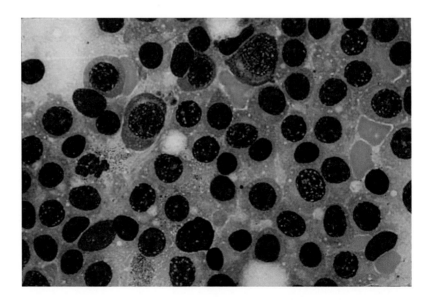

Fig. 11.1 Marrow film from a patient with Waldenström macroglobulinemia. Note infiltrate of mature lymphocytes, lymphoplasmacytic cells, and plasma cells (Used with permission from Marvin J. Stone, MD)

et al. 2013). In a series of 174 untreated WM patients, 6q deletions, followed by trisomy 18, 13q deletions, 17p deletions, trisomy 4, and 11q deletions were observed (Nguyen-Khac et al. 2013). Deletion of 6q and trisomy 4 were associated with adverse prognostic markers in this series. As 6q deletions represent the most recurrent cytogenetic finding in WM cases, there has been great interest in identifying the region of minimal deletion and possible target genes within this region. Two putative gene candidates within this region include TNFAIP3, a negative regulator of nuclear factor kappa B signaling (NFκB), and PRDM1, a master regulator of B-cell differentiation (Hunter et al. 2014; Braggio et al. 2009b). The removal of an NFκB negative regulator is of particular interest as the phosphorylation and translocation of NFκB into the nucleus is a crucial event for WM cell survival (Leleu et al. 2008). The success of proteasome inhibitor therapy in WM has been postulated to occur because the degradation of negative regulators of NFκB such as the Inhibitor of kappa B (IκB) is blocked (Treon et al. 2007; Treon et al. 2014a).

11.2.2 Mutation in MYD88

A highly recurrent somatic mutation (MYD88^{L265P}) was first identified in WM patients by whole genome sequencing (WGS), and confirmed by multiple studies through Sanger sequencing and/or allele-specific polymerase chain reaction assays (Treon et al. 2012; Xu et al. 2013; Varettoni et al. 2013; Jiménez et al. 2013; Poulain et al. 2013; Ansell et al. 2014). MYD88^{L265P} is expressed in 90–95% of WM cases when more sensitive allele-specific PCR has been employed using both CD19-sorted and unsorted bone marrow (BM) cells (Xu et al. 2013; Varettoni et al. 2013; Jiménez et al. 2013; Poulain et al. 2013; Ansell et al. 2014). By comparison, MYD88^{L265P} was absent in myeloma samples, including IgM myeloma, and was expressed in a small subset (6–10%) of MZL patients, who surprisingly have WM-related features (Xu et al. 2013; Varettoni et al. 2013; Jiménez et al. 2013; Ngo et al. 2011). By

polymerase chain reaction assays, 50–80% of IgM MGUS patients also express MYD88^{L265P}, and expression of this mutation was associated with increased risk for malignant progression (Xu et al. 2013; Varettoni et al. 2013; Jiménez et al. 2013; Landgren and Staudt 2012). The presence of MYD88^{L265P} in IgM MGUS patient suggests a role for this mutation as an early oncogenic driver, and other mutations and/or copy number alterations leading to abnormal gene expression are likely to promote disease progression (Hunter et al. 2014).

The impact of MYD88^{L265P} to growth and survival signaling in WM cells has been addressed in several studies (Fig. 11.2). Knockdown of MYD88 decreased survival of MYD88^{L265P}-expressing WM cells, whereas survival was enhanced by knock-in of MYD88^{L265P} versus wild-type MYD88 (Yang et al. 2013). The discovery of a mutation in MYD88 is of significance given its role as an adaptor molecule in Toll-like receptor (TLR) and interleukin-1 receptor (IL-1R) signaling (Watters et al. 2007). All TLRs except for TLR3 use MYD88 to facilitate their signaling. Following TLR or IL-1R stimulation, MYD88 is recruited to the activated receptor complex as a homodimer which then complexes with IRAK4 and activates IRAK1 and IRAK2 (Cohen et al. 1998; Loiarro et al. 2009; Lin et al. 2010). Tumor necrosis factor receptor-associated factor 6 is then activated by IRAK1 leading to NFκB activation via IκBα phosphorylation (Kawagoe et al. 2008). Use of inhibitors of MYD88 pathway led to decreased IRAK1 and IκBα phosphorylation, as well as survival of MYD88^{L265P}-expressing WM cells. These observations are of particular relevance to WM since NFκB signaling is important for WM growth and survival (Leleu et al. 2008). Bruton's tyrosine kinase (BTK) is also activated by MYD88^{L265P} (Yang et al. 2013). Activated BTK co-immunoprecipates with MYD88 that could be abrogated by use of a BTK kinase inhibitor, and overexpression of MYD88^{L265P} but not wild-type (WT) MYD88 triggers BTK activation. Knockdown of MYD88 by lentiviral transfection or use of a MYD88 homodimerization inhibitor also abrogated BTK activation in

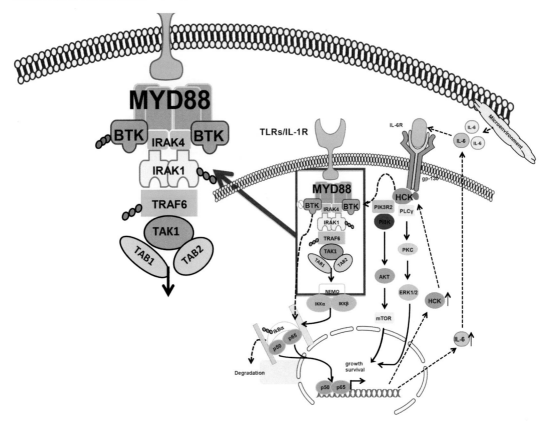

Fig. 11.2 MYD88 activating mutations are highly prevalent in patients with Waldenstrom's macroglobulinemia and trigger multiple growth and survival pathways. Activated MYD88 triggers NF-kB through BTK and IRAK1/IRAK4, as well as HCK that activates BTK, AKT, and ERK

MYD88^{L265P}-mutated WM cells. MYD88 also triggers HCK, a SRC family member that regulates AKT and ERK survival signaling, and also activates BTK itself (Yang et al. 2016). Rarely, non-L265P activating mutations in WM may also occur, and Sanger sequencing of the entire MYD88 gene should be considered in patients suspected of having WM in whom PCR testing for MYD88^{L265P} is negative (Treon et al. 2015a).

11.2.3 CXCR4 WHIM Mutations

The second most common somatic mutation after MYD88^{L265P} revealed by whole genome sequencing was found in the C-terminus of the CXCR4 receptor. These mutations are present in 30–35% of WM patients and impact serine phosphorylation sites that regulate CXCR4 signaling by its only known ligand SDF-1a (CXCL12) (Hunter et al. 2014; Treon et al. 2014b; Roccaro et al. 2014; Stephanie Poulain et al. 2014). The location of somatic mutations found in the C-terminus of CXCR4 in WM is similar to those observed in the germline of patients with WHIM (warts, hypogammaglobulinemia, infections, and myelokathexis) syndrome, a congenital immunodeficiency disorder characterized by chronic noncyclic neutropenia (Busillo et al. 2010). Patients with WHIM syndrome exhibit impaired CXCR4 receptor internalization following SDF-1a stimulation, which results in persistent CXCR4 activation and myelokathexis (Dotta et al. 2011).

In WM patients, two classes of CXCR4 mutations occur in the C-terminus. These include nonsense (CXCR4$^{WHIM/NS}$) mutations that truncate the distal 15–20 amino acid region and frameshift (CXCR4$^{WHIM/FS}$) mutations that compromise a region of up to 40 amino acids in the C-terminal domain (Hunter et al. 2014; Treon et al. 2014b). Nonsense and frameshift mutations are almost equally divided among WM patients with CXCR4 somatic mutations, and over 30 different types of CXCR4^{WHIM} mutations have been identified in WM patients (Hunter et al. 2014; Treon et al. 2014b). In some patients multiple CXCR^{WHIM} mutations may be detected. CXCR4^{WHIM} mutations are usually subclonal to MYD88, with highly variable clonal distribution (Xu et al. 2016). The subclonal nature of these mutations suggests that CXCR4 mutations were likely acquired after MYD88 mutations.

Preclinical studies with WM cells engineered to express nonsense and frameshift CXCR4^{WHIM}-mutated receptors have shown enhanced and sustained AKT and ERK signaling following SDF-1a relative to CXCR4^{WT}, as well increased cell migration, adhesion, growth and survival, and drug resistance (including ibrutinib) in WM cells (Cao et al. 2014; Cao et al. 2015).

11.2.4 Other Somatic Events

Many copy number alterations have been revealed in WM patients that impact growth and survival pathways. Frequent loss of HIVEP2 (80%) and TNAIP3 (50%) genes that are negative regulators of NFkB expression, as well as LYN (70%) and IBTK (40%) that modulate BCR signaling have been revealed by WGS (Hunter et al. 2014). WGS has also revealed common defects in chromatin remodeling with somatic mutations in ARID1A present in 17% and loss of ARID1B in 70% of WM patients. Both ARID1A and ARID1B are members of the SWI/SNF family of proteins and are thought to exert their effects via p53 and CDKN1A regulation. TP53 is mutated in 7% of sequenced WM genomes, while PRDM2 and TOP1 that participate in TP53-related signaling are deleted in 80% and 60% of WM patients, respectively (Hunter et al. 2014). Taken together,

somatic events that contribute to impaired DNA damage response are also common in WM.

11.2.5 Impact of WM Genomics on Clinical Presentation

The importance of MYD88 and CXCR4 mutations in the clinical presentation of WM patients was recently reported. Significantly higher BM disease involvement, serum IgM levels, and symptomatic disease requiring therapy, including hyperviscosity syndrome, was observed in those patients with MYD88^{L265P}CXCR4$^{WHIM/NS}$ mutations (Treon et al. 2014b). Patients with MYD88^{L265P}CXCR4$^{WHIM/FS}$ or MYD88^{L265P}CXCR4^{WT} had intermediate BM and serum IgM levels; those with MYD88^{WT}CXCR4^{WT} showed the lowest BM disease burden. Fewer patients with MYD88^{L265P} and CXCR4$^{WHIM/FS\ or\ NS}$ compared to MYD88^{L265P}CXCR4^{WT} presented with adenopathy, further delineating differences in disease tropism based on CXCR4 status. Despite the more aggressive presentation associated with CXCR4$^{WHIM/NS}$ genotype, risk of death was not impacted by CXCR4 mutation status. Risk of death was found to be tenfold higher in patients with MYD88^{WT} versus MYD88^{L265P} genotype (Treon et al. 2014b).

11.3 Marrow Microenvironment

Increased numbers of mast cells are found in the bone marrow of WM patients, wherein they are usually admixed with tumor cell aggregates (Fig. 11.3) (Swerdlow et al. 2008; San Miguel et al. 2003; Xu et al. 2016). The role of mast cells in WM has been investigated in one study wherein co-culture of primary autologous or mast cell lines with WM LPC resulted in dose-dependent WM cell proliferation and/or tumor colony formation, through CD40 ligand (CD40L) signaling (Tournilhac et al. 2006). WM cells release soluble CD27 (sCD27) which may be triggered by cleavage of membrane-bound CD27 by matrix metalloproteinase-8 (MMP8) (Zhou et al. 2011). sCD27 levels are elevated in the

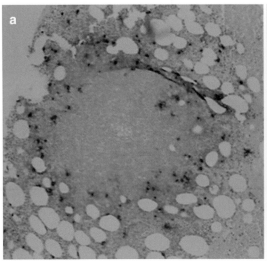
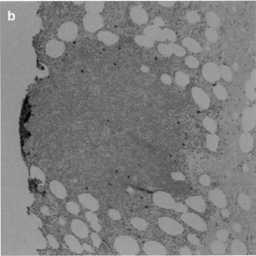

Fig. 11.3 Marrow clot section. (**a**) Tryptase-staining mast cells surrounding a nodule of lymphoplasmacytic cells in a patient with Waldenström macroglobulinemia. (**b**) Mast cells in the same section exhibit strong CD40 ligand signaling, which has been shown to support (at least in part) the growth and survival of lymphoplasmacytic cells

serum of WM patients and follow disease burden in mice engrafted with WM cells, as well as in WM patients (Ngo et al. 2008). sCD27 triggers the upregulation of CD40L as well as A Proliferation Inducing Ligand (APRIL) on mast cells derived from WM patients, as well as mast cell lines through its receptor CD70. Modeling in mice engrafted with a CD70 blocking antibody shows inhibition of tumor cell growth suggesting that WM cells require a microenvironmental support system for their growth and survival (Ho et al. 2008). High levels of CXCR4 and Very Late Antigen-4 (VLA-4) have also been observed in WM cells (Ngo et al. 2008). In blocking experiments studies, CXCR4 was shown to support migration of WM cells, while VLA-4 contributed to adhesion of WM cells to bone marrow stromal cells (Ngo et al. 2008).

lymphadenopathy are uncommon ($\leq 15\%$). Purpura is frequently associated with cryoglobulinemia and in rare circumstances with light-chain (AL) amyloidosis. Hemorrhagic and neuropathic manifestations are multifactorial (see "IgM-Related Neuropathy" below). The morbidity associated with WM is caused by the concurrence of two main components: tissue infiltration by neoplastic cells and, importantly, the physicochemical and immunologic properties of the monoclonal IgM. As shown in Table 11.2, the monoclonal IgM can produce clinical manifestations through several different mechanisms related to its physicochemical properties, nonspecific interactions with other proteins, antibody activity, and tendency to deposit in tissues (Merlini et al. 1986; Farhangi and Merlini 1986; Marmont and Merlini 1991).

11.4 Clinical Features

Table 11.1 presents the clinical and laboratory findings at time of diagnosis of WM in one large institutional study (Treon 2009). Unlike most indolent lymphomas, splenomegaly and

11.4.1 Morbidity Mediated by the Effects of IGM

11.4.1.1 Hyperviscosity Syndrome
The increased plasma IgM levels leads to blood hyperviscosity and its complications (Mackenzie

Table 11.1 Clinical and laboratory findings for 356 consecutive newly diagnosed patients with Waldenström macroglobulinemia (Treon 2009)

	Median	Range	Normal reference range
Age (years)	58	32–91	NA
Gender (male/female)	215/141		NA
Marrow involvement (% of area on slide)	30	5–95	NA
Adenopathy (% of patients)	15		NA
Splenomegaly (% of patients)	10		NA
IgM (mg/dL)	2620	270–12,400	40–230
IgG (mg/dL)	674	80–2770	700–1600
IgA (mg/dL)	58	6–438	70–400
Serum viscosity (cp)	2.0	1.1–7.2	1.4–1.9
Hematocrit (%)	35	17–45	35–44
Platelet count ($\times 10^9$/L)	275	42–675	155–410
White cell count ($\times 10^9$/L)	6.4	1.7–22	3.8–9.2
β_2-M (mg/dL)	2.5	0.9–13.7	0–2.7
LDH (U/mL)	313	61–1701	313–618

β_2M β_2-microglobulin, *cp* centipoise, *LDH* lactic dehydrogenase, *NA* not applicable
Source: Data from patients seen at the Dana-Farber Cancer Institute, Boston, MA

Table 11.2 Physicochemical and immunological properties of the monoclonal IGM protein in Waldenström's macroglobulinemia (Merlini et al. 1986; Farhangi and Merlini 1986; Marmont and Merlini 1991)

Properties of IgM monoclonal protein	Diagnostic condition	Clinical manifestations
Pentameric structure	Hyperviscosity	Headaches, blurred vision, epistaxis, retinal hemorrhages, leg cramps, impaired mentation, intracranial hemorrhage
Precipitation on cooling	Cryoglobulinemia (type I)	Raynaud phenomenon, acrocyanosis, ulcers, purpura, cold urticaria
Autoantibody activity to myelin-associated glycoprotein, ganglioside M₁, sulfatide moieties on peripheral nerve sheaths	Peripheral neuropathies	Sensorimotor neuropathies, painful neuropathies, ataxic gait, bilateral foot drop
Autoantibody activity to IgG	Cryoglobulinemia (type II)	Purpura, arthralgia, renal failure, sensorimotor neuropathies
Autoantibody activity to red blood cell antigens	Cold agglutinins	Hemolytic anemia, Raynaud phenomenon, acrocyanosis, livedo reticularis
Tissue deposition as amorphous aggregates	Organ dysfunction	Skin: Bullous skin disease, papules, Schnitzler syndrome
		Gastrointestinal: Diarrhea, malabsorption, bleeding
		Kidney: Proteinuria, renal failure (light-chain component)
Tissue deposition as amyloid fibrils (light-chain component most commonly)	Organ dysfunction	Fatigue, weight loss, edema, hepatomegaly, macroglossia, organ dysfunction of involved organs (heart, kidney, liver, peripheral sensory and autonomic nerves)

and Babcock 1975). The mechanisms behind the marked increase in the resistance to blood flow and the resulting impaired transit through the microcirculatory system are complex (Mackenzie and Babcock 1975; Gertz and Kyle 1995; Kwaan and Bongu 1999; Singh et al. 1993). The main determinants are (1) a high concentration of monoclonal IgMs, which may form aggregates and may bind water through their carbohydrate component, and (2) their interaction with blood cells. Monoclonal IgM increases red cell aggregation (rouleaux formation) and red cell internal viscosity while reducing red cell deformability. The presence of cryoglobulins contributes to increasing blood viscosity, as well as to the tendency to induce erythrocyte aggregation. Serum viscosity is proportional to IgM concentration up to 30 g/L and then increases sharply at higher levels. Increased plasma viscosity may also contribute to inappropriately low erythropoietin production, which is the major reason for anemia in these patients (Singh et al. 1993). Renal synthesis of erythropoietin is inversely correlated with plasma viscosity. Clinical manifestations are related to circulatory disturbances that can be best appreciated by ophthalmoscopy, which shows distended and tortuous retinal veins, hemorrhages, and papilledema (Fig. 11.4) (Menke et al. 2006). Symptoms usually occur when the monoclonal IgM concentration exceeds 50 g/L or when serum viscosity is >4.0 centipoises (cp), but there is individual variability, with some patients showing no evidence of hyperviscosity even at 10 cp (Mackenzie and Babcock 1975). The most common symptoms are oronasal mucosal bleeding, visual disturbances because of retinal bleeding, and dizziness that rarely may lead to stupor or coma. Heart failure can be aggravated, particularly in the elderly, owing to increased blood viscosity, expanded plasma

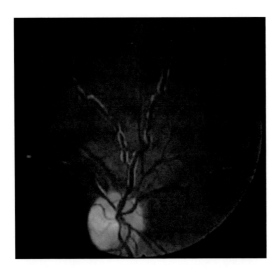

Fig. 11.4 Funduscopic examination of a patient with Waldenström macroglobulinemia with hyperviscosity-related changes, including dilated retinal vessels, hemorrhages, and "venous sausaging." The white material at the edge of the veins may be cryoglobulin (Used with permission from Marvin J. Stone, MD)

volume, and anemia. Inappropriate red cell transfusion can exacerbate hyperviscosity and may precipitate cardiac failure.

11.4.1.2 Cryoglobulinemia

The monoclonal IgM can behave as a cryoglobulin in up to 20% of patients and is usually type I and asymptomatic in most cases (Treon 2009; Mackenzie and Babcock 1975; Stone 2009). Cryoprecipitation is mainly dependent on the concentration of monoclonal IgM; for this reason plasmapheresis or plasma exchange is commonly effective in this condition. Symptoms result from impaired blood flow in small vessels and include Raynaud phenomenon, acrocyanosis, and necrosis of the regions most exposed to cold, such as the tip of the nose, ears, fingers, and toes (Fig. 11.5), malleolar ulcers, purpura, and cold urticaria. Renal manifestations are infrequent. Mixed cryoglobulins (type II) consisting of IgM-IgG complexes may be associated with hepatitis C infections (Stone 2009).

11.4.1.3 Autoantibody Activity

Monoclonal IgM may exert its pathogenic effects through specific recognition of autologous antigens, the most notable being nerve constituents, immunoglobulin determinants, and red blood cell antigens.

11.4.1.4 IgM-Related Neuropathy

IgM-related peripheral neuropathy is common in WM patients, with estimated prevalence rates of 5–40% (Dellagi et al. 1983; Nobile-Orazio et al. 1987; Treon et al. 2010). Approximately 8% of idiopathic neuropathies are associated with a monoclonal gammopathy, with a preponderance of IgM (60%) followed by IgG (30%) and IgA (10%) (Nemni et al. 1994; Ropper and Gorson 1998). The nerve damage is mediated by diverse pathogenetic mechanisms: (1) IgM antibody activity toward nerve constituents causing demyelinating polyneuropathies; (2) endoneurial granulofibrillar deposits of IgM without antibody activity, associated with axonal polyneuropathy; (3) occasionally by tubular deposits in the endoneurium associated with IgM cryoglobulin; and, rarely, (4) by amyloid deposits or by

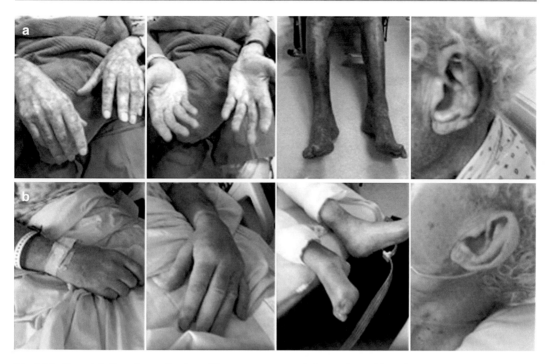

Fig. 11.5 Cryoglobulinemia manifesting with severe acrocyanosis in a patient with Waldenström macroglobulinemia before (**a**) and following warming and plasmapheresis (**b**)

neoplastic cell infiltration of nerve structures (Treon et al. 2010; Vital 2001).

Half of the patients with IgM neuropathy have a distinctive clinical syndrome that is associated with antibodies against a minor 100-kDa glycoprotein component of nerve known as the myelin-associated glycoprotein (MAG). Anti-MAG antibodies are generally monoclonal IgMκ and usually also exhibit reactivity with other glycoproteins or glycolipids that share antigenic determinants with MAG (Latov et al. 1981; Chassande et al. 1998; Weiss et al. 1999). The anti-MAG-related neuropathy is typically distal and symmetrical, affecting both motor and sensory functions; it is slowly progressive with a long period of stability (Nobile-Orazio et al. 1987; Latov et al. 1988). Most patients present with sensory complaints (paresthesias, aching discomfort, dysesthesias, or lancinating pains), imbalance and gait ataxia, owing to lack proprioception; leg muscles atrophy in advanced stage. Patients with predominantly demyelinating sensory neuropathy in association with monoclonal IgM to

gangliosides with disialosyl moieties, such as GD1b, GD3, GD2, GT1b, and GQ1b, have also been reported (Dalakas and Quarles 1996; Eurelings et al. 2001). Anti-GD1b and anti-GQ1b antibodies were associated with sensory ataxic neuropathy. These antiganglioside monoclonal IgMs present core clinical features of chronic ataxic neuropathy sometimes with present ophthalmoplegia and/or red blood cell cold agglutinating activity. The disialosyl epitope is also present on red blood cell glycophorins, thereby accounting for the red cell cold agglutinin activity of anti-Pr2 specificity (Ilyas et al. 1985; Willison et al. 2001). Monoclonal IgM proteins that bind to gangliosides with a terminal trisaccharide moiety, including ganglioside M_2 (GM_2) and GalNac-GD1A, are associated with chronic demyelinating neuropathy and severe sensory ataxia, unresponsive to glucocorticoids (Lopate et al. 2002). Antiganglioside IgM proteins may also cross-react with lipopolysaccharides of *Campylobacter jejuni*, whose infection is known to precipitate the Miller-Fisher syndrome, a variant of the Guillain-Barré syndrome (Jacobs et al. 1997). Thus, molecular mimicry may play a role in this condition. Antisulfatide monoclonal IgM proteins, associated with sensory-sensorimotor neuropathy, have been detected in 5% of patients with IgM monoclonal gammopathy and neuropathy (Nobile-Orazio et al. 1994). Motor neuron disease has been reported in patients with WM and monoclonal IgM with anti-GM$_1$ and sulfoglucuronyl paragloboside activity (Gordon et al. 1997). Polyneuropathy, organomegaly, endocrinopathy, M protein, and skin changes (the POEMS syndrome) are rare in patients with WM (Pavord et al. 1996).

11.4.1.5 Cold Agglutinin Hemolytic Anemia

Monoclonal IgM may have cold agglutinin activity, that is, it can recognize specific red cell antigens at temperatures below 37 °C, producing chronic hemolytic anemia. This disorder occurs in <10% of WM patients and is associated with cold agglutinin titers greater than 1:1000 in most cases (Crisp and Pruzanski 1982). The monoclonal component is usually an IgMκ and reacts most commonly with red cell I/i antigens, resulting in complement fixation and activation (Pruzanski and Shumak 1977a, b). Mild to moderate chronic hemolytic anemia can be exacerbated after cold exposure. Hemoglobin usually remains above 70 g/L. The hemolysis is usually extravascular, mediated by removal of C3b-opsonized red cells by the mononuclear phagocyte system, primarily in the liver. Intravascular hemolysis from complement destruction of red blood cell membrane is infrequent. The agglutination of red cells in the skin circulation also causes Raynaud syndrome, acrocyanosis, and livedo reticularis. Macroglobulins with the properties of both cryoglobulins and cold agglutinins with anti-Pr specificity can occur. These properties may have as a common basis the binding of the sialic acid-containing carbohydrate present on red blood cell glycophorins and on Ig molecules. Several other macroglobulins with antibody activity toward autologous antigens (i.e., phospholipids, tissue and plasma proteins, etc.) and foreign ligands have also been described.

11.4.1.6 IgM Tissue Deposition

The monoclonal protein can deposit in several tissues as amorphous aggregates. Linear deposition of monoclonal IgM along the skin basement membrane is associated with bullous skin disease (Whittaker et al. 1996). Amorphous IgM deposits in the dermis result in IgM storage papules on the extensor surface of the extremities, referred to as macroglobulinemia cutis (Daoud et al. 1999). Deposition of monoclonal IgM in the lamina propria and/or submucosa of the intestine may be associated with diarrhea, malabsorption, and gastrointestinal bleeding (Gad et al. 1995; Amrein and Compton 1990). Kidney involvement is less common and less severe in WM than in myeloma, probably because the amount of light chain excreted in the urine is generally lower in WM than in myeloma and because of the absence of contributing factors, such as hypercalcemia. Urinary cast nephropathy, however, has occurred in WM (Isaac and Herrera 2002). On the other hand, the IgM macromolecule is more susceptible to being trapped in the glomerular loops where ultrafiltration presumably contributes to its precipitation, forming subendothelial deposits of aggregated IgM proteins that occlude the glomerular capillaries (Morel-Maroger et al. 1970). Mild and reversible proteinuria may result and most patients are asymptomatic. The deposition of monoclonal light chain as fibrillar amyloid deposits (AL amyloidosis) is uncommon in patients with WM (Gertz et al. 1993). Clinical expression and prognosis are similar to those of other AL amyloidosis patients with involvement of the heart (44%), kidneys (32%), liver (14%), lungs (10%), peripheral or autonomic nerves (38%), and soft tissues (18%). The incidence of cardiac and pulmonary involvement is higher in patients with monoclonal IgM than with other immunoglobulin isotypes. The association of WM with reactive amyloidosis has been documented rarely (Moyner et al. 1980; Gardyn et al. 2001). Simultaneous occurrence of fibrillary glomerulopathy, characterized by glomerular deposits of wide noncongophilic fibrils and amyloid deposits, has been described (Dussol et al. 1998).

11.4.2 Manifestations Related to Tissue Infiltration by Neoplastic Cells

Tissue infiltration by neoplastic cells is uncommon but can involve various organs and tissues, including the liver, spleen, lymph nodes, lungs, gastrointestinal tract, kidneys, skin, eyes, and central nervous system.

11.4.2.1 Lung

Pulmonary involvement in the form of masses, nodules, diffuse infiltrate, or pleural effusions is uncommon; the overall incidence of pulmonary and pleural findings is approximately 4% (Rausch and Herion 1980; Fadil and Taylor 1998; Kyrtsonis et al. 2001). Cough is the most common presenting symptom, followed by dyspnea and chest pain. Chest radiographic findings include parenchymal infiltrates, confluent masses, and effusions.

11.4.2.2 Gastrointestinal Tract

Malabsorption, diarrhea, bleeding, or obstruction may indicate involvement of the gastrointestinal tract at the level of the stomach, duodenum, or small intestine (Kaila et al. 1996; Yasui et al. 1997; Rosenthal et al. 1998; Recine et al. 2001).

11.4.2.3 Renal System

In contrast to myeloma, infiltration of the kidney interstitium with lymphoplasmacytoid cell can occur in WM, and renal or perirenal masses are not uncommon (Veltman et al. 1997; Moore et al. 1995).

11.4.2.4 Skin

The skin can be the site of dense lymphoplasmacytic infiltrates, similar to that seen in the liver, spleen, and lymph nodes, forming cutaneous plaques and, rarely, nodules (Mascaro et al. 1982). Chronic urticaria and IgM gammopathy are the two cardinal features of the Schnitzler syndrome, which is not usually associated initially with clinical features of WM, although evolution to WM is not uncommon (Schnitzler et al. 1974). Thus, close follow-up of these patients is important.

11.4.2.5 Joints

Invasion of articular and periarticular structures by WM malignant cells is rarely reported (Roux et al. 1996).

11.4.2.6 Eye

The neoplastic cells can infiltrate the periorbital structures, lacrimal gland, and retro-orbital lymphoid tissues, resulting in ocular nerve palsies (Orellana and Friedman 1981; Ettl et al. 1992).

11.4.2.7 Central Nervous System

Direct infiltration of the central nervous system by monoclonal lymphoplasmacytic cells as infiltrates or as tumors constitutes the rarely observed Bing-Neel syndrome, characterized clinically by confusion, memory loss, disorientation, and motor dysfunction. The diagnosis and management of Bing-Neel Syndrome is reviewed in Minnema et al. 2017).

11.5 Laboratory Findings

11.5.1 Blood Abnormalities

Anemia is the most common finding in patients with symptomatic WM and is caused by a combination of factors: decrease in red cell survival, impaired erythropoiesis, moderate plasma volume expansion, hepcidin production leading to iron re-utilization defect, and blood loss from the gastrointestinal tract (Treon 2009; Ciccarelli et al. 2011; Treon et al. 2013). Blood films are usually normocytic and normochromic, and rouleaux formation is often pronounced. Mean red cell volume may be elevated spuriously owing to erythrocyte aggregation. In addition, the hemoglobin estimate can be inaccurate, that is, falsely high, because of interaction between the monoclonal protein and the diluent used in some automated analyzers (Owen et al. 2001). Leukocyte and platelet counts are usually within the reference range at presentation, although patients may occasionally present with severe thrombocytopenia. Monoclonal B lymphocytes expressing surface IgM and late-differentiation B-cell markers are uncommonly detected in blood by flow cytometry. A raised erythrocyte sedimentation rate is almost always present and may be the first clue to the presence of the macroglobulinemia. The clotting abnormality detected most frequently is prolongation of thrombin time. AL amyloidosis should be suspected in all patients with nephrotic syndrome, cardiomyopathy, hepatomegaly, or peripheral neuropathy. Diagnosis requires the demonstration of green birefringence under polarized light of amyloid deposits stained with Congo red.

11.5.2 Marrow Findings

Central to the diagnosis of WM is the demonstration, by trephine biopsy, of marrow infiltration by a lymphoplasmacytic cell population characterized by small lymphocytes with evidence of plasmacytoid and plasma cell maturation (Fig. 11.1) (Owen et al. 2003; Swerdlow et al. 2008). The pattern of marrow infiltration may be diffuse, interstitial, or nodular, usually with an intertrabecular pattern of infiltration. A solely paratrabecular pattern of infiltration is unusual and should raise the possibility of follicular lymphoma (Owen et al. 2003). The marrow cell immunophenotype should be confirmed by flow cytometry and/or immunohistochemistry. The cell immunoprofile: $sIgM^{+}CD19^{+}CD20^{+}CD22^{+}CD79^{+}$ is characteristic of WM (Swerdlow et al. 2008; Owen et al. 2001; Feiner et al. 1990). Up to 20% of cases may express either CD5, CD10, or CD23 (Hunter et al. 2005). In these cases, chronic lymphocytic leukemia and mantle cell lymphoma should be excluded. "Intranuclear" periodic acid-Schiff-positive inclusions (Dutcher-Fahey bodies) (Dutcher and Fahey 1959) consisting of IgM deposits in the perinuclear space, and sometimes in intranuclear vacuoles, may be seen occasionally in lymphoid cells. An increased number of mast cells, usually in association with the lymphoid aggregates, are commonly found, and their presence may help in differentiating WM from other B-cell lymphomas (see Fig. 11.3) (Swerdlow et al. 2008). $MYD88^{L265P}$ testing of bone marrow samples has been incorporated into many clinical laboratories and may help in

clarifying the diagnosis of WM from other IgM-secreting entities (Treon et al. 2012; Xu et al. 2013; Varettoni et al. 2013; Jiménez et al. 2013; Poulain et al. 2013). The use of peripheral blood B cells may also permit determination of $MYD88^{L265P}$ status by allele-specific polymerase chain reaction assays, particularly in untreated WM patients. CXCR4 mutation testing may also be useful in patients being considered for ibrutinib therapy (discussed below).

11.5.3 Immunologic Abnormalities

High-resolution electrophoresis combined with immunofixation of serum and urine is recommended for identification and characterization of the IgM monoclonal protein. The light chain of the monoclonal IgM is κ in 75–80% of patients. More than one M component may be present. The concentration of the serum monoclonal protein is very variable but in most cases lies within the range of 15–45 g/L. Densitometry should be adopted to determine IgM levels for serial evaluations because nephelometry is unreliable and shows large laboratory variation. The presence of cold agglutinins or cryoglobulins may affect determination of IgM levels, and, therefore, testing for cold agglutinins and cryoglobulins should be performed at diagnosis. If present, subsequent serum samples should be analyzed at 37 °C for determination of serum monoclonal IgM level. Although Bence Jones proteinuria is frequently present, it exceeds 1 g/24 h in only 3% of cases. Whereas IgM levels are elevated in WM patients, IgA and IgG levels are most often depressed and do not recover after successful treatment (Hunter et al. 2010).

11.5.4 Serum Viscosity

Because of its large size (almost 1,000,000 daltons), most IgM molecules are retained within the intravascular compartment and can exert an undue effect on serum viscosity (Mackenzie and Babcock 1975). Serum viscosity can be measured if the patient has signs or symptoms of hyperviscosity syndrome, though levels often slow to be resulted and erratic due to a lack of standardization in most clinical laboratories (Treon 2009). As such, serum IgM levels may be more expedient and relied upon. Patients typically become symptomatic at serum viscosity levels of 4.0 centipoise and above that relates to serum IgM levels above 6000 mg/dL (Stone and Bogen 2012; Menke and Treon 2007). Patients may be symptomatic at lower serum viscosity and IgM levels, and in these patients cryoglobulins may be present. Recurring nosebleeds, headaches, and visual disturbances are common symptoms in patients with symptomatic hyperviscosity (Treon 2009). Funduscopy is an important indicator of clinically relevant hyperviscosity. Among the first clinical signs of hyperviscosity are the appearance of peripheral and midperipheral dot and blot-like hemorrhages in the retina, which are best appreciated with indirect ophthalmoscopy and scleral depression (Menke et al. 2006). In more severe cases of hyperviscosity, dot, blot, and flame-shaped hemorrhages can appear in the macular area along with markedly dilated and tortuous veins with focal constrictions resulting in "venous sausaging," as well as papilledema (Fig. 11.4).

11.5.5 Imaging

Magnetic resonance imaging (MRI) of the spine in conjunction with computed tomography (CT) of the abdomen and pelvis is useful in evaluating the disease status (Moulopoulos et al. 1993). Marrow involvement can be documented by MRI studies of the spine in more than 90% of patients; CT of the abdomen and pelvis demonstrates enlarged nodes in approximately 20% of WM patients at diagnosis but may be higher at relapse (Moulopoulos et al. 1993).

11.5.6 Lymph Node Biopsy

Lymph node biopsy may show preserved architecture or replacement by infiltration of neoplastic cells with lymphoplasmacytoid, lymphoplasmacytic, or polymorphous cytologic patterns. Testing for MYD88 mutations may help.

11.6 Treatment

11.6.1 Initiating Treatment

As part of the Second International Workshop on Waldenström's Macroglobulinemia, a consensus panel was organized to recommend criteria for the initiation of therapy in patients with WM (Kyle et al. 2003). The panel recommended that initiation of therapy should not be based on the IgM level per se, as this may not correlate with the clinical manifestations of WM. The consensus panel did, however, agree that initiation of therapy is appropriate for patients with constitutional symptoms, such as recurrent fever, night sweats, fatigue as a consequence of anemia, or weight loss. Progressive symptomatic lymphadenopathy and/or splenomegaly provide additional reasons to begin therapy. Anemia with a hemoglobin value of ≤ 10 g/dL or a platelet count of $\leq 100 \times 10^9$/L owing to marrow infiltration also justifies treatment. Certain complications, such as hyperviscosity syndrome, symptomatic sensorimotor peripheral neuropathy, systemic amyloidosis, renal insufficiency, or symptomatic cryoglobulinemia, may also be indications for therapy (Treon 2009; Kyle et al. 2003).

11.6.2 Initial Therapy

The International Workshops on Waldenström Macroglobulinemia have also formulated consensus recommendations for both initial therapy and therapy for refractory disease based on the best available evidence. The most recent recommendations emerged from the Eighth International Workshop on WM (Leblond et al. 2016). Individual patient considerations, including the presence of cytopenias, need for more rapid disease control, age, and candidacy for autologous transplant therapy, should be taken into account in making the choice of the drugs to use. For patients who are candidates for autologous stem cell transplantation, which typically is reserved for those patients younger than 70 years of age, the panel recommended that exposure to alkylating agents or nucleoside analogues should be limited. The use of nucleoside analogues should be approached cautiously in WM patients as there appears to be an increased risk for the development of disease transformation as well as myelodysplasia and acute myelogenous leukemia.

11.6.2.1 Oral Alkylating Agents

Oral alkylating drugs, alone and in combination therapy with glucocorticoids, have been extensively evaluated in the treatment of WM. Chlorambucil has been administered on both a continuous (i.e., daily dose schedule) and an intermittent schedule. Patients receiving chlorambucil on a continuous schedule typically receive 0.1 mg/kg per day, whereas on the intermittent schedule patients typically receive 0.3 mg/kg for 7 days, every 6 weeks. In a prospective randomized study, no significant difference in the overall response rate between these schedules was observed (Kyle et al. 2000), although the median response duration was greater for patients receiving intermittent- versus continuous-dose chlorambucil (46 vs. 26 months). Despite the favorable median response duration in this study for use of the intermittent schedule, no difference in the median overall survival was observed. Moreover, an increased incidence for development of myelodysplasia and acute myelogenous leukemia with the intermittent (3 of 22 patients) versus the continuous (0 of 24 patients) chlorambucil schedule prompted the preference for use of continuous chlorambucil dosing. The use of glucocorticoids in combination with alkylating agent therapy has also been explored. Chlorambucil (8 mg/m²) plus prednisone (40 mg/m²) given orally for 10 days, every 6 weeks, resulted in a major response (i.e., reduction of IgM by more than 50%) in 72% of patients (Dimopoulos and Alexanian 1994). Alkylating agent regimens employing melphalan and cyclophosphamide in combination with glucocorticoids have also been examined (Petrucci et al.

1989; Case et al. 1991). This approach produced slightly higher overall response rates and response durations, although the benefit of these more complex regimens over chlorambucil remains to be demonstrated. Pretreatment factors associated with shorter survival in the entire population of patients receiving single-agent chlorambucil were age older than 60 years, male sex, hemoglobin less than 10 g/dL, leukocytes less than 4×10^9/L, and platelets less than 150×10^9/L. Organomegaly, signs of hyperviscosity, renal failure, monoclonal IgM level, blood lymphocytosis, and percentage of marrow lymphoid cells were not significantly correlated with survival (Facon et al. 1993). Additional factors to be taken into account in considering alkylating agent therapy for patients with WM include necessity for more rapid disease control given the slow response, as well as consideration for preserving stem cells in patients who are candidates for autologous stem cell transplantation therapy. A large randomized study showed an inferior response rate and time to progression in WM patients receiving chlorambucil versus fludarabine, as well as a higher incidence of secondary malignancies in the former. Neutropenia was however more pronounced in those patients on fludarabine (Leblond et al. 2013).

11.6.2.2 Nucleoside Analogue Therapy

Cladribine administered as a single agent by continuous intravenous infusion, by 2-h daily infusion, or by subcutaneous bolus injections for 5–7 days has resulted in major responses in 40–90% of patients who received primary therapy, whereas in the previously treated patients, responses have ranged from 38% to 54% (Dimopoulos et al. 1994a; Delannoy et al. 1994; Fridrik et al. 1997; Liu et al. 1998; Hellmann et al. 1999; Betticher et al. 1997; Dimopoulos et al. 1995). Median time to achievement of response in responding patients following cladribine ranged from 1.2 to 5 months. The overall response rate with daily infusion of fludarabine, administered mainly on 5-day schedules, in previously untreated and treated patients ranged from 38 to 100% and 30 to 40%, respectively (Dimopoulos et al. 1993; Foran et al. 1999; Thalhammer-Scherrer et al. 2000; Dhodapkar et al. 2001; Zinzani et al. 1995; Leblond et al. 1998), similar to the responses to cladribine. Median time to achievement of response for fludarabine (3–6 months) was also similar to cladribine. In general, response rates and durations of responses have been greater for patients receiving nucleoside analogues as initial therapy; although in several studies in which both untreated and previously treated patients were enrolled, no difference in the overall response rate was reported.

Myelosuppression commonly occurs following prolonged exposure to either of the nucleoside analogues. A sustained decrease in both CD4+ and CD8+ T lymphocytes, measured 1 year following initiation of therapy, is notable (Dimopoulos et al. 1994a; Delannoy et al. 1994; Fridrik et al. 1997). Treatment-related mortality as a consequence of myelosuppression and/or opportunistic infections attributable to immunosuppression occurred in up to 5% of all treated patients in some series with nucleoside analogues.

Factors predicting for a better response to nucleoside analogues include younger age at start of treatment (<70 years), higher pretreatment hemoglobin (>95 g/L), higher platelet count (>75 × 10^9/L), disease relapsing off therapy, and a long interval between first-line therapy and initiation of a nucleoside analogue in relapsing patients (Dimopoulos et al. 1994a; Betticher et al. 1997; Zinzani et al. 1995). There are limited data on the use of an alternate nucleoside analogue in previously treated patients among whom disease relapsed or who had resistance when not on cladribine or fludarabine therapy (Dimopoulos et al. 1994b; Lewandowski et al. 2002). Three of four (75%) patients responded to cladribine after progression following an unmaintained remission to fludarabine, whereas only one of ten (10%) with disease resistant to fludarabine responded to cladribine (Dimopoulos et al. 1994b). A response in two of six patients (33%) and disease stabilization in the remaining patients to fludarabine, in spite of an inadequate response or progressive disease, following cladribine

therapy has been reported (Lewandowski et al. 2002).

Harvesting autologous blood stem cells succeeded on the first attempt in 14 of 15 patients who did not receive nucleoside analogue therapy as compared to 2 of 6 patients who received a nucleoside analogue (Popat et al. 2009). A sevenfold increase in transformation to an aggressive lymphoma and a threefold increase in the development of myelodysplasia or acute myelogenous leukemia were observed among patients who received a nucleoside analogue versus other therapies for their WM (Leleu et al. 2009a). A meta-analysis of several trials in which patients were treated with nucleoside analogues in WM patients, included patients who had previously received an alkylating agent, and showed a crude incidence of approximately 8% for development of disease transformation and of approximately 5% for development of myelodysplasia or acute myelogenous leukemia (Leleu et al. 2009b). None of the risk factors—that is, gender, age, family history of WM, or B-cell malignancies, typical markers of tumor burden and prognosis, type of nucleoside analogue therapy (cladribine vs fludarabine), time from diagnosis to nucleoside analogue use, nucleoside analogue treatment as primary or salvage therapy, or treatment with an oral alkylator (i.e., chlorambucil)—predicted for the occurrence of transformation or development of myelodysplasia or acute myelogenous leukemia in patients treated with a nucleoside analogue (Leleu et al. 2009b).

11.6.2.3 CD20-Directed Antibody Therapy

Rituximab is a chimeric monoclonal antibody that targets CD20, a widely expressed antigen on lymphoplasmacytic cells in WM (Treon et al. 2003). Several retrospective and prospective studies have indicated that rituximab, when used at standard doses (i.e., four weekly infusions of 375 mg/m^2), induced major responses in approximately 30% of previously treated and untreated patients (Treon et al. 2001; Gertz et al. 2004). Even patients who achieved minor responses benefited from rituximab by improved hemoglobin and platelet counts and reduction of lymphadenopathy and/or splenomegaly (Treon et al. 2001). The median time to treatment failure in these studies was found to range from 8 to 27+ months. Patients on an extended rituximab schedule consisting of four weekly courses at 375 mg/m^2 per week, repeated 3 months later by another 4-week course, have demonstrated major response rates of approximately 45%, with time to progression estimates of 16+ to 29+ months (Dimopoulos et al. 2002; Treon et al. 2005a).

In many WM patients, a transient increase or flare of the serum IgM may occur immediately following initiation of rituximab treatment (Dimopoulos et al. 2002; Treon et al. 2004; Ghobrial et al. 2004). Such an increase does not herald treatment failure, and most patients will return to their baseline serum IgM level by 12 weeks. Some patients continue to show a prolonged increase in IgM despite an apparent reduction in their marrow tumor cells. However, patients with baseline serum IgM levels of >50 g/dL or serum viscosity of >3.5 cp may be particularly at risk for a hyperviscosity-related event, and plasmapheresis should be considered in these patients in advance of rituximab therapy (Treon et al. 2004). Because of the decreased likelihood of response in patients with higher IgM levels, as well as the possibility that serum IgM and blood viscosity levels may abruptly rise, rituximab monotherapy should not be used as sole therapy for the treatment of patients at risk for hyperviscosity symptoms (Leblond et al. 2016; Dimopoulos et al. 2002; Treon et al. 2005a).

Time to response after rituximab is slow and exceeds 3 months on the average. The time to best response in one study was 18 months (Treon et al. 2005a). Patients with baseline serum IgM levels of <60 g/dL are more likely to respond, regardless of the underlying marrow involvement by tumor cells (Dimopoulos et al. 2002; Treon et al. 2005a). An analysis of 52 patients who were treated with single-agent rituximab found the objective response rate was significantly lower in patients who had either low serum albumin (<35 g/L) or a serum monoclonal protein greater than 40 g/L (Dimopoulos et al. 2005a). The presence of both adverse prognostic factors was associated with a short time to progression

(3.6 months). Patients who had normal serum albumin and relatively low serum monoclonal protein levels derived a substantial benefit from rituximab with a time to progression exceeding 40 months.

A correlation between polymorphisms at position 158 in the FcγRIIIa receptor (CD16), an activating Fc receptor on important effector cells that mediate antibody-dependent cell-mediated cytotoxicity, and rituximab response was observed in WM patients (Treon et al. 2005b). Individuals may encode either the amino acid valine or phenylalanine at position 158 in the FcγRIIIa receptor. WM patients who carried the valine amino acid (either in a homozygous or heterozygous pattern) had a fourfold higher major response rate (i.e., 50% decline in serum IgM levels) to rituximab versus those patients who expressed phenylalanine in a homozygous pattern.

11.6.2.4 Proteasome Inhibitors

Both bortezomib and carfilzomib have been evaluated in prospective studies in patients with WM, though the latter only in combination therapy (discussed below). In a retrospective study, ten patients with refractory or relapsed WM were treated with bortezomib administered intravenously at a dose of 1.3 mg/m^2 on days 1, 4, 8 and 11 in a 21-day cycle for a total of four cycles. Most patients had been exposed to all active agents for WM, and eight patients had received three or more regimens. Six of these patients achieved a partial response which occurred at a median of 1 month. The median time to progression in the responding patients is expected to exceed 11 months. Peripheral neuropathy occurred in three patients, and one patient developed severe paralytic ileus in this series (Dimopoulos et al. 2005b). In a prospective study among 27 relapsed or refractory patients who received up to 8 cycles of bortezomib at 1.3 mg/m^2 on days 1, 4, 8, and 11, median serum IgM levels declined significantly from 4.7 to 2.1 g/dL (Treon et al. 2007). The overall response rate was 85%, with 10 and 13 patients achieving a minor (<25%) and major (<50%) decrease in IgM level. Responses occurred at median of 1.4 months. The median time to progression for all responding patients in this study was 7.9 (range, 3–21.4+) months, and the most common grade III/IV toxicities were sensory neuropathies (22.2%), leukopenia (18.5%), neutropenia (14.8%), dizziness (11.1%), and thrombocytopenia (7.4%). Sensory neuropathies resolved or improved in nearly all patients following cessation of therapy. Twenty-seven patients with both untreated (44%) and previously treated (56%) disease received bortezomib, utilizing the standard schedule until they either demonstrated progressive disease or two cycles beyond a complete response or stable disease (Chen et al. 2007). The overall response rate was 78%, with major responses observed in 44% of patients. Sensory neuropathy occurred in 20 patients following 2–4 cycles of therapy. Among the 20 patients developing a neuropathy, 14 showed resolution or improvement 2–13 months after therapy.

11.6.2.5 Combination Therapies

Because rituximab is not myelosuppressive, its combination with chemotherapy has been explored. A regimen of rituximab, cladribine, and cyclophosphamide used in 17 previously untreated patients resulted in a partial response in 94% of WM patients, including a complete response in 18% (Treon et al. 2005b). No patient had relapsed with a median follow-up of 21 months. The combination of rituximab and fludarabine used in 43 patients of whom 32 (75%) were previously untreated led to an overall response rate of 95.3%, with 83% of patients achieving a major response (i.e., 50% reduction in disease burden) (Treon et al. 2009a). The median time to progression was 51.2 months in this series and was longer for those patients who were previously untreated and for those achieving a very good partial remission (i.e., 90% reduction in disease) or better. Hematologic toxicity was common: grade 3 neutropenia and thrombocytopenia observed in 27 and 4 patients, respectively. Two deaths occurred in this study from pneumonia. Secondary malignancies including transformation to aggressive lymphoma and development of myelodysplasia or acute myelogenous leukemia were observed in six patients in this series. The addition of

rituximab to fludarabine and cyclophosphamide has also been explored in previously treated patients, of whom four of five patients had a response (Tam et al. 2005). In another combination study, rituximab along with pentostatin and cyclophosphamide given to 13 patients with untreated and previously treated WM or lymphoplasmacytic lymphoma resulted in a major response in 77% of patients (Hensel et al. 2005). The combination of rituximab, dexamethasone, and cyclophosphamide was used as primary therapy to treat 72 patients with WM in whom a major response was observed in 74% of patients in this study, and the 2-year progression-free survival was 67% (Dimopoulos et al. 2007). Therapy was well tolerated, although one patient died of interstitial pneumonia.

Two studies have examined cyclophosphamide, doxorubicin, vincristine, prednisone (CHOP) in combination with rituximab (R-CHOP). In a randomized trial involving 69 patients, most of whom had WM, the addition of rituximab to CHOP resulted in a higher overall response rate (94% vs. 67%) and median time to progression (63 vs. 22 months) in comparison with patients treated with CHOP alone (Buske et al. 2009). R-CHOP was also used in 13 WM patients, 10 of whom had relapsed or refractory disease (Treon et al. 2005c). Among 13 evaluable patients, 10 patients achieved a major response (77%), including 3 complete and 7 partial remissions. Two other patients achieved a minor response. In a retrospective study of symptomatic WM patients who received either R-CHOP; rituximab, cyclophosphamide, vincristine, and prednisone (R-CVP); or cyclophosphamide, prednisone, and rituximab (CPR) and were similar in most pretreatment variables, the overall response rates to therapy were comparable among all three treatment groups—R-CHOP (96%), R-CVP (88%), and CPR (95%)—although there was a trend for more complete remissions among patients treated with R-CVP and R-CHOP (Ioakimidis et al. 2009). Adverse events attributed to therapy showed a higher incidence for neutropenic fever and treatment-related neuropathy for R-CHOP and R-CVP versus CPR. The results of this study suggest that in WM, the use of CPR may provide analogous treatment responses to more intense cyclophosphamide-based regimens while minimizing treatment-related complications. The extended alkylator bendamustine has also been evaluated in combination with rituximab in both untreated and previously treated WM patients. A randomized study by the German STiL Group examined bendamustine plus rituximab (Benda-R) versus R-CHOP in patients with untreated, indolent B-cell lymphomas including WM (Rummel et al. 2013). Patients with WM in this study showed similar overall responses (96% versus 94%), though progression-free survival was significantly longer (69 versus 29 months) in patients who received Benda-R versus R-CHOP. Treatment was also better tolerated in patients receiving Benda-R. In the relapsed or refractory setting, an overall response rate of 83% was observed with bendamustine in combination with a CD20 monoclonal antibody (Treon et al. 2011a). The median time to progression was 13 months in this study. Prolonged myelosuppression was more common in patients who received prior nucleoside analogues.

The use of two cycles of oral cyclophosphamide along with subcutaneous cladribine to 37 patients with previously untreated WM led to a partial response in 84% of patients, and the median duration of response was 36 months (Weber et al. 2003). Fludarabine in combination with intravenous cyclophosphamide resulted in partial responses in 6 of 11 (55%) WM patients with either primary refractory disease or who had relapsed on treatment (Dimopoulos et al. 2003). The combination of fludarabine plus cyclophosphamide was also evaluated in 49 patients, 35 of whom were previously treated. Seventy-eight percent of the patients achieved a response, and the median time to treatment failure was 27 months (Tamburini et al. 2005). Hematological toxicity was frequent, and three patients died of treatment-related toxicities. Two important findings in this study were the development of acute leukemia in two patients, histologic transformation to diffuse large B-cell lymphoma in one patient, and two cases of solid malignancies (prostate and melanoma), as well as failure to mobilize stem cells in four of six patients.

The combination of bortezomib, dexamethasone, and rituximab (BDR) as primary therapy in 23 patients with WM resulted in an overall response rate of 96% and a major response rate of 83% (Treon et al. 2009b). Maintenance therapy with BDR was used in this study. The incidence of grade 3 neuropathy was approximately 30% and led to discontinuance of bortezomib in 60% of patients on BDR. An increased incidence of herpes zoster was also observed prompting the prophylactic use of antiviral therapy. The median progression-free survival in this study was 66 months, and resolution of treatment-related neuropathy to at least grade 1 or less was observed in most 13/16; 81%) of patients with prolonged follow-up (Treon et al. 2015b).

Alternative schedules for administration of bortezomib (i.e., once weekly at higher doses) in combination with rituximab in patients with WM have achieved overall response rates of 80–90% (Ghobrial et al. 2008; Agathocleous et al. 2010). The European Myeloma Network (EMN) recently showed that transitioning bortezomib from twice weekly intravenous dosing during the first cycle to weekly administration thereafter reduced grade 3 neuropathy to under 10% in patients treated with BDR (Dimopoulos et al. 2013). Overall, treatment was well tolerated, and the overall response rate was 85% that included 68% major responders. The median PFS in this study was 43 months (Gavriatopoulou et al. 2017). While subcutaneous bortezomib is also used to decrease risk of treatment-related neuropathy with bortezomib, no formal studies addressing the safety and efficacy of subcutaneous bortezomib use in WM have been reported.

Carfilzomib is a proteasome inhibitor that is associated with a low risk of treatment-related peripheral neuropathy. The combination of carfilzomib with rituximab and dexamethasone (CaRD) was evaluated in WM patients (Treon et al. 2014a). Carfilzomib was administered intravenously at 20 mg/m^2 (cycle 1), then 36 mg/m^2 (cycles 2–6), together with dexamethasone (20 mg) on days 1, 2, 8, 9 as part of a 21-day cycle. As part of this regimen, rituximab 375 mg/m^2 was given on days 2 and 9 every 21 days. Maintenance therapy was given 8 weeks following induction therapy with intravenous carfilzomib (36 mg/m^2) and dexamethasone (20 mg) administered on days 1, 2 and rituximab 375 mg/m^2 on day 2 every 8 weeks for up to eight cycles. Overall response rate with this regimen was 87% with major responses observed in 68% of patients and was not impacted by MYD88^{L265P} or CXCR4^{WHIM} mutation status. With a median follow-up of 15.4 months, 20 patients remained progression-free. Grade ≥2 toxicities included asymptomatic hyperlipasemia (41.9%), reversible neutropenia (12.9%), and cardiomyopathy in one patient (3.2%) with multiple risk factors. Treatment-related neuropathy occurred in one patient (3.2%) that was grade 2. Declines in serum IgA and IgG were common, and some patients required intravenous gamma globulin therapy for recurring sinus and bronchial infections.

11.6.2.6 Novel Therapeutics

The use of ibrutinib was recently approved by the US Food and Drug Administration and the European Medicines Agency for the treatment of symptomatic patients with WM. Ibrutinib targets BTK and HCK, both targets of ibrutinib that are transactivated by MYD88^{L265P} (Yang et al. 2013; Yang et al. 2016). In a multicenter study that examined the role of ibrutinib in previously treated (median 2 prior therapies, 40% refractory) WM patients, the overall response rate was 91% (Treon et al. 2015c). Patients on this study received 420 mg a day of ibrutinib by mouth. Post-therapy, median serum IgM levels declined from 3610 to 880 mg/dL, hemoglobin rose from 10.5 to 13.8 g/dL, and bone marrow involvement declined from 60% to 25%. Decreased or resolved adenopathy was observed in 60% of patients with extramedullary disease, and five of nine patients with IgM-related PN had symptomatic improvement. At a median of 37 months of follow-up, the median progression-free and overall survival was 68% and 90%, respectively. Major responses were absent in patients with wild-type MYD88, and slower response kinetics were observed in those patients who were both MYD88 and CXCR4 mutated. Major response rates were also lower in those patients with CXCR4 mutations (62%) versus those with wild-type CXCR4 (92%). Grade ≥2 treatment-related toxicities

included neutropenia (25%) and thrombocytopenia (14%) that were more common in heavily pretreated patients, atrial fibrillation associated with a prior history of arrhythmia (5%), and bleeding associated with procedures and marine oil supplements (3%). Serum IgA and IgG levels were unchanged following treatment with ibrutinib, and treatment-related infections were infrequent. A multicenter trial also examined the activity of ibrutinib in rituximab-refractory WM patients who had a median of four prior therapies. The overall response rate in this study was 90%, with major responses observed in 71% of patients. With a median follow-up of 18 months, the median progression-free and overall survival was 86% and 97% (Dimopoulos et al. 2016). Delays in serum IgM and hemoglobin responses were observed among MYD88-mutated patients with CXCR4 mutations, versus those who were wild type for CXCR4. One patient with wild-type MYD88 did not respond. A clinical study of the CXCR4 antagonist ulocuplumab with ibrutinib is being initiated in symptomatic WM patients with CXCR4 mutations.

Everolimus is an oral inhibitor of the mTOR pathway that is active in WM. A multicenter study examined everolimus in 60 previously treated patients that showed an ORR of 73%, with 50% of patients attaining a major response (Ghobrial et al. 2014). The median progression-free survival in this study was 21 months. Grade 3 or higher related toxicities were observed in 67% of patients with cytopenias constituting the most common toxicity. Pulmonary toxicity occurred in 5% of patients, and dose reductions due to toxicity occurred in 52% of patients. A clinical trial examining the activity of everolimus in 33 previously untreated patients with WM has also been reported that included serial bone marrow biopsies in response assessment (Treon et al. 2016). The ORR in this study was 72%, including partial or better responses in 60% of patients. Among genotyped patients, nonresponders associated with wild-type MYD88 and mutated CXCR4 status. Median time to response was 4 weeks. Discordance between serum IgM levels and bone marrow disease burden was remarkable. The median time to progression was 21 months for all patients and 33 months for major responders. Discontinuation of everolimus led to rapid serum IgM rebound in seven patients and symptomatic hyperviscosity in two patients. Toxicity led to treatment discontinuation in 27% of patients, including 18% for pneumonitis which appeared more pronounced versus previously treated WM patients.

11.6.2.7 Maintenance Therapy

The outcome of rituximab-naïve patients who were either observed or received maintenance rituximab categorical responses was examined in a large retrospective study (Treon et al. 2011b). Categorical responses improved after induction therapy in 42% of patients who received maintenance rituximab versus 10% in patients on observation. Additionally, both progression-free (56.3 vs. 28.6 months) and overall survival (>120 vs. 116 months) were longer in patients who received maintenance rituximab. Improved progression-free survival was evident despite previous treatment status, induction with rituximab alone or in combination therapy. Best serum IgM response was also lower and hematocrit higher in those patients who received maintenance rituximab. Among patients who received maintenance rituximab therapy, an increased number of infectious events, predominantly grade 1 or 2 sinusitis and bronchitis, were observed, along with lower serum IgA and IgG levels. A prospective study examining the role of maintenance rituximab has also been initiated by the German STiL group (Rummel et al. 2012). In this study, patients received up to six cycles of bendamustine and rituximab, and responders randomized to either observation or maintenance rituximab every 2 months for 2 years. Enrollment for this study is complete, and response outcome for maintenance rituximab therapy is awaited.

11.6.3 High-Dose Therapy and Stem Cell Transplantation

The European Bone Marrow Transplant Registry reported the largest experience for both autologous and allogeneic SCT in WM (Kyriakou et al. 2010a, b). Among 158 WM patients receiving an autologous SCT, which included primarily relapsed or refractory patients, the 5-year progression-free and overall survival rate was 39.7% and 68.5%, respectively (Kyriakou et al. 2010a). Non-relapse mortality at 1 year was 3.8%. Chemorefractory disease and the number of prior lines of therapy at time of the autologous SCT were the most important prognostic factors for progression-free and overall survival. In the allogeneic SCT experience from the EBMT, the long-term outcome of 86 WM patients was reported (Kyriakou et al. 2010b). A total of 86 patients received allograft by either myeloablative or reduced-intensity conditioning. The median age of patients in this series was 49 years, and 47 patients had three or more previous lines of therapy. Eight patients failed prior autologous SCT. Fifty-nine patients (68.6%) had chemotherapy-sensitive disease at the time of allogeneic SCT. Non-relapse mortality at 3 years was 33% for patients receiving a myeloablative transplant and 23% for those who received reduced-intensity conditioning. The overall response rate was 75.6%. The relapse rates at 3 years were 11% for myeloablative and 25% for reduced-intensity conditioning recipients. Five-year progression-free and overall survival for WM patients who received a myeloablative allogeneic SCT were 56% and 62% and for patients who received reduced-intensity conditioning were 49% and 64%, respectively. The occurrence of chronic graft-versus-host disease was associated with improved progression-free survival and suggested the existence of a clinically relevant graft-versus-WM effect in this study.

11.7 Response Criteria in Waldenström Macroglobulinemia

Table 11.3 summarizes the response categories and criteria for progressive disease in WM based on the most recent consensus recommendations (Owen et al. 2013). The term "overall response" is used to characterize all responses, including minor responses. "Major responses" only include partial, very good partial, and complete responses.

Table 11.3 Summary of consensus response criteria for Waldenström's macroglobulinemia (Owen et al. 2013)

Complete response	CR	Absence of serum monoclonal IgM protein by immunofixation
		Normal serum IgM level
		Complete resolution of extramedullary disease, i.e., lymphadenopathy/splenomegaly if present at baseline
		Morphologically normal bone marrow aspirate and trephine biopsy
Very good partial response	VGPR	Monoclonal IgM protein is detectable
		90% reduction in serum IgM level from baseline or normalization of serum IgM level
		Complete resolution of extramedullary disease, i.e., lymphadenopathy/splenomegaly if present at baseline
		No new signs or symptoms of active disease
Partial response	PR	Monoclonal IgM protein is detectable
		$\geq$50% but <90% reduction in serum IgM level from baseline
		Reduction in extramedullary disease, i.e., lymphadenopathy/splenomegaly if present at baseline
		No new signs or symptoms of active disease
Minor response	MR	Monoclonal IgM protein is detectable
		$\geq$25% but <50% reduction in serum IgM level from baseline
		No new signs or symptoms of active disease
Stable disease	SD	Monoclonal IgM protein is detectable
		<25% reduction and <25% increase in serum IgM level from baseline
		No progression in extramedullary disease, i.e., lymphadenopathy/splenomegaly
		No new signs or symptoms of active disease
Progressive disease	PD	>25% increase in serum IgM level from lowest nadir (requires confirmation) and/or progression in clinical features attributable to the disease

The attainment of very good partial or complete responses is associated with improved progression-free survival (Treon et al. 2009a, b, 2011c; Dimopoulos et al. 2013; Kyriakou et al. 2010a). Response assessments in WM rely primarily on serum IgM or IgM paraprotein levels, though complete responses require disappearance of the IgM monoclonal protein and resolution of bone marrow and/or extramedullary WM disease (Owen et al. 2013). An important concern with the use of IgM as a surrogate marker of disease is that it can fluctuate, independent of tumor cell killing with some agents. By way of example, rituximab can induce a flare in serum IgM levels, whereas everolimus, bortezomib, and ibrutinib can suppress IgM levels independent of tumor cell killing in some patients, a finding referred to as IgM discordance (Treon et al. 2007; Dimopoulos et al. 2002; Treon et al. 2004; Ghobrial et al. 2004; Treon et al. 2015c; Treon et al. 2016; Strauss et al. 2006). Moreover, with selective B-cell depleting agents such as

rituximab and alemtuzumab, residual IgM-producing plasma cells are spared and continue to persist, thus potentially skewing the relative response and assessment to treatment (Varghese et al. 2009). Soluble CD27 levels have been investigated as an alternative surrogate marker in WM given their correlation with WM disease burden and may remain a faithful marker of disease in patients experiencing a rituximab-related IgM flare, as well as after plasmapheresis (Ciccarelli et al. 2009). The use of quantitative allele-specific polymerase chain reaction assays to assess serial MYD88^{L265P} burden in WM patients is also under investigation (Xu et al. 2013; Jiménez et al. 2013; Xu et al. 2014).

11.8 Course and Prognosis

WM typically presents as an indolent disease. The presence of 6q deletions may have prognostic significance, but does not appear to impact overall survival (Nguyen-Khac et al. 2013; Ocio et al. 2007; Chang et al. 2009). Age is an important prognostic factor (>65 years) (Gobbi et al. 1994; Morel et al. 2000; Dimopoulos et al. 2004) but is influenced by comorbidities. Anemia that reflects both marrow involvement and the serum level of the IgM monoclonal protein (because of the impact of IgM on intravascular fluid retention) has emerged as a strong adverse prognostic factor with hemoglobin levels of <9–12 g/dL associated with decreased survival in several series (Dhodapkar et al. 2001; Gobbi et al. 1994; Morel et al. 2000; Dimopoulos et al. 2004). Other cytopenias also may be significant predictors of survival, and the number of cytopenias in a given patient has been proposed as a prognostic factor (Morel et al. 2000). Serum albumin levels have also correlated with survival in some studies in WM patients (Morel et al. 2000; Dimopoulos et al. 2004). Elevated serum β_2-microglobulin levels (>3–3.5 g/dL) have also shown strong prognostic correlation in WM (Dhodapkar et al. 2001; Dimopoulos et al. 2004; Anagnostopoulos et al. 2006). Several scoring systems have been proposed based on these analyses (Table 11.4), including the WM International Prognostic Scoring System (WM IPSS) which incorporates five adverse covariates: advanced age (>65 years), hemoglobin less than or equal to 11.5 g/dL, platelet count less than or equal to 100×10^9/L, beta2-microglobulin more than 3 mg/L, and serum monoclonal protein concentration more than 7.0 g/dL (Morel et al. 2009). Among 537 WM patients evaluated in the development of WM

Table 11.4 Prognostic scoring systems in Waldenström macroglobulinemia

Study	Adverse prognostic factors	Number of groups	Survival
Gobbi et al. (1994)	Hgb <9 g/dL	0–1 prognostic factors	Median: 48 months
	Age >70 years	2–4 prognostic factors	Median: 80 months
	Weight loss		
	Cryoglobulinemia		
Morel et al. (2000)	Age ≥65 years	0–1 prognostic factors	5-year: 87% of patients
	Albumin <4 g/dL	2 prognostic factors	5-year: 62%
	Number of cytopenias:	3–4 prognostic factors	5-year: 25%
	Hgb <12 g/dL		
	Platelets <150 × 10⁹/L		
	WBC <4 × 10⁹/L		
Dhodapkar et al. (2001)	β_2M ≥3 g/dL	β_2M <3 mg/dL + Hgb ≥12 g/dL	5-year: 87% of patients
	Hgb <12 g/dL	β_2M <3 mg/dL + Hgb <12 g/dL	5-year: 63%
	IgM <4 g/dL	β_2M ≥3 mg/dL + IgM ≥4 g/dL	5-year: 53%
		β_2M ≥3 mg/dL + IgM <4 g/dL	5-year: 21%
Application of international staging system criteria for myeloma to WM Dimopoulos et al. (2004)	Albumin ≤3.5 g/dL	Albumin ≥3.5 g/dL + β_2M <3.5 mg/dL	Median: NR
	β_2M ≥3.5 mg/L	Albumin ≤3.5 g/dL + β_2M <3.5 or	Median: 116 months
		B_2M 3.5–5.5 mg/dL	Median: 54 months
		β_2M >5.5 mg/dL	
International prognostic scoring system for WM Morel et al. (2009)	Age >65 years	0–1 prognostic factors (excluding age)	5-year: 87% of patients
	Hgb <11.5 g/dL	2 prognostic factors (or age >65 years)	5-year: 68%
	Platelets <100 × 10⁹/L	3–5 prognostic factors	5-year: 36%
	β_2M >3 mg/L		
	IgM >7 g/dL		

β_2M β_2-microbloulin, *Hgb* hemogloulin, *NR* not reported, *WBC* white blood cell count

IPSS, low-risk patients (27%) presented with no or one of the adverse characteristics and advanced age, intermediate-risk patients (38%) with two adverse characteristics or only advanced age, and high-risk patients (35%) with more than two adverse characteristics. Five-year survival rates for these patients were 87%, 68%, and 36%, respectively. Importantly, the WM IPSS retained its prognostic significance in subgroups defined by age, treatment with alkylating agent, and nucleoside analogues. Recent data from the Surveillance, Epidemiology, and End Results (SEER) database involving 7744 WM patients showed that the relative survival of WM patients has improved over time (Castillo et al. 2014). Patients diagnosed during 2001–2010 had higher 5-year (78% versus 67%) and 10-year (66% versus 49%) relative survival rates versus patients diagnosed during 1980–2000. A Greek study that included 345 patients with WM failed to show any overall or cause-specific survival improvement in recent years, though the study might have been underpowered to detect any expected benefit (Castillo et al. 2014). However, a Swedish study of 1555 patients diagnosed with WM between 1980 and 2005 showed that the 5-year relative survival rate improved from 57% in 1980–1985 to 78% in 2001–2005 (Kristinsson et al. 2013).

References

Ackroyd S, O'Connor SJM, Owen RG (2005) Rarity of IgH translocations in Waldenström macroglobulinemia. Cancer Genet Cytogenet 163:77

Agathocleous A, Rohatiner A, Rule S et al (2010) Weekly versus twice weekly bortezomib given in conjunction with rituximab in patients with recurrent follicular lymphoma, mantle cell lymphoma, and Waldenström macroglobulinemia. Br J Haematol 151:346

Amrein PC, Compton CC (1990) Case records of the Massachusetts General Hospital. Weekly clinicopathological exercises. Case 3–1990. A 66-year-old woman with Waldenström's macroglobulinemia, diarrhea, anemia, and persistent gastrointestinal bleeding. N Engl J Med 322:183

Anagnostopoulos A, Zervas K, Kyrtsonis M et al (2006) Prognostic value of serum beta 2-microglobulin in patients with Waldenström's macroglobulinemia requiring therapy. Clin Lymphoma Myeloma 7:205

Ansell SM, Hodge LS, Secreto FJ et al (2014) Activation of TAK1 by MYD88 L265P drives malignant B-cell growth in non-Hodgkin lymphoma. Blood Cancer J 4:e183. https://doi.org/10.1038/bcj.2014.4

Aoki H, Takishita M, Kosaka M, Saito S (1995) Frequent somatic mutations in D and/or JH segments of Ig gene in Waldenström's macroglobulinemia and chronic lymphocytic leukemia (CLL) with Richter's syndrome but not in common CLL. Blood 85:1913

Avet-Loiseau H, Garand R, Lode L, Robillard N, Bataille R (2003) 14q32 translocations discriminate IgM multiple myeloma from Waldenstrom's macroglobulinemia. Semin Oncol 30:153

Betticher DC, Hsu Schmitz SF, Ratschiller D et al (1997) Cladribine (2-CDA) given as subcutaneous bolus injections is active in pretreated Waldenström's macroglobulinaemia. Swiss Group for Clinical Cancer Research (SAKK). Br J Haematol 99:358

Bjornsson OG, Arnason A, Gudmunosson S et al (1978) Macroglobulinaemia in an Icelandic family. Acta Med Scand 203:283

Braggio E, Keats JJ, Leleu X et al (2009a) High-resolution genomic analysis in Waldenström's macroglobulinemia identifies disease-specific and common abnormalities with marginal zone lymphomas. Clin Lymphoma Myeloma 9:39

Braggio E, Keats JJ, Leleu X et al (2009b) Identification of copy number abnormalities and inactivating mutations in two negative regulators of nuclear factor-kappaB signaling pathways in Waldenstrom's macroglobulinemia. Cancer Res 69:3579

Busillo JM, Amando S, Sengupta R et al (2010) Site-specific phosphorylation of CXCR4 is dynamically regulated by multiple kinases and results in differential modulation of CXCR4 signaling. J Biol Chem 285:7805

Buske C, Hoster E, Dreyling MH et al (2009) The addition of rituximab to front-line therapy with CHOP (R-CHOP) results in a higher response rate and longer time to treatment failure in patients with lymphoplasmacytic lymphoma: results of a randomized trial of the German Low-Grade Lymphoma Study Group (GLSG). Leukemia 23:153

Cao Y, Hunter ZR, Liu X et al (2014) The WHIM-like CXCR4S338X somatic mutation activates AKT and ERK, and promotes resistance to ibrutinib and other agents used in the treatment of Waldenstrom's Macroglobulinemia. Leukemia 29(1):169–176. https://doi.org/10.1038/leu.2014.187

Cao Y, Hunter ZR, Liu X et al (2015) CXCR4 WHIM-like frameshift and nonsense mutations promote ibrutinib resistance but do not supplant MYD88 L265P directed signaling in Waldenstrom macroglobulinaemia cells. Br J Haematol 168:701

Case DC Jr, Ervin TJ, Boyd MA, Redfield DL (1991) Waldenström's macroglobulinemia: long-term results with the M-2 protocol. Cancer Investig 9:1

Castillo JJ, Olszewski A, Cronin AM et al (2014) Survival trends in Waldenstrom macroglobulinemia: an analysis of the Surveillance, Epidemiology and End Results database. Blood 123:3999

Chang H, Qi C, Trieu Y et al (2009) Prognostic relevance of 6q deletion in Waldenström's macroglobulinemia: a multicenter study. Clin Lymphoma Myeloma 9(1):36

Chassande B, Leger JM, Younes-Chennoufi AB et al (1998) Peripheral neuropathy associated with IgM monoclonal gammopathy: correlations between M-protein antibody activity and clinical/electrophysiological features in 40 cases. Muscle Nerve 21:55

Chen CI, Kouroukis CT, White D et al (2007) Bortezomib is active in patients with untreated or relapsed Waldenström's macroglobulinemia: a phase II study of the National Cancer Institute of Canada Clinical Trials Group. J Clin Oncol 25:1570

Ciccarelli BT, Yang G, Hatjiharissi E et al (2009) Soluble CD27 is a faithful marker of disease burden and is unaffected by the rituximab induced IgM flare, as well as plasmapheresis in patients with Waldenström's macroglobulinemia. Clin Lymphoma Myeloma 9:56

Ciccarelli BT, Patterson CJ, Hunter ZR et al (2011) Hepcidin is produced by lymphoplasmacytic cells and is associated with anemia in Waldenström's Macroglobulinemia. Clin Lymphoma Myeloma Leuk 11:160

Cohen L, Henzel WJ, Baeuerie PA (1998) IKAP is a scaffold protein of the IkappaB kinase complex. Nature 395:292

Crisp D, Pruzanski W (1982) B-cell neoplasms with homogeneous cold-reacting antibodies (cold agglutinins). Am J Med 72:915

Dalakas MC, Quarles RH (1996) Autoimmune ataxic neuropathies (sensory ganglionopathies): are glycolipids the responsible autoantigens? Ann Neurol 39:419

Daoud MS, Lust JA, Kyle RA, Pittelkow MR (1999) Monoclonal gammopathies and associated skin disorders. J Am Acad Dermatol 40:507

Delannoy A, Ferrant A, Martiat P et al (1994) 2-Chlorodeoxyadenosine therapy in Waldenström's macroglobulinaemia. Nouv Rev Fr Hematol 36:317

Dellagi K, Dupouey P, Brouet JC et al (1983) Waldenström's macroglobulinemia and peripheral neuropathy: a clinical and immunologic study of 25 patients. Blood 62:280

Dhodapkar MV, Jacobson JL, Gertz MA et al (2001) Prognostic factors and response to fludarabine therapy in patients with Waldenström macroglobulinemia: results of United States intergroup trial (Southwest Oncology Group S9003). Blood 98:41

Dimopoulos M, Gika D, Zervas K et al (2004) The international staging system for multiple myeloma is applicable in symptomatic Waldenström's macroglobulinemia. Leuk Lymphoma 45:1809

Dimopoulos MA, Alexanian R (1994) Waldenström's macroglobulinemia. Blood 83:1452

Dimopoulos MA, O'Brien S, Kantarjian H et al (1993) Fludarabine therapy in Waldenström's macroglobulinemia. Am J Med 95:49

Dimopoulos MA, Kantarjian H, Weber D et al (1994a) Primary therapy of Waldenström's macroglobulinemia with 2-chlorodeoxyadenosine. J Clin Oncol 12:2694

Dimopoulos MA, Weber DM, Kantarjian H et al (1994b) 2-Chlorodeoxyadenosine therapy of patients with Waldenström macroglobulinemia previously treated with fludarabine. Ann Oncol 5:288

Dimopoulos MA, Weber D, Delasalle KB et al (1995) Treatment of Waldenström's macroglobulinemia resistant to standard therapy with 2-chlorodeoxyadenosine: identification of prognostic factors. Ann Oncol 6:49

Dimopoulos MA, Zervas C, Zomas A et al (2002) Treatment of Waldenström's macroglobulinemia with rituximab. J Clin Oncol 20:2327

Dimopoulos MA, Hamilos G, Efstathiou E et al (2003) Treatment of Waldenström's macroglobulinemia with the combination of fludarabine and cyclophosphamide. Leuk Lymphoma 44:993

Dimopoulos MA, Anagnostopoulos A, Zervas C et al (2005a) Predictive factors for response to rituximab in Waldenström's macroglobulinemia. Clin Lymphoma 5:270

Dimopoulos MA, Anagnostopulos A, Kyrtsonis MC et al (2005b) Treatment of relapsed or refractory Waldenstrom's macroglobulinemia with bortezomib. Haematologica 90:1655

Dimopoulos MA, Anagnostopoulos A, Kyrtsonis MC et al (2007) Primary treatment of Waldenström's macroglobulinemia with dexamethasone, rituximab and cyclophosphamide. J Clin Oncol 25:3344

Dimopoulos MA, García-Sanz R, Gavriatopoulou M et al (2013) Primary therapy of Waldenstrom macroglobulinemia (WM) with weekly bortezomib, low-dose dexamethasone, and rituximab (BDR): long-term results of a phase 2 study of the European Myeloma Network (EMN). Blood 122:3276

Dimopoulos MA, Trotman J, Tedeschi A et al (2016) Single agent ibrutinib in rituximab-refractory patients with Waldenström's macroglobulinemia: results from a multicenter, open-label phase 3 substudy (iNNO-VATE™). Lancet Oncol 18(2):241

Dotta L, Tassone L, Badolato R (2011) Clinical and genetic features of Warts, Hypogammaglobulinemia, Infections and Myelokathexis (WHIM) syndrome. Curr Mol Med 11:317

Dussol B, Kaplanski G, Daniel L et al (1998) Simultaneous occurrence of fibrillary glomerulopathy and AL amyloid. Nephrol Dial Transplant 13:2630

Dutcher TF, Fahey JL (1959) The histopathology of macroglobulinemia of Waldenström. J Natl Cancer Inst 22:887

Ettl AR, Birbamer GG, Philipp W (1992) Orbital involvement in Waldenström's macroglobulinemia: ultrasound, computed tomography and magnetic resonance findings. Ophthalmologica 205:40

Eurelings M, Ang CW, Notermans NC et al (2001) Antiganglioside antibodies in polyneuropathy associated with monoclonal gammopathy. Neurology 57:1909

Facon T, Brouillard M, Duhamel A et al (1993) Prognostic factors in Waldenström's macroglobulinemia: a report of 167 cases. J Clin Oncol 11:1553

Fadil A, Taylor DE (1998) The lung and Waldenström's macroglobulinemia. South Med J 91:681

Farhangi M, Merlini G (1986) The clinical implications of monoclonal immunoglobulins. Semin Oncol 13:366

Feiner HD, Rizk CC, Finfer MD et al (1990) IgM monoclonal gammopathy/Waldenström's macroglobulinemia: a morphological and immunophenotypic study of the bone marrow. Mod Pathol 3:348

Foran JM, Rohatiner AZ, Coiffier B et al (1999) Multicenter phase II study of fludarabine phosphate for patients with newly diagnosed lymphoplasmacytoid lymphoma, Waldenström's macroglobulinemia, and mantle-cell lymphoma. J Clin Oncol 17:546

Fridrik MA, Jager G, Baldinger C et al (1997) First-line treatment of Waldenström's disease with cladribine. Arbeitsgemeinschaft Medikamentose Tumortherapie. Ann Hematol 74:7

Gad A, Willen R, Carlen B et al (1995) Duodenal involvement in Waldenström's macroglobulinemia. J Clin Gastroenterol 20:174

Gardyn J, Schwartz A, Gal R et al (2001) Waldenström's macroglobulinemia associated with AA amyloidosis. Int J Hematol 74:76

Gavriatopoulou M, Garcia-Sanz R, Kastritis E et al (2017) BDR in newly diagnosed patients with WM: final analysis of a phase 2 study after a minimum follow up of 6 years. Blood 129(4):456

Gertz MA, Kyle RA (1995) Hyperviscosity syndrome. J Intensive Care Med 10:128

Gertz MA, Kyle RA, Noel P (1993) Primary systemic amyloidosis: a rare complication of immunoglobulin M monoclonal gammopathies and Waldenström's macroglobulinemia. J Clin Oncol 11:914

Gertz MA, Rue M, Blood E et al (2004) Multicenter phase 2 trial of rituximab for Waldenström macroglobulinemia (WM): an Eastern Cooperative Oncology Group Study (E3A98). Leuk Lymphoma 45:2047

Ghobrial IM, Fonseca R, Greipp PR et al (2004) Initial immunoglobulin M "flare" after rituximab therapy in patients with Waldenström macroglobulinemia: an Eastern Cooperative Oncology Group Study. Cancer 101:2593

Ghobrial IM, Matous J, Padmanabhan S et al (2008) Phase II trial of combination of bortezomib and rituximab in relapsed and/or refractory Waldenström's macroglobulinemia. Blood 112:832

Ghobrial IM, Witzig TE, Gertz M et al (2014) Long-term results of the phase II trial of the oral mTOR inhibitor everolimus (RAD001) in relapsed or refractory Waldenstrom Macroglobulinemia. Am J Hematol 89(3):237

Gobbi PG, Bettini R, Montecucco C et al (1994) Study of prognosis in Waldenström's macroglobulinemia: a proposal for a simple binary classification with clinical and investigational utility. Blood 83:2939

Gordon PH, Rowland LP, Younger DS et al (1997) Lymphoproliferative disorders and motor neuron disease: an update. Neurology 48:1671

Groves FD, Travis LB, Devesa SS et al (1998) Waldenström's macroglobulinemia: incidence patterns in the United States, 1988–1994. Cancer 82:1078

Hanzis C, Ojha RP, Hunter Z et al (2011) Associated malignancies in patients with Waldenström's macroglobulinemia and their kin. Clin Lymphoma Myeloma Leuk 11:88

Harris NL, Jaffe ES, Stein H et al (1994) A revised European-American classification of lymphoid neoplasms: a proposal from the International Lymphoma Study Group. Blood 84:1361

Harris NL, Jaffe ES, Diebold J et al (1999) The World Health Organization classification of neoplastic diseases of the hematopoietic and lymphoid tissues. Report of the Clinical Advisory Committee meeting, Airlie House, Virginia, November, 1997. Ann Oncol 10:1419

Hellmann A, Lewandowski K, Zaucha JM et al (1999) Effect of a 2-hour infusion of 2-chlorodeoxyadenosine in the treatment of refractory or previously untreated Waldenström's macroglobulinemia. Eur J Haematol 63:35

Hensel M, Villalobos M, Kornacker M et al (2005) Pentostatin/cyclophosphamide with or without rituximab: an effective regimen for patients with Waldenström's macroglobulinemia/lymphoplasmacytic lymphoma. Clin Lymphoma Myeloma 6:131

Herrinton LJ, Weiss NS (1993) Incidence of Waldenström's macroglobulinemia. Blood 82:3148

Ho AW, Hatjiharissi E, Ciccarelli BT et al (2008) CD27-CD70 interactions in the pathogenesis of Waldenstrom macroglobulinemia. Blood 112:4683

Hunter ZR, Branagan AR, Manning R et al (2005) CD5, CD10, and CD23 expression in Waldenstrom's macroglobulinemia. Clin Lymphoma 5:246

Hunter ZR, Manning RJ, Hanzis C et al (2010) IgA and IgG hypogammaglobulinemia in Waldenstrom's Macroglobulinemia. Haematologica 95:470

Hunter ZR, Xu L, Yang G et al (2014) The genomic landscape of Waldenstom's Macroglobulinemia is characterized by highly recurring MYD88 and WHIM-like CXCR4 mutations, and small somatic deletions associated with B-cell lymphomagenesis. Blood 123:1637

Ilyas AA, Quarles RH, Dalakas MC et al (1985) Monoclonal IgM in a patient with paraproteinemic polyneuropathy binds to gangliosides containing disialosyl groups. Ann Neurol 18:655

Ioakimidis L, Patterson CJ, Hunter ZR et al (2009) Comparative outcomes following CP-R, CVP-R and CHOP-R in Waldenström's macroglobulinemia. Clin Lymphoma Myeloma 9:62

Isaac J, Herrera GA (2002) Cast nephropathy in a case of Waldenström's macroglobulinemia. Nephron 91:512

Jacobs BC, O'Hanlon GM, Breedland EG et al (1997) Human IgM paraproteins demonstrate shared reactivity between Campylobacter jejuni lipopolysaccharides and human peripheral nerve disialylated gangliosides. J Neuroimmunol 80:23

Jiménez C, Sebastián E, Del Carmen Chillón M et al (2013) MYD88 L265P is a marker highly characteristic of, but not restricted to, Waldenström's macroglobulinemia. Leukemia 27:1722

Kaila VL, el Newihi HM, Dreiling BJ et al (1996) Waldenström's macroglobulinemia of the stomach presenting with upper gastrointestinal hemorrhage. Gastrointest Endosc 44:73

Kawagoe T, Sato S, Matsushita K et al (2008) Sequential control of Toll-like receptor dependent responses by IRAK1 and IRAK2. Nat Immunol 9:684

Kristinsson SY, Eloranta S, Dickman PW et al (2013) Patterns of survival in lymphoplasmacytic lymphoma/Waldenstrom macroglobulinemia: a population based study of 1,555 patients diagnosed in Sweden from 1980 to 2005. Am J Hematol 88:60

Kwaan HC, Bongu A (1999) The hyperviscosity syndromes. Semin Thromb Hemost 25:199

Kyle RA, Greipp PR, Gertz MA et al (2000) Waldenström's macroglobulinaemia: a prospective study comparing daily with intermittent oral chlorambucil. Br J Haematol 108:737

Kyle RA, Treon SP, Alexanian R et al (2003) Prognostic markers and criteria to initiate therapy in Waldenström's macroglobulinemia: consensus panel recommendations from the Second International Workshop on Waldenström's macroglobulinemia. Semin Oncol 30:116

Kyriakou C, Canals C, Sibon D et al (2010a) High-dose therapy and autologous stem-cell transplantation in Waldenstrom macroglobulinemia: the Lymphoma Working Party of the European Group for Blood and Marrow Transplantation. J Clin Oncol 28:2227

Kyriakou C, Canals C, Cornelissen JJ et al (2010b) Allogeneic stem-cell transplantation in patients with Waldenström macroglobulinemia: report from the Lymphoma Working Party of the European Group for Blood and Marrow Transplantation. J Clin Oncol 28:4926

Kyrtsonis MC, Angelopoulou MK, Kontopidou FN et al (2001) Primary lung involvement in Waldenström's macroglobulinaemia: report of two cases and review of the literature. Acta Haematol 105:92

Landgren O, Staudt L (2012) MYD88 L265P somatic mutation in IgM MGUS. N Engl J Med 367:2255

Latov N, Braun PE, Gross RB et al (1981) Plasma cell dyscrasia and peripheral neuropathy: identification of the myelin antigens that react with human paraproteins. Proc Natl Acad Sci U S A 78:7139

Latov N, Hays AP, Sherman WH (1988) Peripheral neuropathy and anti-MAG antibodies. Crit Rev Neurobiol 3:301

Leblond V, Ben Othman T, Deconinck E et al (1998) Activity of fludarabine in previously treated Waldenström's macroglobulinemia: a report of 71 cases. Groupe Cooperatif Macroglobulinemie. J Clin Oncol 16:2060

Leblond V, Johnson S, Chevret S et al (2013) Results of a randomized trial of chlorambucil versus fludarabine for patients with Waldenstrom macroglobulinemia, marginal zone lymphoma, or lymphoplasmacytic lymphoma. J Clin Oncol 31:301

Leblond V, Kastritis E, Advani R et al (2016) Treatment recommendations for Waldenström macroglobulin-

emia from the Eighth International Workshop on WM. Blood 128:1321

Leleu X, O'Connor K, Ho A et al (2007) Hepatitis C viral infection is not associated with Waldenström's macroglobulinemia. Am J Hematol 82:83

Leleu X, Eeckhoute J, Jia X et al (2008) Targeting NF-kappaB in Waldenstrom macroglobulinemia. Blood 111:5068

Leleu XP, Manning R, Soumerai JD et al (2009a) Increased incidence of transformation and myelodysplasia/acute leukemia in patients with Waldenström macroglobulinemia treated with nucleoside analogs. J Clin Oncol 27:250

Leleu XP, Tamburini J, Roccaro A et al (2009b) Balancing risk versus benefit in the treatment of Waldenström's macroglobulinemia patients with nucleoside analogue based therapy. Clin Lymphoma Myeloma 9:71

Lewandowski K, Halaburda K, Hellmann A (2002) Fludarabine therapy in Waldenström's macroglobulinemia patients treated previously with 2-chlorodeoxyadenosine. Leuk Lymphoma 43:361

Lin SC, Lo YC, Wu H (2010) Helical assembly in the MYD88-IRAK4-IRAK2 complex in TLR/IL-1R signaling. Nature 465:885

Liu ES, Burian C, Miller WE, Saven A (1998) Bolus administration of cladribine in the treatment of Waldenström macroglobulinaemia. Br J Haematol 103:690

Loiarro M, Gallo G, Fanto N et al (2009) Identification of critical residues of the MYD88 death domain involved in the recruitment of downstream kinases. J Biol Chem 284:28093

Lopate G, Choksi R, Pestronk A (2002) Severe sensory ataxia and demyelinating polyneuropathy with IgM anti-GM$_2$ and GalNAc-GD1A antibodies. Muscle Nerve 25:828

Mackenzie MR, Babcock J (1975) Studies of the hyperviscosity syndrome. II: macroglobulinemia. J Lab Clin Med 85:227

Marmont AM, Merlini G (1991) Monoclonal autoimmunity in hematology. Haematologica 76:449

Mascaro JM, Montserrat E, Estrach T et al (1982) Specific cutaneous manifestations of Waldenström's macroglobulinaemia. A report of two cases. Br J Dermatol 106:217

Menke MN, Treon SP (2007) Hyperviscosity syndrome. In: Sekeres, Kalaycio, Bolwell (eds) Clinical malignant hematology. McGraw Hill Publishing, New York, pp 937–941

Menke MN, Feke GT, McMeel JW et al (2006) Hyperviscosity-related retinopathy in Waldenström's macroglobulinemia. Arch Ophthalmol 124:1601

Merlini G, Farhangi M, Osserman EF (1986) Monoclonal immunoglobulins with antibody activity in myeloma, macroglobulinemia and related plasma cell dyscrasias. Semin Oncol 13:350

Minnema MC, Kimby E, D'Sa S et al (2017) Guideline for the diagnosis, treatment and response criteria for Bing-Neel syndrome. Haematologica 102:43–51. https://doi.org/10.3324/haematol.2016.147728

Moore DF Jr, Moulopoulos LA, Dimopoulos MA (1995) Waldenström macroglobulinemia presenting as a renal or perirenal mass: clinical and radiographic features. Leuk Lymphoma 17:331

Morel P, Monconduit M, Jacomy D et al (2000) Prognostic factors in Waldenström macroglobulinemia: a report on 232 patients with the description of a new scoring system and its validation on 253 other patients. Blood 96:852

Morel P, Duhamel A, Gobbi P et al (2009) International prognostic scoring system for Waldenström macroglobulinemia. Blood 113:4163

Morel-Maroger L, Basch A, Danon F et al (1970) Pathology of the kidney in Waldenström's macroglobulinemia. Study of sixteen cases. N Engl J Med 283:123

Moulopoulos LA, Dimopoulos MA, Varma DG et al (1993) Waldenström macroglobulinemia: MR imaging of the spine and CT of the abdomen and pelvis. Radiology 188:669

Moyner K, Sletten K, Husby G, Natvig JB (1980) An unusually large (83 amino acid residues) amyloid fibril protein AA from a patient with Waldenström's macroglobulinaemia and amyloidosis. Scand J Immunol 11:549

Nemni R, Gerosa E, Piccolo G, Merlini G (1994) Neuropathies associated with monoclonal gammopathies. Haematologica 79:557

Ngo HT, Leleu X, Lee J et al (2008) SDF-1/CXCR4 and VLA-4 interaction regulates homing in Waldenstrom macroglobulinemia. Blood 112:150

Ngo VN, Young RM, Schmitz R, Jhavar S, Xiao W, Lim KH et al (2011) Oncogenically active MYD88 mutations in human lymphoma. Nature 470:115

Nguyen-Khac F, Lambert J, Chapiro E et al (2013) Chromosomal aberrations and their prognostic value in a series of 174 untreated patients with Waldenstrom's macroglobulinemia. Haematologica 98:649

Nobile-Orazio E, Marmiroli P, Baldini L et al (1987) Peripheral neuropathy in macroglobulinemia: incidence and antigen-specificity of M proteins. Neurology 37:1506

Nobile-Orazio E, Manfredini E, Carpo M et al (1994) Frequency and clinical correlates of antineural IgM antibodies in neuropathy associated with IgM monoclonal gammopathy. Ann Neurol 36:416

Ocio EM, Schop RF, Gonzalez B et al (2007) 6q deletion in Waldenström macroglobulinemia is associated with features of adverse prognosis. Br J Haematol 136(1):80

Ogmundsdottir HM, Sveinsdottir S, Sigfusson A et al (1999) Enhanced B cell survival in familial macroglobulinaemia is associated with increased expression of Bcl-2. Clin Exp Immunol 117:252

Orellana J, Friedman AH (1981) Ocular manifestations of multiple myeloma, Waldenström's macroglobulinemia and benign monoclonal gammopathy. Surv Ophthalmol 26:157

Owen RG, Barrans SL, Richards SJ et al (2001) Waldenström macroglobulinemia. Development of diagnostic criteria and identification of prognostic factors. Am J Clin Pathol 116:420

Owen RG, Treon SP, Al-Katib A et al (2003) Clinicopathological definition of Waldenström's macroglobulinemia: Consensus Panel Recommendations from the Second International Workshop on Waldenström's macroglobulinemia. Semin Oncol 30:110

Owen RG, Kyle RA, Stone MJ et al (2013) Response assessment in Waldenstrom macroglobulinemia. Br J Haematol 160(2):171

Paiva B, Montes MC, García-Sanz R et al (2013) Multiparameter flow cytometry for the identification of the Waldenström's clone in IgM MGUS and Waldenström's macroglobulinemia: new criteria for differential diagnosis and risk stratification. Leukemia 28:166

Pavord SR, Murphy PT, Mitchell VE (1996) POEMS syndrome and Waldenström's macroglobulinaemia. J Clin Pathol 49:181

Petrucci MT, Avvisati G, Tribalto M et al (1989) Waldenström's macroglobulinaemia: results of a combined oral treatment in 34 newly diagnosed patients. J Intern Med 226:443

Popat U, Saliba R, Thandi R et al (2009) Impairment of filgrastim-induced stem cell mobilization after prior lenalidomide in patients with multiple myeloma. Biol Blood Marrow Transplant 15:718

Poulain S, Roumier C, Decambron A et al (2013) MYD88 L265P mutation in Waldenstrom's macroglobulinemia. Blood 121:4504

Preud'homme JL, Seligmann M (1972) Immunoglobulins on the surface of lymphoid cells in Waldenström's macroglobulinemia. J Clin Invest 51:701

Pruzanski W, Shumak KH (1977a) Biologic activity of cold-reacting autoantibodies (first of two parts). N Engl J Med 297:538

Pruzanski W, Shumak KH (1977b) Biologic activity of cold-reacting autoantibodies (second of two parts). N Engl J Med 297:583

Rausch PG, Herion JC (1980) Pulmonary manifestations of Waldenström macroglobulinemia. Am J Hematol 9:201

Recine MA, Perez MT, Cabello-Inchausti B et al (2001) Extranodal lymphoplasmacytoid lymphoma (immunocytoma) presenting as small intestinal obstruction. Arch Pathol Lab Med 125:677

Renier G, Ifrah N, Chevailler A et al (1989) Four brothers with Waldenström's macroglobulinemia. Cancer 64:1554

Roccaro A, Sacco A, Jiminez C et al (2014) C1013G/CXCR4 acts as a driver mutation of tumor progression and modulator of drug resistance in lymphoplasmacytic lymphoma. Blood 123:4120

Ropper AH, Gorson KC (1998) Neuropathies associated with paraproteinemia. N Engl J Med 338:1601

Rosenthal JA, Curran WJ Jr, Schuster SJ (1998) Waldenström's macroglobulinemia resulting from localized gastric lymphoplasmacytoid lymphoma. Am J Hematol 58:244

Roux S, Fermand JP, Brechignac S et al (1996) Tumoral joint involvement in multiple myeloma and Waldenström's macroglobulinemia—Report of 4 cases. J Rheumatol 23:2175

Rummel M, Niederle N, Maschmeyer G et al (2013) Bendamustine plus rituximab versus CHOP plus rituximab as first-line treatment for patients with indolent and mantle-cell lymphomas: an open-label, multicentre, randomised, phase 3 non-inferiority trial. Lancet 381:1203–1210

Rummel MJ, Lerchenmüller C, Greil R et al (2012) Bendamustine-rituximab induction followed by observation or rituximab maintenance for newly diagnosed patients with Waldenström's Macroglobulinemia: results from a prospective, randomized, multicenter study (StiL NHL 7–2008). Blood 120(21):Abstract 2739

Sahota SS, Forconi F, Ottensmeier CH et al (2002) Typical Waldenstrom macroglobulinemia is derived from a B-cell arrested after cessation of somatic mutation but prior to isotype switch events. Blood 100:1505

San Miguel JF, Vidriales MB, Ocio E et al (2003) Immunophenotypic analysis of Waldenstrom's macroglobulinemia. Semin Oncol 30:187

Santini GF, Crovatto M, Modolo ML et al (1993) Waldenström macroglobulinemia: a role of HCV infection? Blood 82:2932

Schnitzler L, Schubert B, Boasson M et al (1974) Urticaire chronique, lésions osseuses, macroglobulinémie IgM: Maladie de Waldenström? Bull Soc Fr Dermatol Syphiligr 81:363

Schop RF, Kuehl WM, Van Wier SA et al (2002) Waldenström macroglobulinemia neoplastic cells lack immunoglobulin heavy chain locus translocations but have frequent 6q deletions. Blood 100:2996

Shiokawa S, Suehiro Y, Uike N, Muta K, Nishimura J (2001) Sequence and expression analyses of mu and delta transcripts in patients with Waldenström's macroglobulinemia. Am J Hematol 68:139

Silvestri F, Barillari G, Fanin R et al (1996) Risk of hepatitis C virus infection, Waldenström's macroglobulinemia, and monoclonal gammopathies. Blood 88:1125

Singh A, Eckardt KU, Zimmermann A et al (1993) Increased plasma viscosity as a reason for inappropriate erythropoietin formation. J Clin Invest 91:251

Smith BR, Robert NJ, Ault KA (1983) Waldenstrom's macroglobulinemia the quantity of detectable circulating monoclonal B lymphocytes correlates with clinical course. Blood 61:911

Stephanie Poulain S, Roumier C, Doye E, et al (2014) Genomic landscape of CXCR4 mutations in Waldenstrom's Macroglobulinemia. Proc Am Soc Hematol: Abstract 1610

Stone MJ (2009) Waldenström's macroglobulinemia: hyperviscosity syndrome and cryoglobulinemia. Clin Lymphoma Myeloma 9:97

Stone MJ, Bogen SA (2012) Evidence-based focused review of management of hyperviscosity syndrome. Blood 119:2205

Strauss SJ, Maharaj L, Hoare S et al (2006) Bortezomib therapy in patients with relapsed or refractory lymphoma: potential correlation of in vitro sensitivity and tumor necrosis factor alpha response with clinical activity. J Clin Oncol 24:2105

Swerdlow SH, Campo E, Harris NL et al (2008) WHO classification of tumours of haematopoietic and lymphoid tissues, 4th edn. IARC Press, Lyon

Tam CS, Wolf MM, Westerman D et al (2005) Fludarabine combination therapy is highly effective in first-line and salvage treatment of patients with Waldenström's macroglobulinemia. Clin Lymphoma Myeloma 6:136

Tamburini J, Levy V, Chateilex C et al (2005) Fludarabine plus cyclophosphamide in Waldenström's macroglobulinemia: results in 49 patients. Leukemia 19:1831

Thalhammer-Scherrer R, Geissler K, Schwarzinger I et al (2000) Fludarabine therapy in Waldenström's macroglobulinemia. Ann Hematol 79:556

Tournilhac O, Santos DD, Xu L et al (2006) Mast cells in Waldenstrom's macroglobulinemia support lymphoplasmacytic cell growth through CD154/CD40 signaling. Ann Oncol 17:1275

Treon SP (2009) How I treat Waldenstrom's macroglobulinemia. Blood 114:2375

Treon SP, Agus DB, Link B et al (2001) CD20-directed antibody-mediated immunotherapy induces responses and facilitates hematologic recovery in patients with Waldenström's macroglobulinemia. J Immunother 24:272

Treon SP, Kelliher A, Keele B et al (2003) Expression of serotherapy target antigens in Waldenström's macroglobulinemia: therapeutic applications and considerations. Semin Oncol 30:248

Treon SP, Branagan AR, Hunter Z et al (2004) Paradoxical increases in serum IgM and viscosity levels following rituximab in Waldenström's macroglobulinemia. Ann Oncol 15:1481

Treon SP, Emmanouilides C, Kimby E et al (2005a) Extended rituximab therapy in Waldenström's Macroglobulinemia. Ann Oncol 16:132

Treon SP, Hansen M, Branagan AR et al (2005b) Polymorphisms in FcγRIIIA (CD16) receptor expression are associated with clinical responses to rituximab in Waldenström's macroglobulinemia. J Clin Oncol 23:474

Treon SP, Hunter Z, Branagan A (2005c) CHOP plus rituximab therapy in Waldenström's macroglobulinemia. Clin Lymphoma Myeloma 5:273

Treon SP, Hunter ZR, Matous J et al (2007) Multicenter clinical trial of bortezomib in relapsed/refractory Waldenstrom's macroglobulinemia: results of WMCTG Trial 03-248. Clin Cancer Res 13:3320

Treon SP, Branagan AR, Ioakimidis L et al (2009a) Long term outcomes to fludarabine and rituximab in Waldenström's macroglobulinemia. Blood 113:3673

Treon SP, Ioakimidis L, Soumerai JD et al (2009b) Primary therapy of Waldenström's macroglobulinemia with bortezomib, dexamethasone and rituximab. J Clin Oncol 27:3830

Treon SP, Hanzis C, Ioakimidis L et al (2010) Clinical characteristics and treatment outcome of disease-related peripheral neuropathy in Waldenstrom's macroglobulinemia (WM). J Clin Oncol 28:15s. (Abstract 8114)

Treon SP, Hanzis C, Tripsas C et al (2011a) Bendamustine therapy in patients with relapsed or refractory Waldenstrom's macroglobulinemia. Clin Lymphoma Myeloma Leuk 211:133–135

Treon SP, Hanzis C, Manning RJ et al (2011b) Maintenance rituximab is associated with improved clinical outcome in rituximab naïve patients with Waldenstrom's Macroglobulinemia who respond to a Rituximab containing regimen. Br J Haematol 154:357

Treon SP, Yang G, Hanzis C et al (2011c) Attainment of complete/very good partial response following rituximab based therapy is an important determinant to progression-free survival and is impacted by polymorphisms in FCGR3A in Waldenstrom macroglobulinaemia. Br J Haematol 154:223

Treon SP, Xu L, Yang G et al (2012) MYD88 L265P somatic mutation in Waldenstrom's macroglobulinemia. N Engl J Med 367:826

Treon SP, Tripsas C, Ciccarelli BT, Manning RJ, Patterson CJ, Sheehy P, Hunter ZR (2013) Patients with Waldenstrom macroglobulinemia commonly present with iron deficiency and those with severely depressed transferrin saturation levels show response to parenteral iron administration. Clin Lymphoma Myeloma Leuk 13:241

Treon SP, Tripsas CK, Meid K et al (2014a) Carfilzomib, rituximab and dexamethasone (CaRD) is active and offers a neuropathy-sparing approach for proteasome-inhibitor based therapy in Waldenstrom's macroglobulinemia. Blood 124:503

Treon SP, Cao Y, Xu L et al (2014b) Somatic mutations in MYD88 and CXCR4 are determinants of clinical presentation and overall survival in Waldenstrom macroglobulinemia. Blood 123:2791

Treon SP, Xu L, Hunter ZR (2015a) MYD88 mutations and response to ibrutinib in Waldenstrom's macroglobulinemia. N Engl J Med 373:584

Treon SP, Meid K, Gustine J, et al. (2015b) Long-term outcome of a prospective study of bortezomib, dexamethasone and rituximab (BDR) in previously untreated, symptomatic patients with Waldenstrom's macroglobulinemia. Blood 126(23):Abstract 1833

Treon SP, Tripsas CK, Meid K et al (2015c) Ibrutinib in previously treated patients with Waldenström's Macroglobulinemia. N Engl J Med 372(15):1430

Treon SP, Tripsas CK, Meid K et al (2016) Prospective, multicenter study of everolimus as primary therapy in Waldenstrom's Macroglobulinemia. Clin Cancer Res. https://doi.org/10.1158/1078-0432.122:1822

Varettoni M, Arcaini L, Zibellini S et al (2013) Prevalence and clinical significance of the MYD88 L265P somatic mutation in Waldenstrom macroglobulinemia, and related lymphoid neoplasms. Blood 121:2522

Varghese AM, Rawstron AC, Ashcroft J et al (2009) Assessment of bone marrow response in Waldenström's macroglobulinemia. Clin Lymphoma Myeloma 9:53

Veltman GA, van Veen S, Kluin-Nelemans JC et al (1997) Renal disease in Waldenström's macroglobulinaemia. Nephrol Dial Transplant 12:1256

Vital A (2001) Paraproteinemic neuropathies. Brain Pathol 11:399

Wagner SD, Martinelli V, Luzzatto L (1994) Similar patterns of V kappa gene usage but different degrees of somatic mutation in hairy cell leukemia, prolymphocytic leukemia, Waldenstrom's macroglobulinemia, and myeloma. Blood 83:3647

Watters T, Kenny EF, O'Neill LAJ (2007) Structure, function and regulation of the Toll/IL-1 receptor adaptor proteins. Immunol Cell Biol 85:411

Weber DM, Dimopoulos MA, Delasalle K et al (2003) 2-chlorodeoxyadenosine alone and in combination for previously untreated Waldenström's macroglobulinemia. Semin Oncol 30:243

Weiss MD, Dalakas MC, Lauter CJ et al (1999) Variability in the binding of anti-MAG and anti-SGPG antibodies to target antigens in demyelinating neuropathy and IgM paraproteinemia. J Neuroimmunol 95:174

Whittaker SJ, Bhogal BS, Black MM (1996) Acquired immunobullous disease: a cutaneous manifestation of IgM macroglobulinemia. Br J Dermatol 135:283

Willison HJ, O'Leary CP, Veitch J et al (2001) The clinical and laboratory features of chronic sensory ataxic neuropathy with anti-disialosyl IgM antibodies. Brain 124:1968

Xu L, Hunter Z, Yang G et al (2013) MYD88 L265P in Waldenstrom macroglobulinemia, immunoglobulin M monoclonal gammopathy, and other B-cell lymphoproliferative disorders using conventional and quantitative allele-specific polymerase chain reaction. Blood 121:2051

Xu L, Hunter ZR, Yang G et al (2014) Detection of MYD88 L265P in peripheral blood of patients with Waldenström's Macroglobulinemia and IgM Monoclonal Gammopathy by allele-specific PCR. Leukemia 28(8):1698

Xu L, Hunter ZR, Tsakmaklis N et al (2016) Clonal architecture of CXCR4 WHIM-like mutations in Waldenström macroglobulinaemia. Br J Haematol 172:735

Yang G, Zhou Y, Liu X, Xu L, Cao Y, Manning RJ et al (2013) A mutation in MYD88 (L265P) supports the survival of lymphoplasmacytic cells by activation of

Bruton tyrosine kinase in Waldenstrom macroglobulinemia. Blood 122:1222

Yang G, Buhrlage SJ, Tan L et al (2016) HCK is a survival
determinant transactivated by mutated MYD88, and a
direct target of ibrutinib. Blood 127:3237

Yasui O, Tukamoto F, Sasaki N et al (1997) Malignant
lymphoma of the transverse colon associated with
macroglobulinemia. Am J Gastroenterol 92:2299

Zhou Y, Liu X, Xu L et al (2011) Matrix metallopro-
teinase-8 is overexpressed in Waldenström's mac-
roglobulinemi a cells, and specific inhibition of this
metalloproteinase blocks release of soluble CD27.
Clin Lymphoma Myeloma Leuk 11:172

Zinzani PL, Gherlinzoni F, Bendandi M et al (1995)
Fludarabine treatment in resistant Waldenström's
macroglobulinemia. Eur J Haematol 54:120

Primary Systemic Amyloidosis

12

Efstathios Kastritis, Ashutosh Wechalekar, and Giampaolo Merlini

12.1 Introduction

The amyloidoses constitute a large group of diseases in which misfolding of extracellular protein has a prominent role. This dynamic process generates insoluble, toxic protein aggregates that are deposited in tissues in bundles of β-sheet fibrillar protein (Lachmann and Hawkins 2006; Merlini and Bellotti 2003). Amyloid deposition may occur in the presence of an abnormal protein (hereditary amyloidosis and acquired systemic immunoglobulin light chain (AL) amyloidosis) or in association with prolonged excess abundance of a normal protein (reactive systemic (AA) amyloidosis and beta-2-microglobulin dialysis-related amyloidosis); may accompany the ageing process for reasons unknown, for example,

wild-type transthyretin amyloidosis (ATTRwt; senile systemic amyloidosis). More than 35 proteins have been identified to form amyloid in man, either locally or systemically (Sipe et al. 2014), but recent use of mass spectrometry for amyloid diagnosis suggests many more proteins may be amyloidogenic (Brambilla et al. 2013). AL amyloidosis is the most frequently diagnosed type in the western world. Table 12.1 lists the common types and their main clinical features (Table 12.1). Advent of newer technologies has improved diagnosis, enabled accurate fibril typing and better risk stratification. Outcomes have improved, at least in AL type, and a number of novel therapies are on the horizon for various types of amyloidosis including antibody-based therapy and RNA inhibition strategies. However, a major challenge remains in that patients with advanced cardiac involvement at diagnosis, nearly a third of all patients with AL amyloidosis, still die within a few months. Early diagnosis of amyloidosis is vital and requires education of both physicians and patients. We review progress in the field over the last decade.

E. Kastritis
Department of Clinical Therapeutics, National and Kapodistrian University of Athens, Athens, Greece

A. Wechalekar
National Amyloidosis Center, University College London Medical School, London, UK

G. Merlini (✉)
Amyloidosis Research and Treatment Center, Fondazione Istituto di Ricovero e Cura a Carattere Scientifico Policlinico San Matteo, Pavia, Italy

Department of Molecular Medicine, University of Pavia, Pavia, Italy
e-mail: gmerlini@unipv.it

12.2 Incidence and Prevalence

Epidemiological data in amyloidosis are few. The first population-based study of AL in Olmsted County, USA, reported in 1992, reported the incidence of AL amyloidosis of approximately ten cases per million population (Kyle et al. 1992).

© Springer International Publishing Switzerland 2018
M. A. Dimopoulos et al. (eds.), *Multiple Myeloma and Other Plasma Cell Neoplasms*,
Hematologic Malignancies, https://doi.org/10.1007/978-3-319-25586-6_12

Table 12.1 The common types of amyloidosis

Amyloid type	Acquired (A)/ hereditary (H)	Underlying disorders	Precursor protein	Organ involvement				
				Heart	Kidneys	Liver	PN (AN)	Other
AL	A	Plasma cell dyscrasia	Monoclonal immunoglobulin light chain	+++	+++	++	+ (+)	Soft tissue GI
AA	A	Inflammatory disorders	Serum amyloid A protein (SAA)	∓ (late)	++++	+ (late)	(+)	GI (late)
ATTR	A	None	Wild-type TTR	+++	−	−	−	Carpal tunnel syndrome
	H	Mutations in TTR gene	Abnormal TTR	++	−	−	+++ (+++)	−
AFib	H	Mutations in fibrinogen α-chain gene	Abnormal fibrinogen	−	+++	∓	−	−
ALect2	A	Uncertain	Leucocyte chemotactic factor 2	−	+++	++	−	−
AApoA1	H	Mutations in apolipoprotein A1 gene	Abnormal ApoA1	+	++	++	± (−)	Testis
ALys	H	Mutations in lysozyme gene	Abnormal lysozyme	−	+	++	−	GI/skin
AGel	H	Mutations in gelsolin gene	Abnormal gelsolin	−	∓	−	++ (−) cranial	−
Aβ2M	A/H	Long-term dialysis	B-2 microglobulin	−	−	−	− (+[a])	Carpal tunnel syndrome, arthropathy

+, indicated relative frequency (+++, very common: ++, common; +, less common; ∓, rare); *AN* autonomic neuropathy, *PN* peripheral neuropathy, *SAA* serum amyloid A, *TTR* transthyretin, *GI* gastrointestinal, *CHF* congestive heart failure
[a]Autonomic neuropathy only in familial Aβ2M amyloidosis (Valleix et al. 2012)

UK death certificate data indicates amyloidosis is the cause of death in 0.58/1000 individuals, and the incidence of amyloidosis is about ten per million population (Pinney et al. 2013). Analysis of Swedish hospital discharge and outpatient registers gave an incidence of nonhereditary amyloidosis of 8.29 per million person-years and of AL amyloidosis of 3.2 per million (Hemminki et al. 2012). The pattern of amyloid patients seen at tertiary referral centres has changed over the last decade. Frequency of AL amyloidosis, as a proportion of total referrals each year, has remained essentially stable over the decades (about two thirds of all cases). Conversely, there has been a remarkable progressive decrease in the proportion of patients referred with AA amyloidosis from a third to less than a tenth from 1987–1995 to 2009–2012, likely reflecting better recent

treatment of inflammatory arthropathies with biologic therapies. Recognition of patients with ATTRwt amyloid-related cardiomyopathy has increased strikingly from hardly any patients to a tenth of the entire case load from 1988–1999 to 2009–2012, respectively. This has led to a substantial diagnostic challenge in these elderly patients with amyloidosis, where the incidence of monoclonal gammopathy is high (up to 30%), to differentiate AL from ATTRwt in an elderly (particularly male) patient with predominant cardiac amyloid deposition. Amyloidosis of the recently described leucocyte chemotactic factor-2 (ALect2) type (Benson et al. 2008) is the third most common cause of acquired renal amyloidosis occurring predominantly in patients from South Asia, North Africa, the Middle East and Mexico (Murphy et al. 2011; Murphy et al. 2010;

Larsen et al. 2010), another important diagnosis to be considered in a patient with isolated renal or liver amyloidosis in absence of a monoclonal protein in the appropriate epidemiological setting.

12.3 Amyloid Fibrils

All amyloid deposits are composed of protein fibrils of remarkably similar structure with a diameter of 7–13 nm and sharing a common core structure consisting of antiparallel β-strands (or less commonly parallel β-strands) forming sheets (Sawaya et al. 2007; Bonar et al. 1969; Glenner and Terry 1974; Sunde et al. 1997). All amyloid deposits also contain a number of minor non-fibrillary constituents including glycosaminoglycans and serum amyloid P component (SAP) (Pepys et al. 1994; Tan and Pepys 1994). The specific highly ordered ultrastructure of amyloid fibrils accounts for their characteristic property of binding Congo red dye in a spatial manner that produces green birefringence when viewed under cross-polarized light, and this remains the histological gold standard for confirming the presence of amyloid in tissue samples.

The universal presence of common non-fibrillary constituents within amyloid deposits is the basis for specific imaging (SAP scintigraphy) and novel therapeutic approaches (targeting the glycosaminoglycans (Dember et al. 2007) or amyloid-associated SAP (Bodin et al. 2010)).

12.4 Clinical Features of Amyloidosis

The clinical features of systemic amyloidosis are diverse given the potential for amyloid deposits to affect almost any organ system, with the exception of brain, and are rarely type specific leading to diagnostic difficulties and delays of over a year from the first physician visit in a third of all patients with over five different specialities consulted before the diagnosis was made (Lousada et al. 2015). Clinical features that are virtually pathognomonic of AL amyloidosis include a combination of macroglossia and periorbital purpura; however, they occur in less than a third of all cases. Isolated periorbital purpura is occasionally seen in other types of amyloidosis.

Cardiac involvement is the leading cause of morbidity and mortality in amyloidosis (Falk 2005; Merlini and Palladini 2013) and occurs in about 70% of patients with AL amyloidosis (Merlini 2012). Amyloid cardiomyopathy presents with heart failure and preserved ejection fraction, typically with echocardiography of restrictive cardiomyopathy, often with disproportionate signs of right ventricular failure (oedema, raised jugular vein distension and congestive hepatomegaly); low cardiac output and hypotension are features of advanced disease. Patients with AL cardiomyopathy are often more symptomatic compared to patients with other types given an apparently similar degree of amyloid deposition in the heart, supporting in vitro evidence of myocardial cell toxicity of amyloidogenic light chains in AL type (Liao et al. 2001; Shi et al. 2010; Lavatelli et al. 2015).

Kidneys are the next most common organ involved in AL amyloidosis presenting with albuminuria, which typically has progressed to nephrotic syndrome in majority of cases. Renal dysfunction may remain asymptomatic until it is very advanced. Liver involvement is seen in 15–20% of all patients. ^{123}I-labelled serum amyloid P component scintigraphy identifies asymptomatic liver involvement in another 10–20% of patients. Liver amyloidosis, although less common, is still the commonest cause of morbidity and mortality in patients with otherwise early-stage disease.

Although mild neuropathy is not uncommon, significant neuropathy (peripheral and/or autonomic neuropathy) as presenting feature of AL amyloidosis occurs in 10–20% of patients. Amyloid peripheral neuropathy is a predominantly axonal length-dependent neuropathy causing both small and large fibre involvement. It begins with loss of the small fibre-mediated sensations of heat or cold, may be painful (Reilly and Staunton 1996) and can be difficult to differentiate from the more common chronic inflammatory demyelinating polyneuropathy. Autonomic neuropathy causes impotence as an early symptom in men followed by postural hypotension, early satiety, diarrhoea and/or constipation. Other than amyloidosis and severe diabetic neuropathy, diseases causing a combination of progressive sensory motor peripheral neuropathy and autonomic neuropathy are rare. Isolated neuropathy in absence of other organ involvement is uncommon in AL amyloidosis—thus most patients with monoclonal gammopathy and an isolated neuropathy do not have amyloidosis although this remains a differential diagnosis.

Involvement of soft tissues, apart from carpal tunnel syndrome, is almost unique to AL amyloidosis. Macroglossia, muscular pseudohypertrophy, "shoulder pad" sign, salivary gland enlargement and submandibular soft tissue infiltration are common.

Localized AL amyloidosis is associated with in situ production of amyloidogenic light chains by clonal B cells in the affected tissue. Common sites include the respiratory tract, bladder, eyelids and skin. This form of amyloidosis is an indolent disease that almost never evolves systemically, but it can nevertheless have serious space occupying and other consequences. Local surgical measures to control symptoms are usually appropriate, and radiotherapy may have a role in selected cases (Gertz et al. 2005).

12.5   Diagnosis

A stepwise approach to diagnosis and staging of amyloidosis is critical (Fig. 12.1). This involves confirmation of amyloid deposition, identification of fibril type, assessment of the underlying clonal disorder and evaluation of the extent and severity of amyloidotic organ involvement. Serum cardiac biomarkers are an important validated tool for risk stratification/staging in AL amyloidosis (Dispenzieri et al. 2004).

Advanced and irreversible organ dysfunction has often ensued by the time a clinical diagnosis of amyloidosis is made. Specific symptom combinations in a patient with a monoclonal gammopathy should trigger suspicion for a diagnosis of amyloidosis such as nephrotic syndrome and heart failure, a combination of peripheral and autonomic neuropathy, thick-walled heart failure with normal- or low-voltage ECG, recurrent carpal tunnel syndrome and a combination of carpal tunnel syndrome and heart failure. Since the

outcome of patients treated prior to development of clinical symptoms is significantly better, keeping a high index of suspicion and making an early diagnosis is critical. Addition of regular testing for NTproBNP and urine sample for albuminuria in a patient with monoclonal gammopathy of uncertain significance with abnormal free light chain ratio will identify over 95% of patients with AL amyloidosis and should become a part of standard practice (Merlini et al. 2013).

12.5.1   Histological Confirmation of Diagnosis and Type of Amyloid Fibril Protein

Demonstration of characteristic green birefringence under cross-polarized light following Congo red staining of a tissue biopsy remains the gold standard for confirming amyloid deposition. Novel fluorescent dyes show promise for both identifying and typing amyloid deposits (Sipe et al. 2012; Nilsson et al. 2010). Biopsy of an organ suspected to be involved by amyloid is the commonest approach, but there is a risk of bleeding, and biopsy should only be considered if other methods do not reveal amyloid deposits. Abdominal fat aspiration is a simple and innocuous test with high rates of detection in systemic AL amyloidosis. A negative fat aspirate does not exclude amyloidosis, and rectal or labial salivary glands biopsy are alternatives with reasonable diagnostic sensitivity (Foli et al. 2011).

The critical next step is to confirm the amyloid fibril type—this is crucial to avoid catastrophic treatment errors. Immunohistochemistry with antibodies to amyloid fibril protein was the most widely available method for fibril typing. When using specifically developed panel of antibodies (Schonland et al. 2012) or used as immune-electron microscopy (Arbustini et al. 1997; Fernandez de Larrea et al. 2015), this has a very high diagnostic accuracy. However, using commercially available antibodies, which are not optimized for amyloid fibril detection, risks misdiagnosis. The proteomic method of mass spectrometric analysis of amyloidotic material captured by laser microdissection from tissue sections or from abdominal fat aspirates is the new gold standard for fibril typing (Tan and Pepys 1994;

Dember et al. 2007). Although a robust and reliable technique, it requires validation in each laboratory prior to routine clinical use. Gene sequencing must be performed when there is any suspicion of hereditary amyloidosis. An online database (www.amyloidosismutations.com) provides an updated list of amyloidogenic mutations and an outline of phenotype in hereditary amyloidosis (Fig. 12.2).

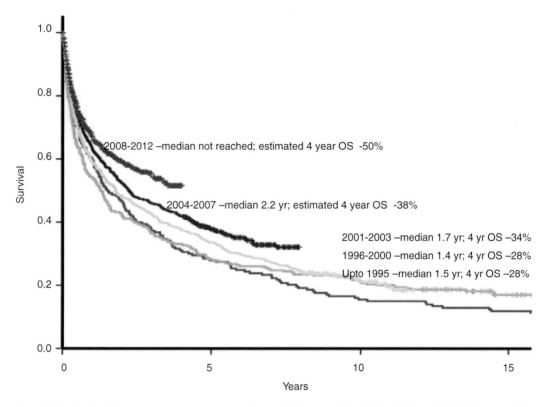

Fig. 12.1 Kaplan-Meier survival curve showing improvement in overall survival of patients with systemic AL amyloidosis seen at the UK National Amyloidosis Centre (n = 3486). The estimated 4-year survival has improved from 28% for patients diagnosed in early part of the last decade to nearly 50% for patients diagnosed in the last 4 years (log rank p values: 2008–2012 vs 2004–2007, p = 0.008; 2004–2007 vs 2001– 2003, p = 0.03; 2001–2003 vs 1996–2000, p = 0.29; 1996–2000 vs up to 1995, p = 0.64). This improvement in survival has coincided with availability of novel agents like thalidomide and bortezomib for the treatment of AL amyloidosis. However, over the last two decades, there has been no improvement in the early mortality in the first few months after diagnosis of AL amyloidosis (Reproduced from Lancet 2015)

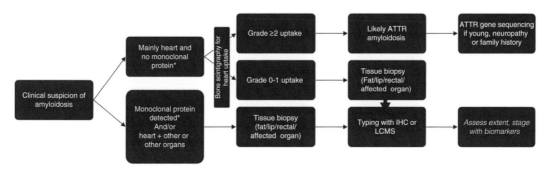

Fig. 12.2 Approach to a patient with suspected systemic amyloidosis. *Monoclonal protein—serum and urine immunofixation + serum free light chain measurement. *ATTR* transthyretin amyloidosis, *IHC* immunohistochemistry, *LCMS* laser capture mass spectrometry

12.5.2 Monoclonal Protein Detection and Assessment of the Underlying Clonal Disorder

Assessment or identification of the underlying disorder is the next step in patients with AL amyloidosis. Detection and accurate quantification of the monoclonal protein, particularly of the monoclonal amyloidogenic light chains, is crucial at diagnosis especially prior to starting any treatment. All patients need combination of serum and urine testing with electrophoresis, immunofixation (IFE) and measurement of serum free light chain (FLC) (Palladini et al. 2009). Each technique in isolation will miss a substantial number of patients but when used together will be informative in over 98% cases (Lachmann et al. 2003). AL fibrils are four times more often of lambda than kappa light chain type, in contrast with MGUS and myeloma. The plasma cell infiltrate in the bone marrow is usually very modest with a median of 10% (Deshmukh et al. 2009; Paiva et al. 2009). Chromosomal translocations (such as $t(11;14)$) or deletions (del 1p or 17p) appear to negatively influence outcomes with chemotherapy in AL amyloidosis (Bochtler et al. 2014). Baseline testing should be considered although data is not forthcoming about utility of such markers in selection of therapy. Whole body imaging with low-dose CT, PET-CT or MRI is needed to detect presence of myeloma-related bone disease. Patients with AL amyloidosis with additional features of myeloma-related end organ damage have worse outcomes.

12.5.3 Increasingly Important Role of Imaging

Assessment of amyloid-related end organ damage informs prognosis, supportive care needs and formulation of a risk-adapted treatment plan. Until recently, serum amyloid P component (SAP) scintigraphy was the only specific imaging method available and enables the amyloid load in the liver, kidneys, spleen, adrenal glands, bones and various other sites to be ascertained and monitored serially (Hawkins et al. 1990). SAP scintigraphy shows that there is a poor correlation between the quantity of amyloid present in a given organ and the level of organ dysfunction, and that regression of amyloid deposits occurs at different rates in different organs. Lately, bone scintigraphy tracers (^{99m}Tc-labelled DPD, PYP or HMDP), which show high-affinity uptake in cardiac amyloidosis (mainly ATTR but about half all cases with AL amyloidosis), and thioflavin-like tracers (carbon-11-labelled Pittsburgh compound-B (^{11}C-PIB) (Antoni et al. 2013), florbetapir (Dorbala et al. 2014) and florbetaben (Law et al. 2016) which have been extensively used in Alzheimer's disease) appear to have a role in amyloid-specific imaging (Fig. 12.3).

Cross-sectional imaging has been used for defining the anatomical characteristics of organs in amyloidosis—particularly in the heart—with echocardiography and, more recently, by cardiac magnetic resonance imaging. Echocardiography, including tissue Doppler and strain imaging, is important to document baseline cardiac structure and function (Falk 2005; Buss et al. 2012). Echocardiography shows "pan-cardiac" thickening (increased thickness of left and right ventricular free walls, septum, valves and intra-atrial septum with dilation of the atria) which is rare in other infiltrative cardiomyopathies. A thick-walled heart on echocardiogram with normal- or low-voltage electrocardiogram remains a diagnostic hallmark of amyloidosis with a high sensitivity (72–79%) and specificity (91–100%) for the diagnosis (Selvanayagam et al. 2007). 2-D strain mapping shows relative preservation of apical function which can be an early clue to amyloidosis—this gives rise to a "bull's-eye" pattern on plotting the segmental stain, which is rare in other cardiomyopathies (Fig. 12.3).

Cardiac MRI for amyloid imaging has been a major advance over echocardiography providing an easily available diagnostic tool with a high specificity for diagnosis of cardiac amyloidosis

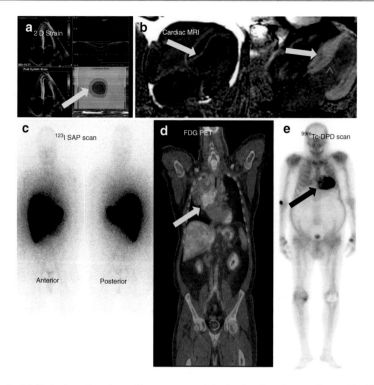

Fig. 12.3 (**a**) Typical 2-D strain pattern in cardiac amyloidosis showing marked impairment of function at the base compared to the apex giving a typical "bull's-eye" pattern in mapping. (**b**) Cardiac MRI scan after gadolinium contrast showing a rim on late subendocardial enhancement in the left picture and extensive transmural enhancement in the right panel. (**c**) 123I-labelled serum amyloid P component scintigraphy showing extensive uptake in the liver in a patient with AL amyloidosis **c**. 18F-FDG PET scan in a patient with localized amyloidosis showing FDG uptake in the amyloidotic mass **d**. 99mTc-DPD scan in a patient with transthyretin amyloidosis showing marked cardiac uptake with attenuation of the bone signal—grade 2 uptake which in the absence of a detectable monoclonal protein is characteristic of ATTR amyloidosis

(Maceira et al. 2005; Mekinian et al. 2010). Amyloid cardiomyopathy demonstrates a typical pattern of late subendocardial or diffuse enhancement after gadolinium contrast injection (Lachmann et al. 2003; Deshmukh et al. 2009). CMR can give accurate anatomical information including the wall thickness and LV mass. Equilibrium contrast MRI (Eq-CMR) is a technique using a low-dose gadolinium infusion for contrast and allows accurate quantification of the myocardial interstitial volume fraction which is greatly expanded in amyloidosis (Banypersad et al. 2013) and therefore provides a novel tool for monitoring cardiac amyloid load.

99mTc-3,3-diphosphono-1,2-propanodicarboxylic acid (99mTc-DPD), 99mTc-hydroxymethylene diphosphonate (99mTc-HMDP) and 99mTc-pyrophosphate (99mTc-PYP) are bone-seeking radionuclide tracers that appear to also localize in cardiac ATTR amyloid deposits with remarkable sensitivity (Bokhari et al. 2013; Chen and Dilsizian 2012; Castano et al. 2012; Rapezzi et al. 2011; Rapezzi et al. 2008; Perugini et al. 2005; Galat et al. 2017; Galat et al. 2015) (Fig. 12.3). 99mTc-DPD scans appear to show asymptomatic ATTR cardiac deposits before any other imaging modality (Hutt et al. 2014). Uptake into other types of cardiac amyloid may occur but is usually minor (Rapezzi et al. 2008). 99mTc-DPD/HMDP/PYP scintigraphy may have a potential role for screening for cardiac ATTR amyloidosis in elderly patients with cardiac failure of unclear aetiology. An algorithm for non-invasively diagnosing ATTR cardiac amyloidosis has recently been published (Gillmore et al. 2016). ^{123}I-mIBG (metaiodobenzylguanidine) scintigraphy can provide information on cardiac autonomic neuropathy, but its place in clinical practice remains to be established (Hongo et al. 2002; Lekakis et al. 2003).

12.6 Treatment Approach to Patients with AL Amyloidosis

The ultimate goal of therapy in AL amyloidosis is to improve organ function and to extend survival of the patient. Until recently, no effective therapies targeting directly amyloid deposits existed, and the treatment strategy was solely based on the elimination of light chain production and supportive care for the complications of the disease and therapy. Several lines of evidence have shown that reducing the amount of the pro-amyloidogenic protein results in stabilization and regression of amyloid deposits in the tissues and organs and in many cases in organ function improvement and extended survival (van Gameren et al. 2009; Wechalekar et al. 2016; Dispenzieri and Merlini 2016). In fact, AL amyloidosis represents, among all amyloid diseases, the most successful example of the effect of therapy on organ recovery providing substantial survival improvement. This is due to the fact that in AL amyloidosis it is possible to suppress the synthesis of the amyloid protein. Therefore, in AL amyloidosis, the mainstay of therapy is the rapid reduction and, even better, the elimination of the light chain-producing plasma cell or B-cell clone by means of chemotherapy.

Defining an effective and safe treatment strategy requires assessment of treatment efficacy based on objective criteria. Both the clonal disease and the organ function should be assessed by reproducible and objectively measurable biomarkers which are associated with clinically meaningful endpoints. Hematologic response represents the reduction of the amount of clonal free light chains. Organ response assesses the improvement of involved organ function. There

is a close association of hematologic and organ response: improvement of organ function follows clonal light chain reduction.

12.7 Hematologic Response

According to the updated criteria, the evaluation of hematologic response is based on the measurement of serum free light chains (sFLCs): a partial hematologic response requires the reduction of the dFLC (difference of involved and uninvolved light chain) by 50%, a very good partial response (VGPR) requires dFLC <40 mg/L and a complete hematologic response requires a normal FLC concentration and ratio and negative serum and urine immunofixation (Palladini et al. 2012a). However, a significant minority of patients with AL may have sFLCs levels that are below the threshold that is considered as "measurable" (defined as a dFLC ≥50 mg/L with abnormal ratio). In these patients the reduction of the circulating FLCs is still the goal of therapy, but there are difficulties in the evaluation of hematologic response (PR and VGPR while there is no problem in assessing the CR). In most centres the FLCs are measured using a polyclonal antisera-based assay (Freelite), and the current criteria have been developed using this assay (Palladini et al. 2012a). Two new assays using monoclonal antisera (N Latex and Seralite) have been introduced and may give different results (Lock et al. 2013; Campbell et al. 2017; Te Velthuis et al. 2016). Both Freelite and N Latex assays have shown good correlation in detecting the abnormal light chain subtype, but there is significant discordance in absolute values between the assays, and thus they are not interchangeable (Mahmood et al. 2016). Patients should be followed using the same assay, and an extensive evaluation of the new assays should be performed before introducing their results in the response criteria. Most patients with AL amyloidosis have serum monoclonal protein below the levels that are considered as measurable by SPEP criteria, but in those with measurable M-spikes (≥0.5 gr/dl), the reduction of the monoclonal peak may be

Table 12.2 Evaluation of risk in patients with AL amyloidosis based on Mayo staging system based on NTproBNP and cTnT (Dispenzieri et al. 2004) and the revised system based on NTproBNP, cTnT and dFLC (Kumar et al. 2012a)

	Stage	% of patients with AL amyloidosis	Median survival (months)
Good/low risk	Mayo stage I	15–20%	26–94
	Modified Mayo stage I		
Intermediate risk	Mayo stage II	25–30%	12–40
	Modified Mayo stage II or some III		
High risk	Mayo stage III	25–30%	9–26
	Modified Mayo stage III, some IV and few II		
Very high risk	Mayo stage III with NTproBNP >8500 pg/ml	10–15%	3–6
	Modified Mayo stage IV and some III		

used to assess the quality of response, if serum FLCs are below "measurable" (Table 12.2).

12.8 Organ Response

Organ response criteria have been developed and modified with the addition of biomarkers for cardiac assessment (Gertz et al. 2005; Palladini et al. 2012b). According to these criteria, at least 30% reduction of NTproBNP (provided that at baseline was ≥650 ng/L and the absolute of reduction is at least 300 ng/L) from baseline defines a cardiac response (Palladini et al. 2012b). This response, at 3 and 6 months post initiation of therapy, has been strongly associated with functional improvement and survival benefit in a large cohort and validated in an independent cohort of patients with AL amyloidosis. However, specific therapies (thalidomide, lenalidomide or pomalidomide) (Dispenzieri et al. 2010) may

disproportionally increase NTproBNP; renal dysfunction (especially if eGFR <30 ml/min) also increases NTproBNP. Until recently, renal response criteria required the reduction of proteinuria by ≥50% without increase in serum creatinine (Gertz et al. 2005). In a collaborative project, the Pavia and Heidelberg groups evaluated renal outcomes in 732 patients and identified that a >25% eGFR decrease predicted poor renal survival, while a decrease in proteinuria by ≥30% or below 0.5 g/24 h without renal progression at 6 months was associated with longer renal survival and was proposed as criterion for renal response (Palladini et al. 2014a). Improvement of proteinuria is closely associated to hematologic response, with the greatest probability for renal response among patients who achieve at least a VGPR (Palladini et al. 2014a; Pinney et al. 2011).

12.9 Risk Assessment

Patients with AL amyloidosis are often frail due to multiorgan involvement and prone to treatment-related toxicities. The design of an effective treatment strategy requires the evaluation of the risks that are associated with a specific treatment and the potential benefits in the short and long term. Cardiac biomarkers (NTproBNP and cardiac troponins) are powerful risk stratification tools, and a cardiobiomarker-based staging system proposed by the Mayo Clinic investigators (Mayo Clinic cardiac staging system) has been adopted (Dispenzieri et al. 2004). A refinement of risk stratification by including the level of the free light chains has also been proposed (Kumar et al. 2012a) (Table 12.3). However, a subgroup of patients, those with stage III by the Mayo stage system and with NTproBNP level >8500 pg/ml (stage 3B) seem to have the poorest survival despite any recent treatment advances (Palladini et al. 2015; Wechalekar et al. 2013; Merlini and Palladini 2013); this prognosis is even poorer if systolic blood pressure is low (Wechalekar et al. 2013). Markers of endothelial dysfunction as reflected by increased levels of von Willebrand factor seem to identify patients with very poor outcomes even among stage 3B patients (Kastritis

Table 12.3 Clonal and organ response and progression criteria (Palladini et al. 2012a, 2014a; Gertz et al. 2005)

	Response	Progression
Clonal disease (hematologic assessment)	Complete response: Normalization of FLC levels and κ to λ ratio, with negative serum and urine immunofixation Very good partial response: Decrease of dFLC to <40 mg/l Partial response: >50% reduction of dFLC	From a complete response: Any detectable monoclonal protein or abnormal FLC ratio (amyloidogenic FLC levels must double) From a partial response: ≥50% increase in serum M protein levels to >0.5 g/dl or ≥50% increase in urine M protein levels to >200 mg per day (a visible peak must be present) or ≥50% increase in involved FLC levels to >100 mg/l
Heart	>30% and >300 ng/l decrease in NTproBNP levels in patients with NTproBNP levels ≥650 ng/l at baseline or ≥2-class decrease in NYHA class in patients with NYHA class 3 or 4 at baseline	>30% and >300 ng/l increase in NTproBNP levels or ≥33% increase in cardiac troponin levels or ≥10% decrease in ejection fraction
Kidney	>50% (≥0.5 g per day) decrease in 24 h urine protein levels in patients with urine protein levels >0.5 g per day at baseline without ≥25% increase in serum creatinine levels or decrease in creatinine clearance from baseline Proposed modification: Decrease in proteinuria by ≥30% or below 0.5 g/24 h without renal progression	≥50% (≥1 g per day) increase in 24 h urine protein levels or ≥25% increase in serum creatinine levels or ≥25% decrease in creatinine clearance from baseline
Liver	≥50% decrease in alkaline phosphatase levels and/or ≥2 cm decrease in liver size (assessed by radiography)	≥50% increase in alkaline phosphatase levels from the lowest recorded value
Peripheral nervous system	Improvement in electromyogram nerve conduction velocity (such a response is rare)	Progressive neuropathy by electromyography or nerve conduction velocity

et al. 2016). Both the "tumour burden", as reflected by the bone marrow plasma cell infiltration, and the presence of specific cytogenetic abnormalities of the plasma cells are also affecting prognosis; however, this effect is mostly observed in those patients which have less severe cardiac involvement (Bochtler et al. 2014; Bochtler et al. 2015). In most patients with AL amyloidosis, plasma cell clones are small (median bone marrow infiltration is 7–10%) with low proliferative activity (Gertz et al. 1989), expressing λ-light chains in 75%. A minority of patients with extensive infiltration (more than 30% of plasma cells) present with symptoms of amyloidotic organ involvement and not with classical myeloma CRAB criteria. More extensive marrow infiltration is associated with inferior survival, independently of other disease characteristics (Kourelis et al. 2013). High-risk cytogenetic abnormalities, such as t(4;14) and del17p, are uncommon in AL amyloidosis (Bochtler et al. 2011), but t(11;14) is more common and, in contrast to what has been observed in MM, is associated with adverse prognosis in patients treated with conventional chemotherapy or high-dose therapy (Bryce et al. 2009) or bortezomib-based regimens (Bochtler et al. 2015). In a large series from Mayo Clinic, the presence of FISH-detected abnormalities was associated with poor prognosis and cardiac involvement (Warsame et al. 2015). Regarding specific abnormalities, when plasma cell burden was ≤10%, then trisomies predicted for worse survival (44 vs 19 months), and when it was ≤10%, then t(11;14) predicted for worse survival (53 months vs not reached); abnormal cIg-FISH remained a prognostic factor on multivariate analysis (Warsame et al. 2015). Amplification of chromosome 1q21 has been associated with less favourable prognosis in patients treated with melphalan and dexamethasone (Bochtler et al. 2014). IgM-related amyloidosis may have distinct characteristic regarding the B-cell clone and pattern of organ involvement (Sachchithanantham et al. 2016).

12.10 Therapies Targeting the Light Chain-Producing Clone

AL amyloidosis is a rare disease, and only few prospective randomized phase III studies have been conducted. Thus, most treatment recommendations are based on phase II studies, retrospective comparisons and case series (Tables 12.4 and 12.5). The effort to reduce or eliminate the light chain production is based on chemotherapy approaches, based on regimens that were developed for the treatment of myeloma, with adaptations in terms of dose and schedule. In the case of IgM-related AL amyloidosis, regimens used for the treatment of lymphoplasmacytic lymphoma/Waldenström's macroglobulinemia are commonly used (Wechalekar et al. 2008). The most commonly used drugs, in various combinations, include alkylators, proteasome inhibitors, IMiDs and in most regimens steroids.

12.10.1 Alkylators

Alkylator-based therapy, either standard or high dose (i.e. high-dose melphalan with ASCT), has been the mainstay of therapy of AL for decades. Standard-dose oral melphalan with high-dose dexamethasone (MDex) (Palladini et al. 2004) has been associated with favourable long-term outcomes in patients at good or intermediate risk, with low toxicity (Palladini et al. 2014b). However, patients with high-risk disease have poor outcomes with MDex (Palladini et al. 2014b). In a prospective randomized multicentre phase III trial, MDex was not inferior to high-dose melphalan with ASCT (Jaccard et al. 2007), but this study was conducted before the availability of cardiac biomarkers and included also patients that would be considered ineligible for ASCT with the current selection criteria. Melphalan dose also needs adjustment for renal dysfunction. Cyclophosphamide has also been used, especially in combination with the new drugs (thalidomide, lenalidomide, bortezomib), and at the standard dosing may be easier to use in patients with renal dysfunction. Bendamustine has been used in patients with AL amyloidosis who have relapsed after previous therapy, but the experience is not very extensive (Palladini et al. 2012b); however, in patients with IgM-related AL amyloidosis, bendamustine-based regimens in combination with rituximab may be the preferable treatment (Leblond et al. 2016).

12.10.1.1 High-Dose Melphalan with ASCT

High-dose melphalan supported by ASCT induces high rates of long maintained complete hematologic responses which are followed by organ responses. In the USA, HDM with ASCT

Table 12.4 Outcome of high-dose melphalan followed by autologous stem cell transplantation

Author	N	HR (CR)	Organ responses	TRM	PFS/OS (years)
Boston University (Sanchorawala 2014) (1994–2013)	607	34%	NR	9%	Median OS: 6.7 years Median OS for those in CR >12 years
Mayo Clinic (Gertz et al. 2010) (1996–2010)	434	39%	47%	10%	CR >10 years PR: 8.9 years NR: 2.7 years
MD Anderson (Parmar et al. 2014) (1998–2011)	80	31%	39%	12.5%	OS >10 years (56% at 10 years)
Heidelberg (Hegenbart et al. 2014) (1998–2014)	174	38%	40%	2%	Median OS: 11. 3 years
CIBMTR registry (D'Souza et al. 2015)	1536	2001–2006: 30% 2007–2012: 37% (*n* = 354 with full data)	2001–2006: 31% 2007–2012: 32% (renal only)	1995–2000: 4% 2001–2006: 11% 2007–2012: 19%	5 year OS: 1995–2000: 55% 2001–2006: 61% 2007–2012: 77%

Table 12.5 Conventional dose regimens for patients with AL amyloidosis

Regimen	N of patients	Treatment naive	Cardiac involvement	Hematologic response	Organ responses	3-month mortality	OS (years)
Melphalan, dexamethasone (Palladini et al. 2004)	46	46	32 (70%)	67% (Cr: 33%)	48% 6/32 (19%) cardiac 16/29 (55%) renal	NR	5.1 years
Melphalan, dexamethasone (Palladini et al. 2014b)	119	119	67 (56%)	76% (Cr: 31%)	36% 25/67 (37%) cardiac 20/82 (24%) renal	0	7.3 years
Melphalan, attenuated-dose dexamethasone (Palladini et al. 2014b)	140	140	122 (87%)	51% (Cr: 12%)	21% 24/122 (20%) cardiac 15/87 (17%) renal	18%	1.7 years
Bortezomib (Reece et al. 2011)	70	0	39/70 (56%)	68% (Cr: 29%)	5/39 (13%) cardiac 14/49 (29%) renal	3%	1-year OS 94%
Bortezomib ± dexamethasone (Kastritis et al. 2010)	94	18	69/94 (73%)	71% (Cr: 25%)	30% 20/69 (29%) cardiac 13/70 (19%) renal 4/18 (22%) liver	3%	1-year OS 76%
Bortezomib, dexamethasone (Kastritis et al. 2015)	49	49	38/49 (77%)	77% (Cr: 39%)	49% 17/38 (45%) cardiac 16/35 (46%) renal	13%	1-year OS 67%
Bortezomib, cyclophosphamide, dexamethasone (Venner et al. 2012)	43	20	32/43 (74%)	83% (Cr: 42%)	46% 11% cardiac responses (33% NTproBNP response), 29% renal responses, 40% liver response	0	98% at 2 years
Bortezomib, cyclophosphamide, dexamethasone (Mikhael et al. 2012)	17	10	10/17 (58%)	94%/71%	5/7 cardiac response 6/12 renal response	NR	70% at 21 months
Bortezomib, cyclophosphamide, dexamethasone (Palladini et al. 2015)	230	230	168 (73%)	62% (Cr: 21%, VGPR: 22%)	29/167 (17%) cardiac 40/157 (25%) renal	12.6%	1-year OS ~70%
Bortezomib, cyclophosphamide, dexamethasone (Jaccard et al. 2014)	60	60	60/60 (100%)	68% (Cr: 17%, VGPR: 25%)	19/60 (32%) cardiac	30%	1-year OS 57%
Cyclophosphamide, Thalidomide, Dexamethasone (CTD) (Wechalekar et al. 2007)	75	31	44 (59%)	74% (Cr: 21%)	11/48 (23%) renal	4%	3.4 years
Lenalidomide, dexamethasone (Dispenzieri et al. 2007)	22	9	14/22 (64%)	41% (Cr: Nr)	23% 2/14 (14%) cardiac 4/16 (25%) renal 2/5 (40%) liver	18%	NR
Lenalidomide, dexamethasone (Sanchorawala et al. 2007)	34	3	17/34 (50%)	67% (Cr:29%)	6/17 (35%) renal 1/17 (6%): Cardiac	3%	NR

(continued)

Table 12.5 (continued)

Regimen	N of patients	Treatment naive	Cardiac involvement	Hematologic response	Organ responses	3-month mortality	OS (years)
Lenalidomide, cyclophosphamide, dexamethasone (Kastritis et al. 2012)	37	24	21/37 (57%)	55% (Cr: 8%)	22% 1/21 (5%) cardiac 8/24 (33%) renal	19%	1.5 years
Lenalidomide, cyclophosphamide, dexamethasone (Cibeira et al. 2015)	28	28	23 (82%)	46% (Cr: 25%)	46% 6/23 (26%) cardiac 10/23 (43%) Renal	35%	2-year OS 59%
Lenalidomide, cyclophosphamide, dexamethasone (Kumar et al. 2012b)	35	11	22 (63%)	44% (Cr:11%)	32% 5/22 (23%) cardiac 8/26 (31%) renal	9%	2-year OS 59%
Lenalidomide, melphalan, dexamethasone (Moreau et al. 2010)	26	26	15 (58%)	58% (Cr: 23%)	50% 6/15 (40%) cardiac 11/15 (73%) renal 3/7 (43%) liver	15%	2-year OS 81%
Lenalidomide, melphalan, dexamethasone (Dinner et al. 2013)	25	23	23 (92%)	58% (Cr: 8%)	8% 2/23 (8%) cardiac	40%	1-year OS 58%
Pomalidomide, dexamethasone (Dispenzieri et al. 2012)	33	0	27 (82%)	48% (Cr: 3%)	15% 4/27 (15%) cardiac 2/12 (17%) renal	3%	1-year OS 76%

is used more extensively than in Europe (Cibeira et al. 2011; Gertz et al. 2010; D'Souza et al. 2015). Large case series from specialized tertiary centres have shown consistently a CR rate of 34–49% with organ responses in 26–53% of patients (Cibeira et al. 2011; Dispenzieri et al. 2013) (Table 12.5). More importantly, 10-year rates of sustained CR are high, especially compared to myeloma patients, probably because the small plasma cell clone may be exterminated by HDM; 10-year survival exceeds 40%(Cibeira et al. 2011; Dispenzieri et al. 2013). However, HDM was associated with significant treatment-related mortality, reaching 10–12% especially before the era of cardiac biomarkers (Cibeira et al. 2011). The introduction of objective risk stratification tools, mainly of cardiac biomarkers, has improved the selection of those patients who have a low risk of fatal complications, and a significant reduction of TRM by about 40%, near the TRM rate for ASCT in patients with MM, has been observed (Gertz et al. 2013). It has been proposed that patients with NTproBNP >5000 pg/ml or troponin-T >0.06 µg/ml should not be considered for ASCT because of high risk of TRM (Gertz et al. 2013). Other exclusion criteria may include age, systolic blood pressure <100 mmHg, positive tests for faecal blood, inadequate liver function and severe autonomic neuropathy (Dingli et al. 2010). Adjustments in the intensity of conditioning with melphalan should be weighed against the probability of reduced effectiveness (Gertz et al. 2004). A strategy incorporating consolidation with bortezomib for patients with less than optimal response after HDM may however improve overall efficacy and deepen responses (Landau et al. 2017). It must be emphasized, however, that the proposed selection criteria (NTproBNP <5000 pg/ml and troponin-T <0.06 µg/ml) rate as "eligible for ASCT" even patients with severe cardiac dysfunction. Also, data on safety of ASCT in such patients derive from highly specialized centres and should be interpreted cautiously in less experienced centres with lower volumes of patients with AL amyloidosis (Table 12.4). Data on maintenance after HDM-ASCT are very limited; whether a maintenance phase could improve outcomes of patients not in CR should be prospectively examined.

12.10.2 Thalidomide and IMiDs

Thalidomide, in combination with dexamethasone, is active but poorly tolerated (Palladini et al. 2005). Given at low doses, and in combination with cyclophosphamide and dexamethasone (CTD) is efficient and better tolerated (Wechalekar et al. 2007) (Table 12.4), however, neurotoxicity and constipation may be significant problems. There is significant experience with the all oral CTD especially in the UK, but today it has been widely replaced by bortezomib-based regimens.

Lenalidomide with dexamethasone (Sanchorawala et al. 2007; Dispenzieri et al. 2007) or with the addition of alkylators (either melphalan (Moreau et al. 2010; Dinner et al. 2013) or cyclophosphamide (Kastritis et al. 2012; Kumar et al. 2012b; Cibeira et al. 2015) has shown efficacy in patients with newly diagnosed or relapsed AL amyloidosis (Table 12.4). However, the toxicity of lenalidomide is higher in patients with AL than in patients with myeloma and lower doses are used (usually no more than 15 mg). Skin rash (Sviggum et al. 2006) and pneumonitis (Zagouri et al. 2011) may be more common in patients with AL than in myeloma patients. Hematologic responses may take a median of 2–3 months to occur; complete hematologic responses are achieved in 10–20% of patients and are durable. In patients with cardiac involvement, the results are poor (Dinner et al. 2013) but for patients at low risk, lenalidomide-based therapy is a safe, effective and convenient option (Kastritis et al. 2012; Cibeira et al. 2015). Pomalidomide has promising activity, mainly in terms of hematologic responses and with a toxicity profile similar to that of lenalidomide. Data from the Pavia and Mayo groups indicate that pomalidomide with dexamethasone may be a very effective salvage therapy for several patients with relapsed or refractory AL amyloidosis,

especially if they have preserved organ function (Dispenzieri et al. 2012; Milani et al. 2013).

12.10.3 Proteasome Inhibitors

Bortezomib is the first-in-class proteasome inhibitor in clinical use and, either alone or in combination with dexamethasone, induces rapid and deep hematologic responses in patients with AL amyloidosis (Kastritis et al. 2010; Reece et al. 2011). Alkylating agents (cyclophosphamide or melphalan) have been added to bortezomib-dexamethasone backbone. Bortezomib-dexamethasone with cyclophosphamide (CyBorD or VCD) is a widely used frontline regimen for AL amyloidosis, but there are no prospective randomized phase III data (Venner et al. 2012; Mikhael et al. 2012) (Table 12.4). In an analysis of 230 patients who received primary therapy with VCD, hematologic responses were recorded in 62%, with 43% of patients achieving at least VGPR. Organ response rates were less impressive (cardiac response in 17% and renal response in 25%). The greatest benefit was obtained by patients at good or intermediate risk, although a subgroup of high-risk patients achieved a long survival (Palladini et al. 2015); patients with stage 3B disease had poor outcome with a median survival of ~6 months. In a retrospective comparison of upfront VCD vs CTD, hematologic response rates were similar between the two regimens, but VGPR (or better) was more common with VCD (40.5% vs 24.6%). Progression-free survival was longer with VCD, but the overall survival was similar (Venner et al. 2014), and both regimens failed to reduce early deaths. In a case-matched-case, retrospective, comparison of bortezomib with MDex (BMDex) vs MDex, triplet combination showed higher rates of complete hematologic responses (42% vs 19%) but without an improvement in overall survival rates (Palladini et al. 2014c). However, in patients with NTproBNP <8500 ng/l, there was a survival benefit, probably reflecting the poor outcome of high-risk patients which is probably independent of treatment. Also, the addition of bortezomib seemed to improve outcomes of patients who could not receive full-dose dexamethasone. Recently, a prospective randomized multicentre study comparing MDex to BMDex in newly diagnosed ASCT ineligible patients (NCT01277016) completed accrual. Interim results showed that BMDex improves responses rates and quality of responses at the expense of increased toxicity (Kastritis et al. 2014); a progression-free survival benefit may also exist. Bortezomib is neurotoxic and many patients with AL have amyloidosis-related neuropathy. Hypotension after bortezomib administration has been reported (Dubrey et al. 2011; Kastritis et al. 2007) and pre-hydration may reduce this complication, but in patients with peripheral oedema or severe cardiac dysfunction, it may not be feasible. Although there are no prospective data in patients with AL amyloidosis, the administration of bortezomib subcutaneously may reduce toxicity without significant reduction of efficacy and is currently used by most centres. Weekly administration is also favoured by most physicians (Palladini et al. 2015; Kastritis et al. 2015). These strategies may reduce toxicity and maintain activity (Kastritis et al. 2015).

Ixazomib is an orally available proteasome inhibitor, structurally similar to bortezomib, and was recently approved for relapsed myeloma. In a phase I study, ixazomib induced hematologic responses in 52% of patients with relapsed or refractory AL, which were higher in bortezomib-naive (100%) than in bortezomib-exposed patients (38%) (Merlini et al. 2014). Cardiac and renal responses were observed in 50% and 18% of patients, respectively, and toxicities were generally mild (mostly diarrhoea, nausea, fatigue, thrombocytopenia, peripheral neuropathy, fever and rash). An ongoing phase III study compares ixazomib with dexamethasone to standard non-PI-containing regimens in patients with relapsed or refractory AL (NCT01659658). Carfilzomib is a second-generation PI, has different structure than bortezomib and ixazomib (it is an epoxyketone), is given as IV infusion and lacks the neurotoxicity of bortezomib, but its use has been associated with a low but reproducible signal of reversible cardiotoxicity. In a phase I study in patients with relapsed or refractory AL, carfilzomib monotherapy (at a dose of 20/36 mg/m^2) was associated with a hematologic response in 78%

(67% VGPR) of nine evaluable patients, most of which were previously treated with bortezomib (Cohen et al. 2014). Cardiac events were common, but it was difficult to assess whether related to carfilzomib toxicity or to the underlying disease. More data are needed regarding the safety of carfilzomib.

12.10.4 Monoclonal Antibodies Targeting Plasma Cell Clone

Daratumumab is a monoclonal anti-CD38 antibody that has shown efficacy in myeloma patients refractory to all available therapies (Lokhorst et al. 2015). The unique mechanism of action of this drug makes it an ideal therapy for patients with AL amyloidosis. There is only limited experience with daratumumab in AL amyloidosis, since it has only recently been approved in the USA. Small series of patients with refractory disease have shown that it is safe and can induce deep hematologic remission in patients with AL amyloidosis (Kaufman et al. 2016; Weiss et al. 2016; Sher et al. 2016). However, more data are needed for the use of daratumumab, safety and the optimal combinations. The cost of daratumumab therapy is also a major issue.

12.10.5 Strategies of Therapy in AL Amyloidosis

Delayed diagnosis and delayed initiation of therapy may lead to irreversible organ damage. The goal of therapy is to rapidly "shut down" the production of the precursor protein (i.e. the clonal light chain), by targeting the underlying plasma cell (or B-cell) clone. The attainment of at least VGPR is associated with a survival benefit, even compared to a PR and a higher probability of organ response (Palladini et al. 2012a, 2014a). Thus, at least a VGPR, within a few months from start of therapy, should be the goal for hematologic response. If a deep hematologic response (i.e. at least VGPR) has not been reached or only a plateau response (i.e. a PR) has been achieved after three to four cycles of therapy, it is probably better to change treatment regimen (either add a drug or switch drug class), in order to achieve the target of hematologic VGPR or CR. However this may not be feasible in many patients.

High-dose melphalan with ASCT is a reasonable primary option, but less than one quarter of patients with AL amyloidosis is eligible. Bortezomib-based combinations are the major primary treatment option for most patients, although no prospective randomized data exist, and it seems that the greatest benefit is obtained by those patients at lower risk (Palladini et al. 2015; Palladini et al. 2014b), although a significant proportion (20–30%) of patients in cardiac stage 3B can still benefit from bortezomib (Palladini et al. 2015). Most centres follow a risk-adapted dosing and schedule strategy, in which lower doses and weekly administrations of bortezomib and dexamethasone are given in patients at intermediate or high risk. A strategy for bortezomib and dexamethasone dosing, based on cardiac biomarkers, age, systolic blood pressure and presence of neuropathy, may reduce early mortality in high-risk patients, without compromising efficacy, but long-term outcomes may not improve significantly (Kastritis et al. 2015). MDex has been considered the standard of care

and remains a reasonable choice for patients at low risk and is associated with low toxicity. The efficacy and outcomes of MDex have not been convincingly outperformed by either ASCT (Jaccard et al. 2007) or bortezomib-based combinations so far (Palladini et al. 2014c); the results of the prospective randomized comparison of BMDex to MDex in newly diagnosed, transplant-ineligible patients are awaited. For patients with low-risk disease, additional options may also include lenalidomide-based combinations especially in patients who present with neuropathy or with renal involvement without severe cardiac dysfunction (Table 12.6), although the potential nephrotoxicity of lenalidomide should be considered (Specter et al. 2011). Patients with IgM-related amyloidosis are usually treated with lymphoma regimens (dexamethasone, rituximab and cyclophosphamide (DRC); rituximab, cyclophosphamide, vincristine and prednisone (R-COP); bendamustine-rituximab), although vincristine should be used cautiously in patients with neuropathy. Ibrutinib may be quite effective in reducing IgM but cannot induce CRs (Leblond et al. 2016; Treon et al. 2015). Patients who present with hematologic relapse may be treated with

Table 12.6 Risk-adapted treatment strategy for patients with AL amyloidosis

Risk category	Primary options	Secondary options
Stage I, PS 0–1, eGFR >60 ml/min/1.73 m², Age <65	1. HDM with ASCT (induction with bortezomib-based therapy before HDM may be considered)	• VCD • BMDex • MDex • Lenalidomide-based
Stage II/III with NTproBNP <5000 ng/L and cTnT <0.06 ng/L, PS 0–1, eGFR >50 ml/min/1.73 m², Age <65	1. HDM with ASCT (if experienced centre) 2. VCD (full or adjusted dose)	• BMDex • MDex
Stage I/II, NTproBNP <5000 ng/L, PS 0–1, no neuropathy, Age >65	1. VCD (full or adjusted dose) 2. BMDex 3. MDex	• Lenalidomide-based
Stage II, NTproBNP >5000 ng/l but <8500 ng/L, PS 1–2, age >65	1. VCD (adjusted dose) 2. BMDex (adjusted dose) 3. MDex (full Dexa dose)	• VD (adjusted dose) • MDex (adjusted Dexa dose)
Stage I/II, AL-related neuropathy	1. MDex 2. Lenalidomide-based	• VCD adjusted dose
High risk: Stage III (but NTproBNP <8500 ng/L)	1. VCD adjusted dose 2. BMDex (adjusted dose)	• MDex
Stage III, NTproBNP >8500 ng/L, low SBP	1. Low-dose VCD (consider in-hospital administration of therapy)	• Low-dose VD

drugs or combinations in which they have not been exposed (lenalidomide-based therapy in bortezomib-treated patients, pomalidomide in lenalidomide- and bortezomib-exposed patients, bortezomib in non-bortezomib-exposed patients, bendamustine combinations). Re-challenge with a regimen which was associated with a durable response may be reasonable for selected patients.

12.11 Therapies Targeting the Amyloid Deposits

Recently, passive immunotherapy has entered the clinical arena; the aim is to accelerate the recovery of the organ function by promoting the clearance of the amyloid deposits. The obligate combination of a small molecule, CPHPC, clearing circulating SAP, followed by monoclonal antibodies directed to SAP present in amyloid deposits, has been shown, in a phase I–II study, to be able to dramatically reduce the amyloid burden in visceral organs (estimated by SAP scintigraphy) in several types of amyloidosis, including AL amyloidosis (Richards et al. 2015; Pepys et al. 2015). Another humanized monoclonal antibody (NEOD001) has been shown, in a phase I–II study in patients with AL amyloidosis, who achieved partial response or better, to improve cardiac and renal biomarkers (Gertz et al. 2016a, b). Based on these very promising results, a phase IIb study in previously treated AL patients and a phase III study in previously untreated patients are ongoing. A third monoclonal antibody targeting AL amyloid deposits has been tested in clinic. Preliminary results, on a very small patient population, show improvement in cardiac and renal biomarkers in some patients (Langer et al. 2015).

Small molecules may promote the reabsorption of amyloid deposits. An anthracycline analogue, iododoxorubicin, has been shown in a phase I–II study to facilitate the clearance of amyloid deposits (Merlini et al. 1995; Gianni et al. 1995). A common antibiotic with the same tetracyclic structure, doxycycline, has been shown to provide some clinical benefit, when used as infection prophylaxis in patients undergoing ASCT (Mayo Clinic ASH abstract). More recently a case-matched study has shown that the addition of doxycycline to chemotherapy reduces significantly the early mortality (within the first 6 months) in patients with cardiac involvement (Wechalekar et al. 2015). A phase III study is warranted in order to determine the clinical utility of this small molecule in improving the outcome of patients with cardiac involvement.

Epigallocatechin gallate has been also claimed to have anti-amyloid activity (Hunstein 2007). Preliminary data suggest that this compound may benefit patients with AL amyloidosis with cardiac involvement (Mereles et al. 2010), but a controlled trial is needed.

12.12 Supportive Care

Treatment may further complicate the management of multisystemic organ dysfunction. Nephrotic syndrome is associated with oedema, anasarca, orthostatic hypotension, syncope and a risk for infections and thrombosis. Albumin infusion with IV diuretics and monitoring of renal function and electrolytes may be used until some improvement in oedema occurs followed by oral diuretics at high doses if blood pressure allows. Nutritional support and counselling is necessary (Caccialanza et al. 2015). There is a risk of infections due to loss of immunoglobulins and the use of immunosuppressive drugs, so that prophylactic antibiotics should be considered, and antiviral prophylaxis with acyclovir is recommended during treatment with proteasome inhibitors. There is also an increased risk of thrombosis due to loss of antithrombotic proteins, but given the potential bleeding tendency due to reduced factor X levels in some patients with AL amyloidosis (Choufani et al. 2001), the decisions for antithrombotic prophylaxis should be individualized.

Diuretic therapy is the mainstay of supportive care for patients with cardiac amyloidosis, but due to restrictive pattern of haemodynamics, it may not be well tolerated. Loop diuretics should be titrated to maintain systolic blood pressure preferably >90 mmHg. Close follow-up of patient's weight is required. Addition of low doses of spironolactone may help some patients.

Angiotensin-converting enzyme inhibitors or angiotensin receptor blockers are poorly tolerated and often cause severe hypotension. Beta blockers are also poorly tolerated, but in some patients, very low doses may be helpful if rate control is required. Calcium channel blockers may cause hypotension and conduction abnormalities. Atrial fibrillation is common and may further compromise haemodynamic stability. Ventricular arrhythmias are frequent findings, especially in 24-h ECGs (Palladini et al. 2001). Amiodarone may reduce the risk of fatal VT, but no controlled studies have been reported. The efficacy of implantable cardioverter-defibrillators has not been demonstrated (Hamon et al. 2016). In a report of 33 patients with AL amyloidosis who received an ICD (12 of which underwent ASCT), three patients died of a sustained VT/VF that could not be terminated by the ICD, and four died of asystolic arrest or pulseless electrical activity (Lin et al. 2013). The median survival was 7.5 months, not different than what is expected in this group of patients without ICDs. Conduction abnormalities and bradyarrhythmias are also common. Among 20 consecutive newly diagnosed patients with severe cardiac AL amyloidosis and symptoms of syncope or pre-syncope who received implantable loop recorders, 13 died, but in each of eight evaluable cases, death was heralded by bradycardia, usually associated with complete atrioventricular block, followed by pulseless electrical activity. Among four patients who received pacemakers, three died of rapid cardiac decompensation (Sayed et al. 2015). Given the failure of pacemaker insertion to salvage patients with bradyarrhythmias, their role must be further investigated before recommending more extensive use.

12.13 Organ Transplantation for AL Amyloidosis

Renal transplantation is associated with a 5- and 10-year probability of graft survival of 54% to 71% and 26%, respectively, in two series (one of 19 patients who received mostly allograft from 18 living donors and one with 21 patients with allograft mostly from deceased donors) (Pinney et al. 2011; Tang et al. 2013). Therapy, including ASCT, was given either before or after renal transplantation, with similar results regarding renal outcomes. Although there were some cases of rejection, there was no allograft loss. Recurrence of renal amyloid was also found either with biopsy or with SAP scintigraphy in some patients. Thus, in carefully selected patients, renal transplantation is associated with long allograft survival, although recurrence of amyloidosis in the kidney allograft may occur.

Cardiac transplantation is the most effective treatment for patients at terminal stage of heart failure. Cardiac transplantation has been reported before or after intensive therapy with HDM or after conventional dose therapy. Patients who receive a heart transplant followed by ASCT seem to have the best outcomes (Gray Gilstrap et al. 2014; Dey et al. 2010; Sattianayagam et al. 2010; Davis et al. 2015), but these results reflect the highly selected patient population but also the reduced risk of relapse in those who achieve a complete hematologic response with ASCT. Unfortunately, many patients die while awaiting a heart allograft. Mechanical support using left or biventricular assist devices may offer the additional time needed in some patients until a heart allograft is available (Swiecicki et al. 2013). Liver transplantation for end-stage liver disease caused by AL amyloidosis has also been used for few selected patients. In a series of nine patients who received orthotopic liver transplantation, 1- and 5-year survival were 33% and 22% (six patients died within the first year). Three patients were unable to receive effective chemotherapy, and those who received subsequently ASCT and achieved a hematologic response had the longer survival (Sattianayagam et al. 2010).

One- and 5-year patient survival from transplantation among those receiving OLT were 33% and 22%, respectively. Causes of death among the six patients who died within the first year were as follows: intraoperative death due to cardiac decompensation (one case), sepsis (three cases), sudden unexplained death (one case) and declining renal function (one case).

Conclusions

During the last decade, impressive advances have occurred in the field of AL amyloidosis that translated into improved quality of life and extended survival. AL amyloidosis represents the most successful example of effective therapy in the whole realm of amyloidosis, due to the possibility to effectively suppress the synthesis of the amyloidogenic precursor, the monoclonal light chains. Newer anti-clone agents, able to improve our capability to annihilate the amyloidogenic clone, and passive immunotherapy targeting the cumbersome amyloid deposits promise to change the face of this disease, making the cure a reachable target. What remains disheartening is the still high rate of late diagnosis, with patients diagnosed when irreversible organ damage has occurred, missing the therapeutic windows. Early diagnosis is therefore imperative. The haematologist should keep a high level of clinical awareness and alertness and use, during the follow-up of patients at risk (with MGUS and abnormal FLC ratio), two simple and extremely powerful biomarkers, NTproBNP, for the early detection of amyloid cardiac involvement, and urinary albumin, for the detection of renal involvement. The use of these two biomarkers allows the identification of 97% of patients with AL amyloidosis (Merlini et al. 2013).

References

Antoni G, Lubberink M, Estrada S, Axelsson J, Carlson K, Lindsjo L et al (2013) In vivo visualization of amyloid deposits in the heart with 11C-PIB and PET. J Nucl Med 54(2):213–220

Arbustini E, Morbini P, Verga L, Concardi M, Porcu E, Pilotto A et al (1997) Light and electron microscopy immunohistochemical characterization of amyloid deposits. Amyloid 4(3):157–170

Banypersad SM, Sado DM, Flett AS, Gibbs SD, Pinney JH, Maestrini V et al (2013) Quantification of myocardial extracellular volume fraction in systemic AL amyloidosis: an equilibrium contrast cardiovascular magnetic resonance study. Circ Cardiovasc Imaging 6(1):34–39

Benson MD, James S, Scott K, Liepnieks JJ, Kluve-Beckerman B (2008) Leukocyte chemotactic factor 2: a novel renal amyloid protein. Kidney Int 74(2):218–222

Bochtler T, Hegenbart U, Heiss C, Benner A, Moos M, Seckinger A et al (2011) Hyperdiploidy is less frequent in AL amyloidosis compared with monoclonal gammopathy of undetermined significance and inversely associated with translocation t(11;14). Blood 117(14):3809–3815

Bochtler T, Hegenbart U, Kunz C, Benner A, Seckinger A, Dietrich S et al (2014) Gain of chromosome 1q21 is an independent adverse prognostic factor in light chain amyloidosis patients treated with melphalan/dexamethasone. Amyloid 21(1):9–17

Bochtler T, Hegenbart U, Kunz C, Granzow M, Benner A, Seckinger A et al (2015) Translocation t(11;14) is associated with adverse outcome in patients with newly diagnosed AL amyloidosis when treated with bortezomib-based regimens. J Clin Oncol 33(12):1371–1378

Bodin K, Ellmerich S, Kahan MC, Tennent GA, Loesch A, Gilbertson JA et al (2010) Antibodies to human serum amyloid P component eliminate visceral amyloid deposits. Nature 468(7320):93–97

Bokhari S, Castano A, Pozniakoff T, Deslisle S, Latif F, Maurer MS (2013) (99m)Tc-pyrophosphate scintigraphy for differentiating light-chain cardiac amyloidosis from the transthyretin-related familial and senile cardiac amyloidoses. Circ Cardiovasc Imaging 6(2):195–201

Bonar L, Cohen AS, Skinner MM (1969) Characterization of the amyloid fibril as a cross-beta protein. Proc Soc Exp Biol Med 131(4):1373–1375

Brambilla F, Lavatelli F, Merlini G, Mauri P (2013) Clinical proteomics for diagnosis and typing of systemic amyloidoses. Proteomics Clin Appl 7(1-2):136–143

Bryce AH, Ketterling RP, Gertz MA, Lacy M, Knudson RA, Zeldenrust S et al (2009) Translocation t(11;14) and survival of patients with light chain (AL) amyloidosis. Haematologica 94(3):380–386

Buss SJ, Emami M, Mereles D, Korosoglou G, Kristen AV, Voss A et al (2012) Longitudinal left ventricular function for prediction of survival in systemic light-chain amyloidosis: incremental value compared with clinical and biochemical markers. J Am Coll Cardiol 60(12):1067–1076

Caccialanza R, Palladini G, Cereda E, Bonardi C, Milani P, Cameletti B et al (2015) Nutritional counseling improves quality of life and preserves body weight in systemic immunoglobulin light-chain (AL) amyloidosis. Nutrition 31(10):1228–1234

Campbell JP, Heaney JL, Shemar M, Baldwin D, Griffin AE, Oldridge E et al (2017) Development of a rapid and quantitative lateral flow assay for the simultaneous measurement of serum kappa and lambda immunoglobulin free light chains (FLC): inception of a new near-patient FLC screening tool. Clin Chem Lab Med 55(3):424–434

Castano A, Bokhari S, Brannagan TH 3rd, Wynn J, Maurer MS (2012) Technetium pyrophosphate myocardial uptake and peripheral neuropathy in a rare variant of familial transthyretin (TTR) amyloidosis (Ser23Asn): a case report and literature review. Amyloid 19(1):41–46

Chen W, Dilsizian V (2012) Molecular imaging of amyloidosis: will the heart be the next target after the brain? Curr Cardiol Rep 14(2):226–233

Choufani EB, Sanchorawala V, Ernst T, Quillen K, Skinner M, Wright DG et al (2001) Acquired factor X deficiency in patients with amyloid light-chain amyloidosis: incidence, bleeding manifestations, and response to high-dose chemotherapy. Blood 97(6):1885–1887

Cibeira MT, Sanchorawala V, Seldin DC, Quillen K, Berk JL, Dember LM et al (2011) Outcome of AL amyloidosis after high-dose melphalan and autologous stem cell transplantation: long-term results in a series of 421 patients. Blood 118(16):4346–4352

Cibeira MT, Oriol A, Lahuerta JJ, Mateos MV, de la Rubia J, Hernandez MT et al (2015) A phase II trial of lenalidomide, dexamethasone and cyclophosphamide for newly diagnosed patients with systemic immunoglobulin light chain amyloidosis. Br J Haematol 170(6):804–813

Cohen AD, Scott EC, Liedtke M, Kaufman JL, Landau H, Vesole DH et al (2014) A phase I dose-escalation study of carfilzomib in patients with previously-treated systemic light-chain (AL) amyloidosis. Blood 124(21):4741

D'Souza A, Dispenzieri A, Wirk B, Zhang MJ, Huang J, Gertz MA et al (2015) Improved outcomes after autologous hematopoietic cell transplantation for light chain amyloidosis: a Center for International Blood and Marrow Transplant Research Study. J Clin Oncol 33(32):3741–3749

Davis M, Kale P, Witteles RM (2015) Outcomes after heart transplantation for amyloid cardiomyopathy in the modern era. J Heart Lung Transplant 33(4):S51

Dember LM, Hawkins PN, Hazenberg BP, Gorevic PD, Merlini G, Butrimiene I et al (2007) Eprodisate for the treatment of renal disease in AA amyloidosis. N Engl J Med 356(23):2349–2360

Deshmukh M, Elderfield K, Rahemtulla A, Naresh KN (2009) Immunophenotype of neoplastic plasma cells in AL amyloidosis. J Clin Pathol 62(8):724–730

Dey BR, Chung SS, Spitzer TR, Zheng H, Macgillivray TE, Seldin DC et al (2010) Cardiac transplantation followed by dose-intensive melphalan and autologous stem-cell transplantation for light chain amyloidosis and heart failure. Transplantation 90(8):905–911

Dingli D, Tan TS, Kumar SK, Buadi FK, Dispenzieri A, Hayman SR et al (2010) Stem cell transplantation in patients with autonomic neuropathy due to primary (AL) amyloidosis. Neurology 74(11):913–918

Dinner S, Witteles W, Afghahi A, Witteles R, Arai S, Lafayette R et al (2013) Lenalidomide, melphalan and dexamethasone in a population of patients with immunoglobulin light chain amyloidosis with high rates of advanced cardiac involvement. Haematologica 98(10):1593–1599

Dispenzieri A, Merlini G (2016) Immunoglobulin light chain systemic amyloidosis. Cancer Treat Res 169:273–318

Dispenzieri A, Gertz MA, Kyle RA, Lacy MQ, Burritt MF, Therneau TM et al (2004) Serum cardiac troponins and N-terminal pro-brain natriuretic peptide: a staging system for primary systemic amyloidosis. J Clin Oncol 22(18):3751–3757

Dispenzieri A, Lacy MQ, Zeldenrust SR, Hayman SR, Kumar SK, Geyer SM et al (2007) The activity of lenalidomide with or without dexamethasone in patients with primary systemic amyloidosis. Blood 109(2):465–470

Dispenzieri A, Dingli D, Kumar SK, Rajkumar SV, Lacy MQ, Hayman S et al (2010) Discordance between serum cardiac biomarker and immunoglobulin-free light-chain response in patients with immunoglobulin light-chain amyloidosis treated with immune modulatory drugs. Am J Hematol 85(10):757–759

Dispenzieri A, Buadi F, Laumann K, LaPlant B, Hayman SR, Kumar SK et al (2012) Activity of pomalidomide in patients with immunoglobulin light-chain amyloidosis. Blood 119(23):5397–5404

Dispenzieri A, Seenithamby K, Lacy MQ, Kumar SK, Buadi FK, Hayman SR et al (2013) Patients with immunoglobulin light chain amyloidosis undergoing autologous stem cell transplantation have superior outcomes compared with patients with multiple myeloma: a retrospective review from a tertiary referral center. Bone Marrow Transplant 48(10):1302–1307

Dorbala S, Vangala D, Semer J, Strader C, Bruyere JR Jr, Di Carli MF et al (2014) Imaging cardiac amyloidosis: a pilot study using (1)(8)F-florbetapir positron emission tomography. Eur J Nucl Med Mol Imaging 41(9):1652–1662

Dubrey SW, Reece DE, Sanchorawala V, Hegenbart U, Merlini G, Palladini G et al (2011) Bortezomib in a phase 1 trial for patients with relapsed AL amyloidosis: cardiac responses and overall effects. QJM 104(11):957–970

Falk RH (2005) Diagnosis and management of the cardiac amyloidoses. Circulation 112(13):2047–2060

Fernandez de Larrea C, Verga L, Morbini P, Klersy C, Lavatelli F, Foli A et al (2015) A practical approach to the diagnosis of systemic amyloidoses. Blood 125(14):2239–2244

Foli A, Palladini G, Caporali R, Verga L, Morbini P, Obici L et al (2011) The role of minor salivary gland biopsy in the diagnosis of systemic amyloidosis: results of a prospective study in 62 patients. Amyloid 18(Suppl 1):80–82

Galat A, Rosso J, Guellich A, Van Der Gucht A, Rappeneau S, Bodez D et al (2015) Usefulness of (99m)Tc-HMDP scintigraphy for the etiologic diagnosis and prognosis of cardiac amyloidosis. Amyloid 22(4):210–220

Galat A, Van der Gucht A, Guellich A, Bodez D, Cottereau AS, Guendouz S et al (2017) Early phase 99Tc-HMDP scintigraphy for the diagnosis and typing of cardiac amyloidosis. JACC Cardiovasc Imaging 10(5):601–603

Gertz MA, Kyle RA, Greipp PR (1989) The plasma cell labeling index: a valuable tool in primary systemic amyloidosis. Blood 74(3):1108–1111

Gertz MA, Lacy MQ, Dispenzieri A, Ansell SM, Elliott MA, Gastineau DA et al (2004) Risk-adjusted manipulation of melphalan dose before stem cell transplantation in patients with amyloidosis is associated with a lower response rate. Bone Marrow Transplant 34(12):1025–1031

Gertz MA, Comenzo R, Falk RH, Fermand JP, Hazenberg BP, Hawkins PN et al (2005) Definition of organ involvement and treatment response in immunoglobulin light chain amyloidosis (AL): a consensus opinion from the 10(th) International Symposium on Amyloid and Amyloidosis. Am J Hematol 79(4):319–328

Gertz MA, Lacy MQ, Dispenzieri A, Hayman SR, Kumar SK, Dingli D et al (2010) Autologous stem cell transplant for immunoglobulin light chain amyloidosis: a status report. Leuk Lymphoma 51(12):2181–2187

Gertz MA, Lacy MQ, Dispenzieri A, Kumar SK, Dingli D, Leung N et al (2013) Refinement in patient selection to reduce treatment-related mortality from autologous stem cell transplantation in amyloidosis. Bone Marrow Transplant 48(4):557–561

Gertz MA, Landau H, Comenzo RL, Seldin D, Weiss B, Zonder J et al (2016a) First-in-human phase I/II study of NEOD001 in patients with light chain amyloidosis and persistent organ dysfunction. J Clin Oncol 34(10):1097–1103

Gertz MA, Landau HJ, Weiss BM (2016b) Organ response in patients with AL amyloidosis treated with NEOD001, an amyloid-directed monoclonal antibody. Am J Hematol 91(12):E506–E508

Gianni L, Bellotti V, Gianni AM, Merlini G (1995) New drug-therapy of amyloidoses—resorption of AL-type deposits with 4′-Iodo-4′-deoxydoxorubicin. Blood 86(3):855–861

Gillmore JD, Maurer MS, Falk RH, Merlini G, Damy T, Dispenzieri A et al (2016) Nonbiopsy diagnosis of cardiac transthyretin amyloidosis. Circulation 133(24):2404–2412

Glenner GG, Terry WD (1974) Characterization of amyloid. Annu Rev Med 25:131–135

Gray Gilstrap L, Niehaus E, Malhotra R, Ton VK, Watts J, Seldin DC et al (2014) Predictors of survival to orthotopic heart transplant in patients with light chain amyloidosis. J Heart Lung Transplant 33(2):149–156

Hamon D, Algalarrondo V, Gandjbakhch E, Extramiana F, Marijon E, Elbaz N et al (2016) Outcome and incidence of appropriate implantable cardioverter-defibrillator therapy in patients with cardiac amyloidosis. Int J Cardiol 222:562–568

Hawkins PN, Lavender JP, Pepys MB (1990) Evaluation of systemic amyloidosis by scintigraphy with 123I-labeled serum amyloid P component. N Engl J Med 323(8):508–513

Hegenbart UB, Dreger T, Kimmich P, Ziehl R, Goldschmidt R, Ho H, Schonland A (2014) Long-term results of 174 patients with systemic AL amyloidosis treated with high-dose melphalan and autologous stem cell transplantation: a single center experience. Haematologica 99:S1305

Hemminki K, Li X, Forsti A, Sundquist J, Sundquist K (2012) Incidence and survival in non-hereditary amyloidosis in Sweden. BMC Public Health 12:974

Hongo M, Urushibata K, Kai R, Takahashi W, Koizumi T, Uchikawa S et al (2002) Iodine-123 metaiodobenzylguanidine scintigraphic analysis of myocardial sympathetic innervation in patients with AL (primary) amyloidosis. Am Heart J 144(1):122–129

Hunstein W (2007) Epigallocatechin-3-gallate in AL amyloidosis: a new therapeutic option? Blood 110(6):2216

Hutt DF, Quigley AM, Page J, Hall ML, Burniston M, Gopaul D et al (2014) Utility and limitations of 3,3-diphosphono-1,2-propanodicarboxylic acid scintigraphy in systemic amyloidosis. Eur Heart J Cardiovasc Imaging 15(11):1289–1298

Jaccard A, Moreau P, Leblond V, Leleu X, Benboubker L, Hermine O et al (2007) High-dose melphalan versus melphalan plus dexamethasone for AL amyloidosis. N Engl J Med 357(11):1083–1093

Jaccard A, Comenzo RL, Hari P, Hawkins PN, Roussel M, Morel P et al (2014) Efficacy of bortezomib, cyclophosphamide and dexamethasone in treatment-naive patients with high-risk cardiac AL amyloidosis (Mayo Clinic stage III). Haematologica 99(9):1479–1485

Kastritis E, Anagnostopoulos A, Roussou M, Toumanidis S, Pamboukas C, Migkou M et al (2007) Treatment of light chain (AL) amyloidosis with the combination of bortezomib and dexamethasone. Haematologica 92(10):1351–1358

Kastritis E, Wechalekar AD, Dimopoulos MA, Merlini G, Hawkins PN, Perfetti V et al (2010) Bortezomib with or without dexamethasone in primary systemic (light chain) amyloidosis. J Clin Oncol 28(6):1031–1037

Kastritis E, Terpos E, Roussou M, Gavriatopoulou M, Pamboukas C, Boletis I et al (2012) A phase 1/2 study of lenalidomide with low-dose oral cyclophosphamide and low-dose dexamethasone (RdC) in AL amyloidosis. Blood 119(23):5384–5390

Kastritis E, Leleu X, Arnulf B, Zamagni E, Mollee P, Cibeira MT et al (2014) A randomized phase III trial of melphalan and dexamethasone (MDex) versus bortezomib, melphalan and dexamethasone (BMDex) for untreated patients with AL amyloidosis. Blood 124(21):35

Kastritis E, Roussou M, Gavriatopoulou M, Migkou M, Kalapanida D, Pamboucas C et al (2015) Long-term outcomes of primary systemic light chain (AL) amyloidosis in patients treated upfront with bortezomib or lenalidomide and the importance of risk adapted strategies. Am J Hematol 90(4):E60–E65

Kastritis E, Papassotiriou I, Terpos E, Roussou M, Gavriatopoulou M, Komitopoulou A et al (2016) Clinical and prognostic significance of serum levels of von Willebrand factor and ADAMTS-13 antigens in AL amyloidosis. Blood 128(3):405–409

Kaufman G, Witteles R, Wheeler M, Ulloa P, Lugtu M, Arai S, et al (2016) The anti-CD38 monoclonal antibody daratumumab produces rapid hematologic responses in patients with heavily pretreated AL amyloidosis. In: XVth International Symposium on Amyloidosis, UPPSALA, p. PB 63

Kourelis TV, Kumar SK, Gertz MA, Lacy MQ, Buadi FK, Hayman SR et al (2013) Coexistent multiple myeloma or increased bone marrow plasma cells define equally high-risk populations in patients with immunoglobulin light chain amyloidosis. J Clin Oncol 31(34):4319–4324

Kumar S, Dispenzieri A, Lacy MQ, Hayman SR, Buadi FK, Colby C et al (2012a) Revised prognostic staging system for light chain amyloidosis incorporating cardiac biomarkers and serum free light chain measurements. J Clin Oncol Off J Am Soc Clin Oncol 30(9):989–995

Kumar SK, Hayman SR, Buadi FK, Roy V, Lacy MQ, Gertz MA et al (2012b) Lenalidomide, cyclophosphamide, and dexamethasone (CRd) for light-chain amyloidosis: long-term results from a phase 2 trial. Blood 119(21):4860–4867

Kyle RA, Linos A, Beard CM, Linke RP, Gertz MA, O'Fallon WM et al (1992) Incidence and natural history of primary systemic amyloidosis in Olmsted County, Minnesota, 1950 through 1989. Blood 79(7):1817–1822

Lachmann HJ, Hawkins PN (2006) Systemic amyloidosis. Curr Opin Pharmacol 6(2):214–220

Lachmann HJ, Gallimore R, Gillmore JD, Carr-Smith HD, Bradwell AR, Pepys MB et al (2003) Outcome in systemic AL amyloidosis in relation to changes in concentration of circulating free immunoglobulin light chains following chemotherapy. Br J Haematol 122(1):78–84

Landau H, Smith M, Landry C, Chou JF, Devlin SM, Hassoun H et al (2017) Long-term event-free and overall survival after risk-adapted melphalan and SCT for systemic light chain amyloidosis. Leukemia 31(1):136–142

Langer AL, Miao S, Mapara M, Radhakrishnan J, Maurer MS, Raza S et al (2015) Results of phase I study of chimeric fibril-reactive monoclonal antibody 11-1F4 in patients with AL amyloidosis. Blood 126(23)

Larsen CP, Walker PD, Weiss DT, Solomon A (2010) Prevalence and morphology of leukocyte chemotactic factor 2-associated amyloid in renal biopsies. Kidney Int 77(9):816–819

Lavatelli F, Imperlini E, Orrù S, Rognoni P, Sarnataro D, Palladini G et al (2015) Novel mitochondrial protein interactors of immunoglobulin light chains causing heart amyloidosis. FASEB J 29(11):4614–4628

Law WP, Wang WY, Moore PT, Mollee PN, Ng AC (2016) Cardiac amyloid imaging with 18F-florbetaben positron emission tomography: a pilot study. J Nucl Med 57(11):1733–1739

Leblond V, Kastritis E, Advani R, Ansell SM, Buske C, Castillo JJ et al (2016) Treatment recommendations from the Eighth International Workshop on Waldenstrom's Macroglobulinemia. Blood 128(10):1321–1328

Lekakis J, Dimopoulos MA, Prassopoulos V, Mavrikakis M, Gerali S, Sifakis N et al (2003) Myocardial adrenergic denervation in patients with primary (AL) amyloidosis. Amyloid 10(2):117–120

Liao R, Jain M, Teller P, Connors LH, Ngoy S, Skinner M et al (2001) Infusion of light chains from patients with cardiac amyloidosis causes diastolic dysfunction in isolated mouse hearts. Circulation 104(14):1594–1597

Lin G, Dispenzieri A, Kyle R, Grogan M, Brady PA (2013) Implantable cardioverter defibrillators in patients with cardiac amyloidosis. J Cardiovasc Electrophysiol 24(7):793–798

Lock RJ, Saleem R, Roberts EG, Wallage MJ, Pesce TJ, Rowbottom A et al (2013) A multicentre study comparing two methods for serum free light chain analysis. Ann Clin Biochem 50(Pt 3):255–261

Lokhorst HM, Plesner T, Laubach JP, Nahi H, Gimsing P, Hansson M et al (2015) Targeting CD38 with daratumumab monotherapy in multiple myeloma. N Engl J Med 373(13):1207–1219

Lousada I, Comenzo RL, Landau H, Guthrie S, Merlini G (2015) Light chain amyloidosis: patient experience survey from the Amyloidosis Research Consortium. Adv Ther 32(10):920–928

Maceira AM, Joshi J, Prasad SK, Moon JC, Perugini E, Harding I et al (2005) Cardiovascular magnetic resonance in cardiac amyloidosis. Circulation 111(2):186–193

Mahmood S, Wassef NL, Salter SJ, Sachchithanantham S, Lane T, Foard D et al (2016) Comparison of free light chain assays: Freelite and N latex in diagnosis, monitoring, and predicting survival in light chain amyloidosis. Am J Clin Pathol 146(1):78–85

Mekinian A, Lions C, Leleu X, Duhamel A, Lamblin N, Coiteux V et al (2010) Prognosis assessment of cardiac involvement in systemic AL amyloidosis by magnetic resonance imaging. Am J Med 123(9):864–868

Mereles D, Buss SJ, Hardt SE, Hunstein W, Katus HA (2010) Effects of the main green tea polyphenol epigallocatechin-3-gallate on cardiac involvement in patients with AL amyloidosis. Clin Res Cardiol 99(8):483–490

Merlini G (2012) CyBorD: stellar response rates in AL amyloidosis. Blood 119(19):4343–4345

Merlini G, Bellotti V (2003) Molecular mechanisms of amyloidosis. N Engl J Med 349(6):583–596

Merlini G, Palladini G (2013) Light chain amyloidosis: the heart of the problem. Haematologica 98(10):1492–1495

Merlini G, Ascari E, Amboldi N, Bellotti V, Arbustini E, Perfetti V et al (1995) Interaction of the anthracycline 4′-iodo-4′-deoxydoxorubicin with amyloid fibrils—inhibition of amyloidogenesis. Proc Natl Acad Sci U S A 92(7):2959–2963

Merlini G, Wechalekar AD, Palladini G (2013) Systemic light chain amyloidosis: an update for treating physicians. Blood 121(26):5124–5130

Merlini G, Sanchorawala V, Jeffrey ZA, Kukreti V, Schoenland SO, Jaccard A et al (2014) Long-term outcome of a phase 1 study of the investigational oral proteasome inhibitor (PI) ixazomib at the recommended phase 3 dose (RP3D) in patients (Pts) with relapsed or refractory systemic light-chain (AL) amyloidosis (RRAL). Blood 124(21):3450

Mikhael JR, Schuster SR, Jimenez-Zepeda VH, Bello N, Spong J, Reeder CB et al (2012) Cyclophosphamide-bortezomib-dexamethasone (CyBorD) produces rapid and complete hematologic response in patients with AL amyloidosis. Blood 119(19):4391–4394

Milani P, Rosin MV, Foli A, Merlini G (2013) High-dose pomalidomide and dexamethasone induce rapid responses in patients with AL amyloidosis exposed to alkylators, immune modulatory drugs, and proteasome inhibitors. Blood 122(21):288

Moreau P, Jaccard A, Benboubker L, Royer B, Leleu X, Bridoux F et al (2010) Lenalidomide in combination with melphalan and dexamethasone in patients with newly diagnosed AL amyloidosis: a multicenter phase 1/2 dose-escalation study. Blood 116(23):4777–4782

Murphy C, Wang S, Kestler D, Larsen C, Benson D, Weiss D et al (2011) Leukocyte chemotactic factor 2 (LECT2)-associated renal amyloidosis. Amyloid 18(Suppl 1):223–225

Murphy CL, Wang S, Kestler D, Larsen C, Benson D, Weiss DT et al (2010) Leukocyte chemotactic factor 2 (LECT2)-associated renal amyloidosis: a case series. Am J Kidney Dis 56(6):1100–1107

Nilsson KP, Ikenberg K, Aslund A, Fransson S, Konradsson P, Rocken C et al (2010) Structural typing of systemic amyloidoses by luminescent-conjugated polymer spectroscopy. Am J Pathol 176(2):563–574

Paiva B, Vidriales MB, Perez JJ, Mateo G, Montalban MA, Mateos MV et al (2009) Multiparameter flow cytometry quantification of bone marrow plasma cells at diagnosis provides more prognostic information than morphological assessment in myeloma patients. Haematologica 94(11):1599–1602

Palladini G, Malamani G, Co F, Pistorio A, Recusani F, Anesi E et al (2001) Holter monitoring in AL amyloidosis: prognostic implications. Pacing Clin Electrophysiol 24(8 Pt 1):1228–1233

Palladini G, Perfetti V, Obici L, Caccialanza R, Semino A, Adami F et al (2004) Association of melphalan and high-dose dexamethasone is effective and well tolerated in patients with AL (primary) amyloidosis who are ineligible for stem cell transplantation. Blood 103(8):2936–2938

Palladini G, Perfetti V, Perlini S, Obici L, Lavatelli F, Caccialanza R et al (2005) The combination of thalidomide and intermediate-dose dexamethasone is an effective but toxic treatment for patients with primary amyloidosis (AL). Blood 105(7):2949–2951

Palladini G, Russo P, Bosoni T, Verga L, Sarais G, Lavatelli F et al (2009) Identification of amyloidogenic light chains requires the combination of serum-free light chain assay with immunofixation of serum and urine. Clin Chem 55(3):499–504

Palladini G, Dispenzieri A, Gertz MA, Kumar S, Wechalekar A, Hawkins PN et al (2012a) New criteria for response to treatment in immunoglobulin light chain amyloidosis based on free light chain measurement and cardiac biomarkers: impact on survival outcomes. J Clin Oncol 30(36):4541–4549

Palladini G, Schonland SO, Milani P, Kimmich C, Foli A, Bochtler T et al (2012b) Treatment of AL amyloidosis with bendamustine. ASH Annu Meet Abstr 120(21):4057

Palladini G, Hegenbart U, Milani P, Kimmich C, Foli A, Ho AD et al (2014a) A staging system for renal outcome and early markers of renal response to chemotherapy in AL amyloidosis. Blood 124(15):2325–2332

Palladini G, Milani P, Foli A, Obici L, Lavatelli F, Nuvolone M et al (2014b) Oral melphalan and dexamethasone grants extended survival with minimal toxicity in AL amyloidosis: long-term results of a risk-adapted approach. Haematologica 99(4):743–750

Palladini G, Milani P, Foli A, Vidus Rosin M, Basset M, Lavatelli F et al (2014c) Melphalan and dexamethasone with or without bortezomib in newly diagnosed AL amyloidosis: a matched case-control study on 174 patients. Leukemia 28(12):2311–2316

Palladini G, Sachchithanantham S, Milani P, Gillmore J, Foli A, Lachmann H et al (2015) A European collaborative study of cyclophosphamide, bortezomib, and dexamethasone in upfront treatment of systemic AL amyloidosis. Blood 126(5):612–615

Parmar S, Kongtim P, Champlin R, Dinh Y, Elgharably Y, Wang M et al (2014) Auto-SCT improves survival in systemic light chain amyloidosis: a retrospective analysis with 14-year follow-up. Bone Marrow Transplant 49(8):1036–1041

Pepys MB, Rademacher TW, Amatayakul-Chantler S, Williams P, Noble GE, Hutchinson WL et al (1994) Human serum amyloid P component is an invariant constituent of amyloid deposits and has a uniquely homogeneous glycostructure. Proc Natl Acad Sci U S A 91:5602–5606

Pepys MB, Cookson LM, Barton SV, Berges AC, Lane T, Hutt D et al (2015) Dose-dependent progressive immunotherapeutic clearance of systemic amyloid deposits by repeated doses of antibody to serum amyloid P component (SAP). Blood 126(23):1836

Perugini E, Guidalotti PL, Salvi F, Cooke RM, Pettinato C, Riva L et al (2005) Noninvasive etiologic diagnosis of cardiac amyloidosis using 99mTc-3,3-diphosphono-1,2-propanodicarboxylic acid scintigraphy. J Am Coll Cardiol 46(6):1076–1084

Pinney JH, Lachmann HJ, Bansi L, Wechalekar AD, Gilbertson JA, Rowczenio D et al (2011) Outcome in renal AL amyloidosis after chemotherapy. J Clin Oncol 29(6):674–681

Pinney JH, Smith CJ, Taube JB, Lachmann HJ, Venner CP, Gibbs SD et al (2013) Systemic amyloidosis in England: an epidemiological study. Br J Haematol 161(4):525–532

Rapezzi C, Guidalotti P, Salvi F, Riva L, Perugini E (2008) Usefulness of 99mTc-DPD scintigraphy in cardiac amyloidosis. J Am Coll Cardiol 51(15):1509–1510. author reply 10

Rapezzi C, Quarta CC, Guidalotti PL, Longhi S, Pettinato C, Leone O et al (2011) Usefulness and limitations of 99mTc-3,3-diphosphono-1,2-propanodicarboxylic acid scintigraphy in the aetiological diagnosis of amyloidotic cardiomyopathy. Eur J Nucl Med Mol Imaging 38(3):470–478

Reece DE, Hegenbart U, Sanchorawala V, Merlini G, Palladini G, Blade J et al (2011) Efficacy and safety of once-weekly and twice-weekly bortezomib in patients with relapsed systemic AL amyloidosis: results of a phase 1/2 study. Blood 118(4):865–873

Reilly MM, Staunton H (1996) Peripheral nerve amyloidosis. Brain Pathol 6(2):163–177

Richards DB, Cookson LM, Berges AC, Barton SV, Lane T, Ritter JM et al (2015) Therapeutic clearance of amyloid by antibodies to serum amyloid P component. N Engl J Med 373(12):1106–1114

Sachchithanantham S, Roussel M, Palladini G, Klersy C, Mahmood S, Venner CP et al (2016) European collaborative study defining clinical profile outcomes and novel prognostic criteria in monoclonal immunoglobulin M-related light chain amyloidosis. J Clin Oncol 34(17):2037–2045

Sanchorawala V (2014) High dose melphalan and autologous peripheral blood stem cell transplantation in AL amyloidosis. Hematol Oncol Clin North Am 28(6):1131–1144

Sanchorawala V, Wright DG, Rosenzweig M, Finn KT, Fennessey S, Zeldis JB et al (2007) Lenalidomide and dexamethasone in the treatment of AL amyloidosis: results of a phase 2 trial. Blood 109(2):492–496

Sattianayagam PT, Gibbs SD, Pinney JH, Wechalekar AD, Lachmann HJ, Whelan CJ et al (2010) Solid organ transplantation in AL amyloidosis. Am J Transplant 10(9):2124–2131

Sawaya MR, Sambashivan S, Nelson R, Ivanova MI, Sievers SA, Apostol MI et al (2007) Atomic structures of amyloid cross-beta spines reveal varied steric zippers. Nature 447(7143):453–457

Sayed RH, Rogers D, Khan F, Wechalekar AD, Lachmann HJ, Fontana M et al (2015) A study of implanted cardiac rhythm recorders in advanced cardiac AL amyloidosis. Eur Heart J 36(18):1098–1105

Schonland SO, Hegenbart U, Bochtler T, Mangatter A, Hansberg M, Ho AD et al (2012) Immunohistochemistry in the classification of systemic forms of amyloidosis: a systematic investigation of 117 patients. Blood 119(2):488–493

Selvanayagam JB, Hawkins PN, Paul B, Myerson SG, Neubauer S (2007) Evaluation and management of the cardiac amyloidosis. J Am Coll Cardiol 50:2101–2110

Sher T, Fenton B, Akhtar A, Gertz MA (2016) First report of safety and efficacy of daratumumab in two cases of advanced immunoglobulin light chain amyloidosis. Blood 128(15):1987–1989

Shi J, Guan J, Jiang B, Brenner DA, Del Monte F, Ward JE et al (2010) Amyloidogenic light chains induce cardiomyocyte contractile dysfunction and apoptosis via a non-canonical p38alpha MAPK pathway. Proc Natl Acad Sci U S A 107(9):4188–4193

Sipe JD, Benson MD, Buxbaum JN, Ikeda S, Merlini G, Saraiva MJ et al (2012) Amyloid fibril protein nomenclature: 2012 recommendations from the Nomenclature Committee of the International Society of Amyloidosis. Amyloid 19(4):167–170

Sipe JD, Benson MD, Buxbaum JN, Ikeda S, Merlini G, Saraiva MJ et al (2014) Nomenclature 2014: amyloid fibril proteins and clinical classification of the amyloidosis. Amyloid 21(4):221–224

Specter R, Sanchorawala V, Seldin DC, Shelton A, Fennessey S, Finn KT et al (2011) Kidney dysfunction during lenalidomide treatment for AL amyloidosis. Nephrol Dial Transplant 26(3):881–886

Sunde M, Serpell LC, Bartlam M, Fraser PE, Pepys MB, Blake CC (1997) Common core structure of amyloid fibrils by synchrotron X-ray diffraction. J Mol Biol 273(3):729–739

Sviggum HP, Davis MD, Rajkumar SV, Dispenzieri A (2006) Dermatologic adverse effects of lenalidomide therapy for amyloidosis and multiple myeloma. Arch Dermatol 142(10):1298–1302

Swiecicki PL, Edwards BS, Kushwaha SS, Dispenzieri A, Park SJ, Gertz MA (2013) Left ventricular device implantation for advanced cardiac amyloidosis. J Heart Lung Transplant 32(5):563–568

Tan SY, Pepys MB (1994) Amyloidosis. Histopathology 25:403–414

Tang W, McDonald SP, Hawley CM, Badve SV, Boudville N, Brown FG et al (2013) End-stage renal failure due to amyloidosis: outcomes in 490 ANZDATA registry cases. Nephrol Dial Transplant 28(2):455–461

Te Velthuis H, Drayson M, Campbell JP (2016) Measurement of free light chains with assays based on monoclonal antibodies. Clin Chem Lab Med 54(6):1005–1014

Treon SP, Tripsas CK, Meid K, Warren D, Varma G, Green R et al (2015) Ibrutinib in previously treated Waldenstrom's macroglobulinemia. N Engl J Med 372(15):1430–1440

Valleix S, Gillmore JD, Bridoux F, Mangione PP, Dogan A, Nedelec B et al (2012) Hereditary systemic amyloidosis due to Asp76Asn variant beta2-microglobulin. N Engl J Med 366(24):2276–2283

van Gameren I, van Rijswijk MH, Bijzet J, Vellenga E, Hazenberg BP (2009) Histological regression of amyloid in AL amyloidosis is exclusively seen after normalization of serum free light chain. Haematologica 94(8):1094–1100

Venner CP, Lane T, Foard D, Rannigan L, Gibbs SD, Pinney JH et al (2012) Cyclophosphamide, bortezomib, and dexamethasone therapy in AL amyloidosis is associated with high clonal response rates and prolonged progression-free survival. Blood 119(19):4387–4390

Venner CP, Gillmore JD, Sachchithanantham S, Mahmood S, Lane T, Foard D et al (2014) A matched comparison of cyclophosphamide, bortezomib and dexamethasone (CVD) versus risk-adapted cyclophosphamide, thalidomide and dexamethasone (CTD) in AL amyloidosis. Leukemia 28(12):2304–2310

Warsame R, Kumar SK, Gertz MA, Lacy MQ, Buadi FK, Hayman SR et al (2015) Abnormal FISH in patients with immunoglobulin light chain amyloidosis is a risk factor for cardiac involvement and for death. Blood Cancer J 5:e310

Wechalekar A, Whelan C, Lachmann H, Fontana M, Mahmood S, Gillmore JD et al (2015) Oral doxycycline improves outcomes of stage III AL amyloidosis—a matched case control study. Blood 126(23):732

Wechalekar AD, Goodman HJ, Lachmann HJ, Offer M, Hawkins PN, Gillmore JD (2007) Safety and efficacy of risk-adapted cyclophosphamide, thalidomide, and dexamethasone in systemic AL amyloidosis. Blood 109(2):457–464

Wechalekar AD, Lachmann HJ, Goodman HJ, Bradwell A, Hawkins PN, Gillmore JD (2008) AL amyloidosis associated with IgM paraproteinemia: clinical profile and treatment outcome. Blood 112(10):4009–4016

Wechalekar AD, Schonland SO, Kastritis E, Gillmore JD, Dimopoulos MA, Lane T et al (2013) A European collaborative study of treatment outcomes in 346 patients with cardiac stage III AL amyloidosis. Blood 121(17):3420–3427

Wechalekar AD, Gillmore JD, Hawkins PN (2016) Systemic amyloidosis. Lancet 387(10038):2641–2654

Weiss B, Waxman A, Cohen A, Dember L, Zonder J (2016) Clinical experience with daratumumab in AL amyloidosis and MM with AL amyloidosis. In: The XVth International Symposium on Amyloidosis, UPPSALA, p PB 98

Zagouri F, Roussou M, Kastritis E, Koureas A, Tsokou E, Migkou M et al (2011) Lenalidomide-associated pneumonitis in patients with plasma cell dyscrasias. Am J Hematol 86(10):882–884

PGSTL